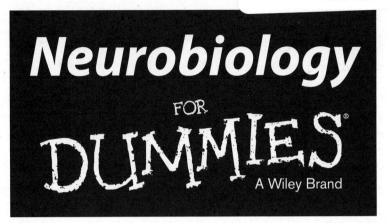

Neurobiology
FOR DUMMIES®
A Wiley Brand

by Frank Amthor, PhD

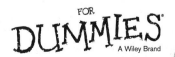

FOR DUMMIES®
A Wiley Brand

Neurobiology For Dummies®

Published by: **John Wiley & Sons, Inc.,** 111 River Street, Hoboken, NJ 07030-5774, www.wiley.com

Copyright © 2014 by John Wiley & Sons, Inc., Hoboken, New Jersey

Published simultaneously in Canada

No part of this publication may be reproduced, stored in a retrieval system or transmitted in any form or by any means, electronic, mechanical, photocopying, recording, scanning or otherwise, except as permitted under Sections 107 or 108 of the 1976 United States Copyright Act, without the prior written permission of the Publisher. Requests to the Publisher for permission should be addressed to the Permissions Department, John Wiley & Sons, Inc., 111 River Street, Hoboken, NJ 07030, (201) 748-6011, fax (201) 748-6008, or online at http://www.wiley.com/go/permissions.

Trademarks: Wiley, For Dummies, the Dummies Man logo, Dummies.com, Making Everything Easier, and related trade dress are trademarks or registered trademarks of John Wiley & Sons, Inc., and may not be used without written permission. All other trademarks are the property of their respective owners. John Wiley & Sons, Inc., is not associated with any product or vendor mentioned in this book.

For general information on our other products and services, please contact our Customer Care Department within the U.S. at 877-762-2974, outside the U.S. at 317-572-3993, or fax 317-572-4002. For technical support, please visit www.wiley.com/techsupport.

Wiley publishes in a variety of print and electronic formats and by print-on-demand. Some material included with standard print versions of this book may not be included in e-books or in print-on-demand. If this book refers to media such as a CD or DVD that is not included in the version you purchased, you may download this material at http://booksupport.wiley.com. For more information about Wiley products, visit www.wiley.com.

Library of Congress Control Number: 2013954238

ISBN 978-1-118-68931-8 (pbk); ISBN 978-1-118-69146-5 (ebk)

Manufactured in the United States of America

10 9 8 7 6 5 4 3 2 1

Contents at a Glance

Table of Contents

Introduction

· ·

*L*ife existed for a long time on earth before human intelligence. Does our planet just happen to be the only one whose conditions make life possible? Or are we one of billions of planets that sustain life? If little green men in flying saucers showed up, we could ask them the answer. But failing that, and without any conclusive evidence, we don't really know.

The data we do have that we can examine is that life originated at least once here on earth very shortly after conditions appeared to be suitable to support it. More than three billion years after that, we humans appeared as a result of an almost uncountable number of life cycles, mutations, and reproductions.

This book is about the essential essence of humans as an intelligent life form — the nervous system. We can and do ask many questions about the nervous system, but here are three of the big ones:

- ✔ What does our nervous system have in common with that of other animals?
- ✔ How is our nervous system different from that of other animals?
- ✔ What differences between humans are associated with differences in their nervous systems?

Neurobiologists have some answers to all three of these questions. We know that neurons are specialized cells with some functions specific to neurons, and others similar to most other cells on earth. We also know that nervous systems have similar organizational themes and methods of communication across all animal species. On the other hand, the nervous systems of mammals and primates are vastly more complicated than those of invertebrates and even of cold-blooded vertebrates. Finally, we know that small genetic differences and life experiences can produce significant changes in the behavior of identical twins that otherwise have almost identical brains.

This book attempts to explain in ordinary language how neurons work, how neurons make nervous systems, and how nervous systems produce intelligence and complex behavior.

About This Book

This book starts with basic concepts and builds off of them. It first discusses cells and their origin and functions, then deals with basic brain anatomy made from those cells, and finally describes specialized systems for sensation, movement, and cognition.

The way this book is organized allows you to find the information you need quickly, whether you want to look up information on a neural dysfunction of a friend or relative who has Alzheimer's or Parkinson's diseases or you want to find out what the brain's thalamus actually does.

Besides being a resource for any non-scientist inquisitive about the brain and nervous system, this book may be a useful accompanying text for students in undergraduate neurobiology courses because it's both modular and functional. For example, many books talk about brain anatomy using massively long lists of obscurely named brain nuclei and tracts, but they don't try to help you understand all these components as a functional system. Perception and behavioral neuroscience courses often neglect important aspects of cognitive processing, while cognitive science texts often give you little information about how neural activity actually supports cognition. This book is different. This book uses plain language and some very simple diagrams to show how important parts of the brain and nervous system function.

Sidebars (text in gray boxes) and anything marked with a Technical Stuff icon are skippable. Also, within this book, you may notice some web addresses breaking across two lines of text. If you're reading this book in print and you want to visit one of these web pages, simply key in the web address exactly as it's noted in the text, pretending as though the line break doesn't exist. If you're reading this as an e-book, you've got it easy — just click the web address to be taken directly to the web page.

Foolish Assumptions

As I wrote this book, I made some assumptions about you, the reader:

- ✔ You may be looking for information about a neurological disease or dysfunction, possibly affecting someone you know. You want access this information quickly in easy-to-understand chunks.

- ✔ You may be taking a college or professional course that covers some aspect of brain function, but the course or the text for the course doesn't provide enough background information.

✔ You may be a beginning student in neuroscience, neurology, or neurosurgery who has already learned what's in this book but you need to look up the basics quickly, maybe to explain it to a layperson. (*Warning:* If your patients notice you rifling through a copy of this book before recommending treatment options, they might request a second opinion.)

Icons Used in This Book

I use icons in this book to help you find specific kinds of information. They include the following:

Anything marked with a Tip icon is a piece of information about an area of neurobiology that's often misunderstood or easily confused.

The Remember icon highlights key concepts and principles that you need to remember to understand other areas of neurobiology.

The Research icon is about key studies that led to our current understanding of neurobiology. Sometimes pieces of research are just beautiful in their own right for their elegance and simplicity. Research info bits are nice to drop in conversations at cocktail parties — if you party with people nerdy enough to know a fair amount of neurobiology, at least.

The Technical Stuff icon is about a recent or surprising finding that is not necessarily crucial to understand the chapter but is interesting or counterintuitive in its own right. You can skip these paragraphs and get by just fine, but you may miss some of the more interesting products of research.

Beyond the Book

In addition to the material in the print or e-book you're reading right now, this product also comes with some access-anywhere goodies on the web. Check out the free Cheat Sheet at www.dummies.com/cheatsheet/neurobiology for interesting information on whether paralysis can be cured, whether the mind can be downloaded, whether cyborgs are possible, and more.

Also, check out www.dummies.com/extras/neurobiology for articles on everything from where consciousness exists in the brain to how vision can be restored to the blind.

Where to Go from Here

You can start reading this book anywhere — you don't have to read it in order from beginning to end. Still, Chapter 1 is a great place to start if you're looking for an introduction to neurobiology. For more on common diseases and disorders, turn to Part IV. And if you're short on time, Chapters 19 and 20 pack a powerful punch in not many pages.

I'm always interested in hearing from readers, so whether you find an error or you'd like to make any other comments about this book, feel free to contact me at amthorfr@gmail.com.

Part I
Getting Started with Neurobiology

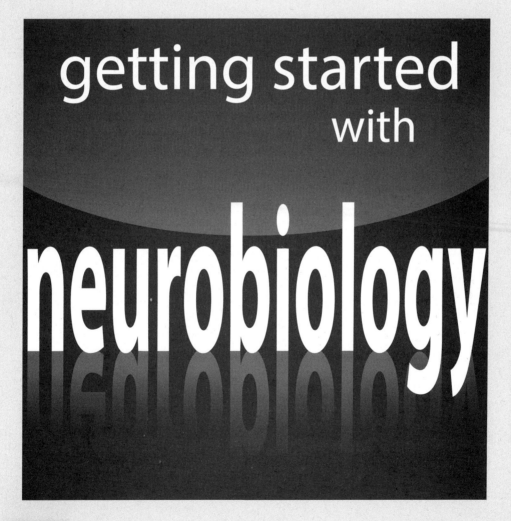

In this part . . .

- ✔ Find out what makes neurons different from other cells in the body.

- ✔ Discover the genetics common to all cells and what happens when neurons have genetic mutations.

- ✔ See what neurons need in order to be able to detect and respond to other neurons, substances in the environment, and energy.

- ✔ Look at how neurons communicate with each other using electrical current flowing through ion channels.

Chapter 1

Welcome to the World of Neurobiology

*W*hat makes you *you?* Your brain, most people would answer. Then what is it about your brain that makes you *you?* The brain is made of neurons. Worms have brains with neurons. So do dogs and monkeys. What about the brain distinguishes these animals from each other, and for that matter, one human from another? Is it more neurons, different neurons, special neural circuits?

Neurobiologists would like to answer all these questions, but they can't yet. Thousands of them at universities all over the world are working on these problems. They have many hypotheses and data sets. This book, in a way, is a progress report on their efforts.

Virtually all neurobiologists believe that intelligence comes from nervous systems that are broadly programmed by genes and fine-tuned by experience. Generally, the human genetic program creates a brain with more neurons than any other animal, allowing for richer experience to produce a unique kind of intelligence.

This chapter gives an overview of the brain, its functions, and its parts. It also looks at why humans are like many other animals, such as primates, because of similarities in our brains, and what differences in the human brain may distinguish us from other species, and from each other.

Introducing Neurons

Neurobiology is the study of neurons and nervous systems, such as brains. *Neurons* are cells. Like other cells, neurons interact with the external world and other cells through specialized receptors in their membranes and through biochemical processes inside their cytoplasm and nucleus.

Neural capabilities evolved from those of single-celled organisms, like bacteria and paramecia, which use membrane sensors to detect food and toxins, and cilia to move toward food and away from toxins. Single-cell organisms may also change their internal metabolism upon ingesting particular substances from the environment.

Multicellular organisms consist of different types of cells that are specialized to do things like secrete hormones or digestive enzymes. They depend on other cells for nutrients, waste removal, and the maintenance of a supportive environment. Neurons are specialized cells in multicellular organisms that, among other things, enable rapid communication across the large distances from one end of an animal to another. This allows the animals to perform coordinated movements and to act upon sensing the surrounding environment.

Evolving cells on early earth

According to astronomers and astrophysicists, the universe as we know it came into existence about 14 billion years ago. After several cycles of star formation, our solar system, including the earth, formed about 4.5 billion years ago. The earth was too hot for life for about a billion years, as it continued to be bombarded by the solar system debris from which it was formed.

Eventually most of the solar system debris stuck to one or another planet, or stabilized in relevantly permanent orbits such as the asteroid belt between Mars and Jupiter. Earth cooled for about 1 billion years, and life arose. No one knows how. Some scientists are suspicious that life arose almost as soon as the earth was cool enough, suggesting either that it must occur almost automatically given the right conditions, or it came from elsewhere and established a foothold as soon as it was possible.

Looking at the origin of single cells

The living things that arose at the 1-billion-year mark were single-celled *prokaryote* cells that lack a nucleus, such as bacteria we have today. Life stayed unicellular for a long time after that. This doesn't mean that no progress was made, though. Undoubtedly the single cells that existed at the time of evolution to multicellularity were more sophisticated and diverse than those that could be found when life originated.

Catalyzing reactions in the primordial soup

All life forms carry out metabolism, using energy to build proteins and other cell constituents. The proteins in all cells are coded for by the same DNA coding scheme (see Chapter 2), one piece of evidence that argues for a common origin of all life. A particularly important type of protein that all cells make is an enzyme. Enzymes cause specific reactions such as cleaving proteins at a particular place or joining proteins to other molecules.

Many of the DNA sequences, proteins, and reactions that exist in multicellular organisms are similar to those in single-celled organisms. This apparent conservation of biochemistry is an important argument for life having a common origin.

Separating inside from out: Membranes

A fundamental property of cells is that they have membranes that separate their insides from the external environment. What makes a cell what it is and does relies significantly on the receptors it has in its membrane and how they respond to external substances and energy inputs.

Cellular responses to substances that bind membrane receptors include biochemical cascades inside the cell, and, in neurons particularly, electrical activity. A significant percentage of all animal genes code for proteins that compose hundreds of different types of membrane receptors.

Comparing eukaryotes to prokaryotes

About 1 to 2 billion years after single-cell life arose, some single-cell life forms developed nuclei and became what are called *eukaryotes* (cells that have a nucleus). Soon after eukaryotes appeared, multicellular organisms came on the scene.

Plant-like multicellular organisms probably arose from aggregations of single cells in shallow ocean areas. These multicellular organisms diversified over more than a billion years. About half a billion years ago, 4 billion years after the earth formed, land plants and animals that we would recognize as such appeared from these multicellular ancestors.

Multicellularity: Sensing and moving

Multicellularity has advantages and disadvantages. Multicellular organisms can be big, have specialized sensors, and move around and ingest single-celled organisms. But movement requires coordination, and the environment of the cells at the periphery of the organisms is quite different from that of those in the middle.

Multicellularity allowed organisms to have cells specialized not only for niches in the external environment, but also for the internal environment created by the structure of the organism itself. Neural cells evolved as sensors, movers (muscles), and communicators.

Detecting food, waste, and toxins

Neurons have some functions that are like all other cells, including those of many single-celled organisms. These include taking in energy through glucose, and oxygen to fuel metabolism. Neurons also excrete metabolic waste products and carbon dioxide. Many of these functions are carried out by membrane receptors and transporters, some of which are highly conserved across the evolution of life on earth. But neurons adapted many functions that single cells use to interact with the environment in order to interact with each other.

Detecting other cells: Hormones and neurotransmitters

Even primitive single-celled and small multicellular organisms respond to the effects of other organisms around them. This happens via their metabolic waste products that signal overcrowding or the depletion of food resources. Neurons evolved the ability to include some specific substances in their waste excretions to signal to other neurons about the state of some part of the organism.

These signaling substances evolved to be secreted specifically into the extra-cellular space around cells in multicellular organisms as hormones. The next step was the extension of a cellular process, such as an axon, from one cell to the vicinity of several distant specific cells where a specific signaling substance, called a *neurotransmitter,* was released. Now, instead of a multicellular signaling soup, there are circuits.

Detecting energy

Although single-celled organisms have membrane receptors that can detect light, heat, and pressure, multicellular organisms devote large, complex cell systems for detecting these and other forms of environmental energy. Cellular systems allow the production of lenses in the visual system for seeing and mechanical amplification in the auditory system for hearing, to name but two examples. Cellular systems in multicellular organisms allow energy detection to be amplified and differentiated, which supports nuanced, complex behavioral outcomes based on the detection.

Cellular motors

Single cells move via cilia, flagella, and other mechanisms such as amoeboid movement. Multicellular organisms use cilia to move substances within the body, but moving the entire body requires other mechanisms.

Cilia and flagella

Cilia are common in multicellular organisms. Motile cilia on cells in the lungs remove debris by carrying it up the windpipe. Immotile or primary cilia have evolved in many multicellular animals into sensory receptors, such as photoreceptor outer segments where the light-absorbing photopigment molecules are located. Auditory hair cells and some olfactory receptors may also be derived from cilia. Flagella are used by sperm cells to propel themselves. However, moving an entire large body via cilia or flagella is not very effective, particularly on land.

Contraction

Animals evolved specialized cells called muscle cells, for movement. Muscle cells work by contracting. In voluntary skeletal muscle, muscle cells contract by being driven by motor neurons. A large group of contracting muscle cells pulls on a tendon that is attached to a bone, moving the joint.

Neurons are necessary for coordinated movement in multicellular animals. Different muscles must be contracted in an organized manner, and information from the senses must be sent to remote parts of the body neurons to coordinate movement.

Neurons accomplish their role of coordinating and communicating activity across the body though chemical communication and electricity. The electrical properties of neurons allow them to communicate information precisely across long distances to specific target cells. In the case of connections to muscles, motor neurons produce movement by inducing their target muscle cells to contract.

Coordinating responses in simple circuits

Nervous systems are complex and hard to study. The human brain has been estimated to contain about 100 billion cells (a recent estimate that used a novel method of counting neural nuclei in emulsified brains produced a figure of 86 billion). All these neurons likely have from 100 trillion to a quadrillion synapses between them. This presents the challenges that we don't know how single cells work, really, and we don't know or cannot even count all the connections between them. So, where do we start?

People often wonder why scientists study the nervous systems of flies, worms, and squids. The reason is that these systems often have advantages in that the cells are fewer, bigger, or more amenable to genetic manipulation. Hodgkin and Huxley won the Nobel Prize for deducing the ionic basis of the action potential in the squid giant axon, which is almost a millimeter in diameter and can be handled and impaled with microelectrodes. It is also possible to squeeze out its internal contents and replace them with a specified salt solution by which it could be determined which ions flow which way through the membrane during electrical activity.

Many invertebrates such as worms and insects have less than a few thousand neurons that are more or less the same from animal to animal. Individual neurons in specific places are even numbered and named in some species. This vastly simplifies the problem of working out a complete neural circuit, including which neurotransmitters are used by which neurons to activate other neurons, and how all the electrical activity is integrated.

Recent progress has been made in making model systems from mammals, using either brain slices or neural tissue cultures that can be mounted on a microscope and recorded and stimulated under well-controlled conditions.

Robotics and bionics

Many scientists feel that we only understand a system when we can simulate it. This involves creating an artificial nervous system that simulates some properties of real ones. In robotics, behavior is simulated. A robot may perform some task, like welding in a car factory, that is otherwise done by intelligent humans. The electronic controllers of such robots can involve the use of neuron-like elements called artificial neural nets (ANNs) that emulate biological control systems. However, most controllers are written in standard computer languages using mathematical algorithms that may function quite differently from biological organizations.

Bionics is the field of applying biological principles of operation to man-made devices. An airplane is a bionic derivative of bird flight, which, however, differs in using engines for thrust rather than flapping wings. A recent use of bionics in computation involves devices called *memristors* that are integrated circuit devices that act like modifiable synapses between neurons. At this point, it's unclear whether memristors devices will have advantages for computing compared to traditional electronic computation done with transistors. They may, however, become a useful tool for simulating complex nervous systems to understand them.

Organizing the Nervous System

The study of the nervous system intrinsically involves many fields. Neurobiology, our focus here, depends on physiology, anatomy, biochemistry, molecular biology, cognitive and behavioral psychology, and artificial intelligence. The basic goals of neurobiology are to describe how the nervous system operates in terms of what the system does, how it's built, and how it works. We try to do these things by considering first various subsystems of the brain and nervous system, and then looking carefully at function in the neural circuitry within those subsystems.

Movement basics: Muscles and motor systems

Chapter 5 deals with the main purpose of the nervous system, the production of movement. Generally, animals move and have nervous systems to control movement, whereas plants don't. Voluntary movement, controlled by the central nervous system, involves the contraction of striated muscle triggered by the receipt of *acetylcholine,* a neurotransmitter released by motor neurons.

Individual muscles are made of thousands of muscle cells innervated by several different types of motor neurons. The contraction of the muscle is produced by the coordinated activity of all these motor neurons that fire in a specified sequence and rate depending on the type of movement programmed, its speed, duration, and variation in load the limb experiences as it moves. Differences or errors between the central commands and actual limb position and acceleration are reported by sensory neurons in the muscles, tendons, and joints that relay this information to the spinal cord in a feedback loop that adjusts the motor neuron output to match the upper-level command goal.

The entire frontal lobe of the brain exists primarily to program and organize goal-directed movement. An abstract goal, such as hitting a tennis ball back into your opponent's court, is translated into a sequence of leg, torso, and arm movements to accomplish this goal. These sequences are programmed into the motor cortex following practice. This practice involves learning sequence timing with the help of the cerebellum. The cerebellum is involved in learning and setting up predictive, feed-forward control for appropriate timing of sequences that transition more rapidly than feedback spinal sensory control could correct.

The spinal cord and autonomic nervous system

The spinal cord is like a subcontractor of the brain that executes the brain's instructions and reports on their progress. The spinal cord is part of the central nervous system, contiguous with it as it merges with the medulla of the brainstem. Chapter 6 discusses its basic organization.

The spinal cord is the transition below the neck between the central and peripheral nervous systems. The peripheral nervous system includes the motor neuron axons that originate within the spinal cord gray area and project from the cord to synapse on muscle cells. Sensory neurons — whose cell bodies are located in dorsal root ganglia just outside the spinal cord — send one axon collateral to the periphery to elaborate into a sensory receptor, while the other collateral makes conventional synapses in the spinal cord gray area for both local circuit spinal feedback control and for relaying sensory information to the brain.

The autonomic and enteric nervous systems are involved in body *homeostasis* (keeping the body's major systems stable and functioning) through controlling glandular secretions, heart rate, respiration, and smooth muscle function. The autonomic nervous system has major subdivisions into sympathetic and parasympathetic branches that tend to oppose each other's actions. The sympathetic system prepares us for action in the fight-or-flight mode, while the parasympathetic system organizes resources for digestion, and the maintenance and conservation of energy.

The brainstem, limbic system, hypothalamus, and reticular formation

When we look at a human brain from above, almost all that we see is neocortex. Students beginning to study the brain often mistakenly think that the neocortex is the real, important part of the brain that has largely superseded phylogenetically older structures that are now almost vestigial and unnecessary (like the appendix).

This is an understandable mistake. However, non-mammalian vertebrates like lizards, frogs, and crocodiles execute complex behavior without any neocortex. Some mammals have very little neocortex as well. The relationship between the neocortex and "lower" brain areas is as much their servant as master, an idea Chapter 7 explores.

The brainstem is not only a transition region between the spinal cord and higher brain centers, but an essential integration and control center by itself. The brainstem includes the medulla at the intersection with the spinal cord, the pons just above the medulla, and the midbrain above that. The cerebellum hangs off the back of the brain behind the pons. The brainstem nuclei convey information between the senses and the spinal cord and higher brain centers. Brainstem nuclei also control essential aspects of homeostasis such as the regulation of heart rate, respiration, and temperature.

Limbic system is an archaic term for a diverse set of subcortical brain areas that are thought to control instinctive behaviors. Areas included in the limbic system's original formation include the hippocampus, amygdala, and cingulate cortex. Chapter 7 discusses how these areas interact with neocortex and other parts of the brain, not as a modular system, but as a set of crucial brain areas each with distinct functions.

The hypothalamus sits just above the pituitary gland and receives sensory input from the autonomic nervous system. It controls many homeostatic processes (such as circadian rhythms — the body's internal "clock") by secretions of hormones into the bloodstream and by projecting to the pituitary, which itself secretes hormones.

The reticular formation is a diffuse network of neurons and axon tracts that runs through the brainstem up into portions of the thalamus. This area controls body state through processes such as controlling wakefulness versus sleep, alertness, and homeostatic mechanisms such as heart rate.

Basal ganglia, cerebellum, motor and premotor cortex, and thalamus

Chapter 8 takes up the basal ganglia, major controllers of behavior. The major basal ganglia nuclei include the caudate and putamen, which together make up the input region called the *striatum*. The globus pallidus is the major basal ganglia output to the motor portion of the thalamus, which projects and receives input from motor areas in the frontal lobe. The basal ganglia nuclei interact extensively with the substantia nigra in the midbrain, and the subthalamic nucleus.

The cerebellum is a motor learning and coordination center. It receives sensory input from spinal sensory neurons and cranial nerves of the vestibular and visual systems. Its major output is to motor thalamus that projects to frontal motor cortex. The cerebellum is necessary for learning coordinated, well-timed movements. It operates as a feed-forward controller that generates error signals used to reprogram motor areas such as premotor cortex to generate appropriate limb movements.

Two frontal areas just anterior to primary motor cortex, the supplementary motor area (SMA) and premotor cortex (PMC), contain motor programs that command and coordinate multi-limb movements to accomplish goals. One main difference between these two areas is that motor programs in SMA tend to be those that we can learn to do with little sensory feedback, such as typing. PMC control tends to occur when sequences are being learned, and depends more on peripheral feedback and cerebellar error signals.

The thalamus is often called the gateway to the neocortex, since all senses — except for some of *olfaction* (the sense of smell) — relay through it. But the neocortex projects back extensively to the thalamus. These back projections come from "higher" cortical areas, as well as from the primary areas that receive inputs from that area of the thalamus.

The gateway metaphor for the thalamus implicitly makes the neocortex the real seat of neural control and computation. The thalamus is the modulator of transmission to the cortex, emphasizing some pathways at the expense of others as a mediator of attention. A different metaphor for thalamic-cortical interactions is that the thalamus is running the "main" program, which makes "subroutine" calls to the neocortex for some detailed neural computations. This makes processing in the thalamus the primary controller of brain activity, including consciousness (see Chapter 14). Activity in the neocortex becomes the content of that consciousness. It's too early to say whether this subroutine metaphor will be as useful as the gateway metaphor has been.

The neocortex

The neocortex is one of the most important "inventions" of mammals. It dominates the mammalian brain in volume, particularly in primates. One of the most remarkable properties of the neocortex is that it has the same six-layered structure virtually everywhere, with the same cell types in what appears to be the same general minicolumn circuit. This is in stark contrast to the rest of the brain, where each area tends to have its own distinct set of cell types and neural circuits.

Mammals became the dominant land animals on earth after the demise of the dinosaurs about 65 million years ago. Some neurobiologists conjecture that mammals were able to rapidly diversify into all the niches abandoned by the extinction of the dinosaurs, as well as many new ones, by expanding the standard neocortex circuit for processing whatever visual, auditory, or fine motor acuity that niche demanded.

Neocortical processing power is primarily a function of area. Increased area in neocortex has two main uses:

- ✓ Increasing "acuity," whereby, for example, a larger area can support a higher density of peripheral receptors, such as retinal ganglion cells in the fovea or mechanoreceptors in the fingertips.
- ✓ Increasing the number of processing stages in a hierarchy of "association" areas that are increasingly specific and powerful with respect to particular features. Examples are the fusiform face area that allows you to instantly identify thousands of faces that all have the same major features (eyes, nose, mouth) in the same relative positions.

TIP

The neocortex goes digital

The expansion of the neocortex is reminiscent of the transition in the 1960s from analog to digital computers. When vacuum tubes and then transistors were made and handled individually, the most efficient control circuits were those in which a small number of devices modeled the control environment and generated a continuous control output from continuous inputs via the model.

But when integrated digital circuits arose using thousands and millions of transistors, it became more efficient to represent the control environment on standard microprocessors using software. This provided the advantages of *acuity* (insensitivity to transistor parameter values) and *adaptability* (software can be changed and augmented easily). The commonality of the representation and transformation of information in the cortical minicolumn appear to be an essential basis of its success in taking over the brain, and in mammals, including humans, taking over the earth.

Perceiving the World, Thinking, Learning, and Remembering

Different parts of the brain do different things. The front of the brain in the frontal lobe controls movement, the back and sides of the brain process sensory information. Specialized memory areas perform certain memory functions — the hippocampus and amygdala, for example. Chapters 10 through 14 deal with pathways and brain areas that process sensory information and memory, and produce motor output and thought.

Looking at vision and audition

The standard list of five major senses consists of vision, hearing, skin sensation, taste, and smell. The senses of limb position (called *proprioception*) and limb movement and acceleration (called *kinesthesis*) are built along similar lines and pathways with skin sensation.

Chapter 10 deals with vision and audition, starting with the peripheral receptors in the eye and ear, and marching up the projection pathways through the thalamus and onto primary, secondary, and higher-order cortical processing areas. In many mammals, particularly primates, visual processing dominates the brain — so much so that just less than 50 percent of the neurons in the brain have their activity modulated by visual input. In both vision and audition, high-order brain areas process complex inputs, such as face-specific neurons in inferotemporal cortex in vision, and language'specific areas in audition such as Wernicke's area.

Feeling, smelling, and tasting

Skin sensation is composed of a group of different types of sensory capabilities controlled by different receptors in the skin and a few other places, such as the mouth and trachea. Mechanoreceptors detect shallow and deep pressure, applied constantly or intermittently. Cold and warm temperature receptors respond to skin temperatures below or above body temperature. Pain receptors respond to mechanical or chemical inputs likely to cause injury.

The sense of smell is mediated by several thousand different receptor types in the olfactory organ in the roof of the nasal cavity. Evolutionary evidence suggests that some of the earliest neocortex in mammals may have been devoted to sorting out and identifying what produced the smells detected by the olfactory receptors.

A dog has about one billion olfactory receptors, a number comparable to the total number of neurons in its entire brain. I'm sure my dogs sniffing around the yard every morning know what was there last night, and probably when, and probably what each critter did, from the smells left over.

The olfactory system is unique in being divided between a pathway that projects (although indirectly) through the thalamus, of which we are aware, and a pathway that is non-thalamic, which influences our behavior, but of which we are not directly aware.

The sense of taste is mediated by salt, sweet, sour, and bitter receptors located mostly on the tongue. Some taste researchers also include the MSG taste, umami, as a fundamental taste.

Learning and memory: Circuits and plasticity

A behavioral hallmark of mammals is they can change their behavior through learning. High-level learning involves a neural representation of both an event and its context. Much of this representation occurs in the lateral prefrontal cortex as what is called *working memory*. This area of cortex has extensive connections with the hippocampus, where modifiable synapses containing NMDA receptors abound. Reciprocal connections between the hippocampus and the neocortical areas that originally represented that which is to be remembered instantiate the memory "trace" back in those areas of the neocortex.

The finding that the neocortex represents both original sensory input and its memory has profound implications for understanding what memory is. Many neuroscientists now believe that memory is intrinsically reconstructive — a hallucination, if you will. This is a very different metaphor from the token look up and address model taken from computer science. One important aspect of the reconstructive aspect of memory is that the act of reconstruction can distort the memory. Suggestions, guesses, and events after the memory can affect the reconstruction such that they become part of, and indistinguishable from, subsequent reconstructions.

The neurobiology of memory depends both on modifiable synaptic weights, such as with NMDA receptors in hippocampus and cortex, and the creation of new neurons in memory areas such as the hippocampus. The discovery of the birth of neurons in the adult hippocampus overturns the old idea of zero neurogenesis in the adult brain. Some senile dementia and even depression appear to be associated with failure of this mechanism.

The frontal lobes and executive brain

The frontal lobes are responsible for planning and executing behavior. Generally speaking, the output of the frontal lobe is in its most posterior portion, the primary motor cortex. Neurons in primary motor cortex send their axons down the spinal cord (or out some cranial nerves) to drive motor neurons that cause muscles throughout the body to contract.

Anterior to the primary motor cortex are the supplementary motor area and pre-motor cortex that organize the firing of groups of muscles. Anterior to those areas are the frontal eye fields and other areas called prefrontal cortex (even though they are in the frontal lobe) that are involved in more abstract aspects of planning.

It is generally held that there is relative expansion of the frontal lobe compared to the rest of the brain in humans compared to other primates, and primates compared to other mammals. Some exceptional non-primate mammals such as the echidna have large frontal lobes, however. This has led to debate among neuroscientists about whether these frontal areas are really homologous across mammalian species. Whatever the result of that debate, we know that damage to prefrontal cortex in humans produces distinctive cognitive deficits such as impulsive behavior and profound changes in affect.

Language, emotions, lateralization, and thought

True grammatically ordered language distinguishes humans from all other species on earth. Recent evidence has suggested an important role for a gene called FOXP2 in generating language capability, although how this gene changes the brain to allow language isn't clear.

The human brain does not contain any distinct anatomical structures or types of neurons associated with language. The human brain areas most crucial for language, Wernicke's and Broca's areas on the left side (in most humans), have homologous areas in other primates, but these areas do not support language. Yet all normal human infants learn, without any explicit instruction, whatever language to which they are exposed, but other animals do not learn grammatical, word-order based language despite extensive instruction.

The capacity for learning language is built in, but neuroscience does not now know how. One clue may be brain lateralization, however. Left- versus right-side specialization for some types of audio processing and production exists in other mammals, and even some birds, but is nowhere near as extensive as in humans.

A similar association exists with right-hand dominance, driven by the left side of the brain, which is more extensive in humans than any other animal. Chimpanzees, for example, may be relatively right- or left-hand preferring, but most have no overall tendency to be strongly right-handed or left-handed, the way humans do.

Neuroscience's view of emotions has changed markedly in the last decades. Earlier views regarded emotions as leftovers from our evolution from non-rational species. *Star Trek*'s Mr. Spock could be taken as a model of a superior, more evolved humanoid. However, we now know that emotions are a means of nonverbal communication within our brains. Hunches and anxiety in certain situations are signs of danger and the need to be cautious.

We see the usefulness of this nonverbal information in people with damage to the orbitofrontal cortex or amygdala. They may gamble recklessly or commit social faux pas because they lack internal feelings about the mistakes they're making.

Developmental, Neurological, and Mental Disorders and Treatments

One of the most important reasons to understand neurobiology is to understand mental disorders and treatments. The good news is that great progress is being made in this field now. We know the genetic bases of many developmental disorders, such as Fragile X and William's syndrome. The bad news is that many disorders remain that we do not know about, and, even among disorders with known genetics, how the gene alteration produces the disorder, and what to do about it, are not clear. Chapters 15 through 18 discuss the background and current treatment approaches (if any) of many common neurological disorders.

Developing the brain and nervous system

The set of genes that define an organism is not a blueprint that is executed by a builder, but a set of procedures that brings about the development of the organism.

A useful metaphor is an ant hill or termite mound. No master ant or termite knows how to build a hill or mound and directs the other insects. Instead, ants and termites respond to each other, and to the environment, by digging holes and gluing arches together. Some holes and arches reach a critical mass that causes nearby insects to concentrate on those structures and related structures, which triggers the completion of the insect home as though its builders were following a design.

Developing cells have genetically coded responses to substances they detect by their membranes or ingest, including cell identity and brain location marker molecules. Cell responses include movement, division, and secretion of other markers and agents. The interactions among cells that have these responses in the embryological environment builds the brain.

Much of the genome is only expressed extensively during development, a time when the organism is also particularly susceptible to toxins that mimic or interfere with these markers and agents. The result of this interference is the construction of an improperly set-up brain, which is typically much worse than inferring temporarily with a properly constructed brain later in life, which often can be reversed.

Movement disorders and symptoms

Movement disorders can originate with brain damage that compromises the control of movement, or neurons that drive muscles, or the muscles themselves. Chapter 16 discusses some of the most common movement disorders. Cerebral palsy and epilepsy typically involve brain damage. Multiple sclerosis is caused by demyelination of axons of motor and other neurons. *Myasthenia gravis* is an autoimmune disease involving the cholinergic receptors on muscle cells.

Some well-known movement disorders, such as Parkinson's and Huntington's diseases, occur only later in life. Neither of these diseases is curable, but a number of treatments can partially alleviate the symptoms of Parkinson's disease. Accidents involving brain or spinal trauma still produce many cases of paralysis every year. Extensive research efforts using stem cells, neural growth factors, and electrical stimulation continue to be made for these problems.

Neural dysfunctions and mental illness

The history of clinical thought on mental illness is a pendulum ride between organic and environmental causes. In the United States, particularly, the dominance of behaviorism in academic psychology and psychiatry was associated with behavioral and cognitive therapeutic strategies based on "undoing" some sort of bad environmental influence or improper response to a relatively normal environment.

Knowledge of genetics, neurotransmitter systems, and the development of neurotransmitter-analog drugs led to pharmacological treatments that were at least partially effective in many psychiatric patients for whom traditional therapy had provided no relief. Schizophrenia and autism are cases in point. In the mid 20th century, the detection of schizophrenia or autism often was treated by family therapy sessions around behavioral theories such as withdrawn, uncaring so-called "refrigerator mothers" being the cause of these disorders.

It is now clear that both schizophrenia and autism have high heritability, although environmental factors are undoubtedly important in the expression and outcome of the disorder. Pharmacological agents deal well with many of the positive symptoms of schizophrenia such as hallucinations. But both schizophrenia and autism have multiple genetic causes, and the relation between the genetic anomaly and the neural dysfunction leading to the phenotype are poorly known. This situation is unfortunately also the case with many other mental disorders, including depression.

Repair and enhancement with artificial brains

Humans increasingly are electronically connected to each other through computers, cellphones, and soon, wearable devices like watches and electronic eyeglasses. It may be a short time before some of this technology is implantable. Brain implants may allow people who are paralyzed to operate computers or control their own or prosthetic limbs.

Deep brain stimulation, originally used widely to relieve Parkinson's disease symptoms, may also be effective in treating some types of depression. Transcranial magnetic stimulation may also mitigate depression without many of the side effects of electroconvulsive therapy (ECT, commonly referred to as "shock treatment"). Transcranial electrical stimulation has been shown in numerous studies to increase learning rates. A new term *electroceuticals* has been introduced for the field of electrical brain stimulation for therapeutic effect. Brain scientists live in exciting times!

Chapter 2

Building Neurons from Molecules

. . . .

In This Chapter

▶ Exploring genetics and inheritance

▶ Investigating cell molecules, important ions, and proteins

▶ Checking out cell architecture

▶ Assembling the cell boundary with membrane lipids

▶ Adjusting cell volume through water channels

▶ Getting to know neurons

▶ Wondering why things go wrong: mutations and illnesses

. . . .

*T*he genes in your body's cells are the reason you have your mother's brown eyes and your father's curly hair. Neurons are cells, and, like all cells in the body, they're controlled by the expression of the DNA within their nuclei. Although the DNA in all non-reproductive cells in the body is the same, how the genes are expressed is what makes the body's 300-plus cell types different from each other.

This chapter covers the basic genetics common to all cells, such as genes, chromosomes, and inheritance. It also discusses the universal genetic code, the expression of genes, and protein synthesis. And if you ever wondered what makes neurons so special compared to other cells, read on to find out about their unique features and functions. Bringing these ideas together, the final sections talk about what happens when neurons have genetic defects, such as mutations that lead to neurological illness. I also look at how science may be able to fix these problems.

Getting into Genetics

Genetics is the study of genes and how they control inheritance. We can typically see the results of inheritance in the features of offspring, which has received genes from each of its parents. *Genes* are sequences of nucleotides (see "Greeting chromosomes and genes," a bit later on for more) located on chromosomes in the cell's nucleus. Genes specify the production of amino acid sequences. (Amino acids are the constituent units that make up proteins.)

Long before genes were known to be located on chromosomes composed of DNA, science had worked out some basic principles of inheritance, such as dominant and recessive traits. The upcoming sections explore these concepts in more detail.

Introducing inheritance

Mendelian inheritance is one of the cornerstones of genetics, based on the famous pea experiments of the monk Gregor Mendel. Genes determine the features, or *traits,* that you inherited from your parents. Some traits you can see, such as height or hair color, and others you can't, such as blood type. Genes are copied and inherited across generations. Different genes cause different traits to present themselves, and each unique form of a single gene is called an *allele.* So, for example, the gene specifying blue eyes comes from a different allele than the gene specifying brown eyes.

Doubling genes

Organisms typically have two copies of each gene, one inherited from each parent. Each parent also has two copies of each gene, and passes along to its offspring a single copy by a (nearly) random selection of their two genes. This gene is found on a chromosome present in either the mother's eggs or the father's sperm. When the egg and sperm join, they form a double set of genes again.

Phenotype and genotype

The set of expressed traits of an organism are called its *phenotype,* whereas the genes within the organism are called its *genotype.* Since Mendel's experiments, we have known that the traits an offspring expresses (phenotype) are not simply a mixing of the traits it got from the two sets of genes it inherited from its parents (genotype).

Determining dominant and recessive traits

One *allele* (that is, one particular form of a gene) may completely override the expression of another, making this the *dominant* allele. The non-expressed allele, or the allele that doesn't show up in the offspring as a trait, is called the *recessive* allele. For a recessive allele to be expressed in an offspring as a trait, the offspring must receive two copies of the same recessive allele. Otherwise, the traits associated with the dominant allele will be expressed.

For example, the O blood type is recessive compared to types A and B. An AO father and BO mother would have A and B blood types, respectively, because the alleles specifying A blood type and B blood type are dominant. However, because these parents both have the recessive O allele, they could potentially produce an OO child. (This happens about 25 percent of the time.)

Most traits, such as height, depend on several genes. These traits have more complicated, mixed inheritance, because each of a number of genes contributes something to the end result. *Mutations,* which are random changes in genes, can also occur. Mutations can convert one allele into another, or even create a totally new allele and corresponding trait. (Go to the end of this chapter for more about mutations.)

Mutations are fundamental to evolution because they allow species to change and adapt over time.

Greeting chromosomes and genes

Genes are made of DNA (DNA stands for deoxyribonucleic acid), a nucleic acid that is composed of long sequences of *nucleotides.* DNA exists in the form of a double helix that is tightly coiled within the nucleus of the cell. Only four types of nucleotides make DNA:

- Adenine (A)
- Cytosine (C)
- Guanine (G)
- Thymine (T)

Mitotic cell division or *mitosis* is the process in which chromosomes are duplicated, segregated, and allocated so that each daughter cell has a complete set of chromosomes derived from the parent. *Eukaryotic organisms* (those whose cells have a nucleus), such as animals and plants, have most of their DNA inside the cell nucleus — although some DNA exists in organelles such as mitochondria. *Prokaryotic organisms* (those whose cells generally do not have a nucleus), such as bacteria, have DNA in their cytoplasm.

Each organism has a unique sequence of DNA. The only exception: identical twins, although even identical twins may differ slightly because of mutations accrued during their development. Humans have 23 pairs of chromosomes that make up a total of over 3 million nucleotides.

The total difference in the DNA sequence between two humans is less than 0.5 percent, whereas the difference between a human and a chimpanzee is about 2 percent.

Replicating DNA and the cell life cycle

Cell division (see the preceding section) involves several additional processes.

DNA replication

DNA replication is the process of copying DNA. It's important for cell division, so that each daughter cell inherits the full genome of its parent cell. The complementary double-stranded DNA molecule splits, and each strand produces a new complement, creating two identical copies of the double-stranded DNA sequence.

Cell division occurs in a cell cycle sequence (which we explore in a moment). A different type of DNA replication occurs in *meiosis,* producing daughter cells that have only half the number of chromosomes as the parent cell. A new chromosome can be created from a combination of both parent chromosomes in a process of breaking and joining, which is called *crossover.*

DNA replication begins when protein complexes sequentially unwind the DNA into two strands. As this unwinding proceeds, new strands that are complementary to each of the single strands are synthesized. The enzyme DNA polymerase is responsible for this process, because it adds nucleotides that are complementary to the nucleotides of the original strand.

The addition of nucleotides is based on the two pairs being complementary: Adenine binds to thymine, and cytosine binds to guanine via hydrogen bonds. One end is called the 3' (three-prime) and the other the 5' (five-prime) end. DNA polymerase (see the upcoming section, "Coding for proteins: RNA and DNA") synthesizes DNA directionally by adding the 5' end of a nucleotide to the free 3' end of a nascent DNA strand. Thus, the DNA strand is elongated in the 5' to 3' direction.

The cell cycle

The *cell cycle* is the process by which one parent cell divides into two daughter cells. This cycle involves both DNA *replication* and cell division. In eukaryotes, the phase when the cell is not dividing is called *interphase.* The division of the cell into two daughter cells occurs during *mitosis,* which is itself divided into different phases: prophase, metaphase, anaphase, and telophase. After telophase, *cytokinesis* occurs, which is the phase when the cytoplasm actually divides into two daughter cells.

Coding for proteins: RNA and DNA

Protein synthesis is the process by which cells generate proteins from the code in the DNA sequence. It occurs in several stages, including *transcription* from DNA to messenger RNA (mRNA), and *translation,* or the assembly of proteins by ribosomes using the mRNA template. (RNA is a nucleotide like DNA, except is has the nucleotide uracil substituted for thymine.) This section explores these stages.

The DNA molecule is a double-stranded helix. It's well suited for storing and replicating biological information because the two strands are complementary. An adenine in one strand is always bound to a thymine in the other, and likewise for guanine and cytosine, called *base pairing.* This complementary structure enables replication by splitting the two DNA strands, so each forms a new complement strand. The double helix is stable and resistant to cleavage, allowing the body's trillions of cells to store the genetic code.

The genetic code

The *genetic code* is a sequence of three nucleotides (called a *codon*) that specifies an amino acid. As I mention earlier in this chapter, four types of nucleotides exist, so a three-nucleotide sequence (such as ACT or TAG) with four choices at each position allows for 64 possible codons (or 4^3). However, only 20 amino acids are used to make proteins. Several different codons specify the same amino acid. This may sound redundant, and the concept is sometimes called *degeneracy,* but this degeneracy does have benefits. One benefit is that some mutations that change one of the nucleotides may not change which amino acid is produced — so the protein's function won't be compromised.

Messenger RNA has a "start" codon that codes for methionine in eukaryotes. Three special codons (TAA, TGA, and TAG), called "stop" codons, signify the end of the coding region for one protein. Start and stop codons allow the biochemical machinery that generates proteins from DNA to begin and end on the right nucleotides. A *frame shift error* occurs when translation doesn't start at the beginning of a codon, but reads the end of one codon and the beginning of another. A frame shift error causes the entire sequence of amino acids to be wrong.

Transcription mechanisms

Transcription occurs in the cell nucleus. The transcription process "reads" the DNA code to create a matching messenger RNA molecular template that will exit the nucleus and be used to synthesize proteins. The RNA strand is complementary to the DNA strand, just like the two single DNA strands are complementary to each other in the double helix, except that in RNA the nucleotide uracil takes the place that thymine occupies in DNA.

In transcription, one strand of the DNA double helix — the template strand — is used to form the complementary mRNA sequence. The transcription process has three stages that are regulated by transcription factors and co-activators:

- **Initiation:** In this first part of transcription, DNA is partially "unzipped" by the enzyme helicase, allowing access to the DNA nucleotide sequence for copying. Transcription factors bind the *promoter* region of the gene, which is a control region immediately preceding the beginning of the gene. *Polymerase,* the molecule that copies DNA into RNA, binds to a complex of transcription factors at the promoter.

- **Elongation:** RNA polymerase unwinds the DNA double helix, moves down it, and elongates the RNA transcript by adding ribonucleotides in a 5' to 3' direction (refer to the earlier section, "DNA replication"). The RNA polymerase "reads" the DNA strand sequentially and produces a single strand of messenger RNA (complementary to the DNA sequence that is its template).

- **Termination:** When the RNA polymerase reaches the end of the gene, the mRNA and polymerase detach from the DNA. The single strand of newly synthesized mRNA leaves the nucleus through nuclear pores and migrates into the cytoplasm.

Protein synthesis

The mRNA sequence is not usually directly *translated* into the amino acid sequence forming a protein. In eukaryotic cells, the mRNA (called *primary transcript*) undergoes post-transcriptional modification to yield what's called heterophilic nuclear RNA (hnRNA). *Spliceosomes* (a combination of nucleoproteins and RNA molecules that help to splice) then remove the *introns* (noncoding parts of the gene) from the hnRNA. This produces the final mRNA — composed of the coding *exons*. (See the section "Introns versus exons," later in this chapter.)

Ribosomes translate the modified messenger RNA and convert its RNA sequence using transfer RNA (tRNA) on ribosomes. Each transfer RNA is a small RNA molecule that is loosely linked to a single amino acid for which it codes. The ribosome binds to the end of an mRNA molecule and then moves along it. As it moves, it sequentially binds to an appropriate tRNA molecule by base-pairing complementary regions of the tRNA with the codon located on the mRNA. The attached amino acid is added to the forming protein, and the tRNA — no longer carrying amino acids — is released. The process then continues to the next mRNA codon.

Within the chromosomes, chromatin proteins such as histones compact and organize DNA. These compact structures guide the interactions between DNA and other proteins, helping control which parts of the DNA are transcribed.

Regulating genes

Cells can modify the rate at which specific gene products (protein or RNA) are produced. This occurs as cells proceed down their developmental pathways, but it also occurs in response to environmental stimuli. Gene expression can be modified at all the stages of transcription, RNA processing, and post-translational protein modification.

One of the main mechanisms of regulating DNA expression is methylation by methyltransferase enzymes (adding methyl groups to adenine or cytosine nucleotides in the DNA), which occurs on cytosine nucleotides. Another important regulation mechanism is *histone acetylation,* when histone acetyl-transferase enzymes (HATs) dissociate the histone complex from a section of DNA. The presence of histones blocks expression, so by removing histones, transcription can proceed. Methylation and histone deacetylation may act simultaneously to control DNA expression.

Introns and exons

The discovery that many genes were interrupted by *introns* (intervening sequences) that were not expressed came as quite a shock to much of the scientific world. Depending on the species, introns may be the majority of the total DNA sequence of the organism. RNA splicing (refer to the earlier section "Protein synthesis") removes introns to produce a final mRNA molecule ready for translation. The term intron refers to both the non-expressed DNA sequence and its corresponding sequence in the unspliced mRNA. After the introns are spliced out of the mRNA, the result is called an *exon.*

The origin of introns is still unclear. Introns were initially viewed as accidental DNA sequences, possibly leftovers from evolution or even parasitic "selfish" DNA. One conjecture has been that introns provide places for the DNA sequence to break during crossover in meiosis, making it less likely that a break will occur in the middle of a needed gene.

Regardless of their origin, introns allow the protein sequences generated from a single gene to vary greatly. This is because the same DNA sequence can generate different proteins by varying how the mRNA is spliced. Environmental factors that get taken up by a cell can modify the control of alternative RNA splicing.

Protein synthesis versus regulation

The classic picture of DNA being transcribed to RNA, and RNA being translated into proteins, was typically thought of as a one-way process. However, this description is not complete. The products of DNA expression, as well as external substances that get taken up by a cell, can also regulate protein production.

One example of the backward flow of information (or *backward synthesis*) is *reverse transcription,* which is the transfer of information from RNA to make new DNA. Reverse transcription occurs in retroviruses such as HIV and is a common feature of the replication cycle for many viruses. The main function of many proteins synthesized from DNA is to regulate DNA expression, typically by modulating methylation and histone acetylation (refer to "Gene regulation," earlier in this chapter). The expression of DNA can even be regulated by sequences within the DNA itself. For example, some introns enhance the expression of the gene in which they dwell through a process called *intron-mediated enhancement.* More generally, introns may have short sequences that are important for efficient splicing by spliceosomes.

Post-translational processing

When proteins are created by ribosomes that translate the mRNA into polypeptide chains, the amino acid polypeptide chains may undergo folding and/or cutting before becoming the final protein. The processes of folding and cutting often occur in the endoplasmic reticulum and may include structural changes based on the formation of disulfide bridges.

Also after translation happens, other biochemical functional groups may be attached to the amino acid sequence of the protein, such as carbohydrates, lipids, and phosphates. Adding phosphate groups is called *phosphorylation.* This is a common mechanism for activating or inactivating an enzyme protein.

Some of the amino acids on a polypeptide can be modified. For example, the amino acid arginine can enzymatically converted to citrulline in a process called *citrullination.* The presence of citrulline residues can alter the protein's structure and thereby change its function. Vesicles containing secretory proteins and some neurotransmitters then pass through the Golgi apparatus, where additional post-translational modifications can occur.

Various enzymes may cut the peptide chain or remove amino acids from the amino end of the protein. Also, most polypeptides initially start with the amino acid methionine because the "start" codon on mRNA codes for it. Methionine is usually taken off during post-translational modification.

Epigenetics

Epigenetics is the change in gene expression (and thus, cell phenotype, which we discuss earlier in this chapter) due to mechanisms *other than changes in the underlying DNA sequence.* The most important epigenetic mechanisms are DNA methylation and histone modification. Other mechanisms include X chromosome inactivation, transvection, and paramutation. *Teratogens* (environmental agents that cause cancer) often act through epigenetic mechanisms.

Epigenetic changes may persist through all cell divisions of a cell and be passed to offspring. If this sounds "Lamarckian" to you, you're partly right. In the original development of the theory of evolution, an alternative theory advanced by French biologist Jean-Baptiste Lamarck was that acquired characteristics could be inherited. Giraffes, for example, by stretching their necks to reach leaves on higher branches would give birth to offspring with longer necks.

However, we know that Lamarck's hypothesis is not the main way that evolution works. An important difference exists between epigenetic and Lamarckian inheritance. The Lamarck hypothesis offers no specific mechanism by which a trait acquired or developed through practice can be inherited. In epigenetics, however, the change in DNA expression may or may not be linked to any behavior, and may or may not actually be selected for in terms of that behavior. Epigenetic changes work according to standard Darwinian evolution.

Epigenetic changes are crucial in the process of cellular differentiation during development, where *totipotent stem cells* (cells that can develop into any cell type) differentiate into hundreds of different cell types such as neurons, muscle cells, or liver cells. This happens because of epigenetic activation and inhibition of relevant genes preserved in subsequent cell divisions of that cell line.

Meeting Cell Molecules: Important Ions and Proteins

What distinguishes neurons from other cells in the body is that they are excellent communicators. Their membranes contain receptors and ion channels that allow them to do the following:

- Sense energy and substances from the environment
- Communicate between distant parts of the same cell
- Communicate with other neurons
- Activate muscles and secretory cells

Most cells in the body have the DNA required to produce the hundreds of ion channel and receptor proteins found in neurons. But the genes that code for many of these neuronal proteins are expressed only in specific types of neurons, and not other cells. Many neuron-specific proteins form receptors or ion channels that either directly or indirectly control the flow of four major ions through the membrane: sodium, potassium, chloride, and calcium. The next section explores these ions in more detail.

Eyeing important ions

The most important ions that flow through neuronal membrane channels are sodium, potassium, chloride, and calcium. A fifth ion, magnesium, is also important because it controls conduction through the NMDA receptor, a glutamate receptor. The following list tells you more about the roles of these ions inside neurons:

- **Sodium:** The concentration of sodium is much higher outside the cell than inside the cell. Sodium entering into cells can trigger action potentials and lead to synaptic release, two crucial neural functions.

- **Potassium:** This ion has a high concentration inside cells compared to fluid outside cells. So, opening potassium channels tends to *hyperpolarize* cells (make the inside more negative) by the exit of the positively charged potassium ions.

- **Chloride:** The concentration of chloride is low inside the cell compared to the outside. Although the tendency exists for diffusion to dissipate this concentration gradient, chloride ions feel a repulsive force from the negative membrane potential inside the cell. Chloride flux tends to occur mostly when the cell is depolarized by an excitatory event. Chloride currents are usually inhibitory.

- **Calcium:** This ion is found in very low (nanomolar to micromolar) concentrations inside neurons because it is heavily buffered by calcium chelating (binding) molecules. Calcium can enter cells through calcium-specific channels and some neurotransmitter channels such as NMDA glutamate receptors and alpha-7 nicotinic acetylcholine receptors. Calcium modulates second messenger cascades inside cells that regulate ion channels from the inside, and may also affect gene expression. The flux of calcium through voltage-dependent calcium channels results in the release of neurotransmitters from *axon* (the part of the neuron that conducts impulses away from the cell) terminals.

- **Magnesium:** Normally magnesium does not pass through neuronal membranes. However, when the neuron is close to the resting potential, magnesium, attracted to the negative charge inside, binds in the extracellular "mouth" of the NMDA glutamate receptor. This receptor will not open unless, in addition to binding glutamate released from a pre-synaptic axon terminal, the membrane is partially depolarized. This depolarization (which is often provided by nearby non-NMDA excitatory receptors) reduces the potential across the membrane and thereby favors the release of the magnesium ion, allowing sodium and some calcium to flow through the channel.

Sizing up proteins

Membrane ion channels and receptors are typically composed of several proteins called *subunits* that, when assembled in the membrane, form a receptor or ion channel. At least 1,000 different receptor types exist in the olfactory (smell) system alone, each with a different combination of protein subunits with varying structures. The majority of ion channels and receptors have from four to six protein subunits.

Going through membrane proteins

Membrane proteins have a three-dimensional configuration. One end of the protein is either in the intracellular or extracellular fluid, the transmembrane region resides within the phospholipid membrane, and the protein terminal, like the beginning, is either in the intracellular or extracellular fluid. Most membrane protein subunits make multiple loops that are embedded in the membrane.

One important chemical distinction among the amino acids that make up proteins is whether the parts of the amino acid jutting out from the polypeptide chain *(residues)* are charged *(hydrophilic* or *lipophobic),* or relatively neutral *(hydrophobic* or *lipophilic).* The two ends of membrane proteins not embedded in the phospholipid bilayer are typically dominated by hydrophilic residues, while the portions of the protein embedded in the phospholipid bilayer are typically dominated by lipophilic residues.

Peeking at the Parts of a Cell

Neurons are cells. Like all eukaryotic cells they have a nucleus with chromosomes made of DNA, surrounded by a nuclear membrane. Outside this nuclear membrane is the cytoplasm, which is surrounded by the cell membrane. The following sections discuss the parts of the neuronal cell that are common with other eukaryotic cells, and later sections discuss the differences.

Cytoplasm and organelles

Within the neuronal cytoplasm are typical eukaryotic *organelles* (or, plainly, parts of the cell). The following organelles reside in the *cytoplasm*:

- ✔ **Mitochondria:** These are self-replicating organelles that generate *adenosine triphosphate* (ATP), the cell's main energy source. ATP is generated by a process called *oxidative phosphorylation,* in which energy from electron transfer involving oxygen adds a phosphate to adenosine diphosphate (ADP). Mitochondria have their own DNA and multiply by cell division on their own, as needed for the cell's energy requirements. Neurons have very high concentrations of mitochondria compared to other cells.

- ✔ **Endoplasmic reticulum (ER):** The ER is an organelle composed of flattened tubes (cisternae) involved in protein synthesis, and carbohydrate and lipid metabolism, among other functions. ER has two forms: rough and smooth. Rough ER contains ribosomes where mRNA is used to synthesize proteins from amino acids. Smooth ER synthesizes steroids, phospholipids, and other lipids. One of its functions in neurons is the modification of cell membrane proteins that will become receptors. It also regulates (sequesters) calcium ion concentration.

- ✔ **Golgi apparatus:** This organelle processes proteins and lipids that are synthesized by the cell. This is also where peptide neurotransmitters may be packaged into vesicles that are suitable to release outside the cell.

- ✔ **Lysosomes and peroxisomes:** These two organelles use enzymes to digest viruses or bacteria that have entered the cell, and non-functioning organelles. Peroxisomes use enzymes to degrade toxic peroxides.

- ✔ **Centrosome:** The centrosome is a cytoskeletal organizer. It consists of two *centrioles* (cylinder-shaped cell structures) that separate during cell division to form the mitotic spindle. Centrosomes are organizing centers for microtubules, which make up a large portion of the overall cytoskeleton. Microtubules are particularly important in extended neural processes such as dendrites and axons. The centrosome also controls transport of proteins through the Golgi apparatus and ER.

Nucleus

The *nucleus* contains the cell's chromosomes and is where DNA replication and RNA transcription occur. The nucleus has a double membrane called the *nuclear envelope* that separates it from the cytoplasm. Many neurons have a prominent *nucleolus,* a small region within the nucleus where ribosome subunits are assembled. There are pores in the nuclear membrane through which mRNA passes to the cytoplasm after being synthesized in the nucleus.

Secretion and hormones

Cellular secretion is the process of releasing substances that cause changes in other cells, usually, or even the secreting cell. Secretion may have evolved from *excretion* (the release of waste products). Although many secretion mechanisms exist, secretion typically involves vesicles transiently docking and fusing with the cell membrane, thereby releasing their contents into the extracellular space. Some secretion occurs from *porosomes,* which are permanent secretory structures at the cell plasma membrane.

Secreted signals are often *hormones* — chemicals released by a cell in one part of the organism that act as messages to cells in other parts of the organism. Hormones may travel in the extracellular space (which is called *paracrine signaling*) or be transported in the blood. Target cells that express a specific hormone receptor can respond when that hormone binds the receptor. This activates a cascade of signals, producing hormone-induced responses. Mechanisms exist to degrade the hormone so the cycle can begin again.

Proteins that are to be secreted are synthesized by ribosomes located on the rough ER. Sugar molecules are then added in a process called *glycosylation,* and the protein begins to fold with the help of special proteins called *molecular chaperones.* Vesicles containing the secretory proteins bud from the ER membrane and travel to the Golgi apparatus. In the Golgi apparatus, where further post-translational modifications may occur, the proteins are encapsulated in secretory vesicles. These vesicles are transported via the cytoskeleton to their destination at the plasma membrane. (Sometimes post-translational modifications occur within the vesicles.) Finally, the vesicle contents are released outside the cell (the process is called *exocytosis*) when the vesicle fuses with the cell membrane.

Secretion probably evolved from excretion when the detection of excreted products from one cell became a signal for other cells whose behavioral changes based on that signal were adaptive to the organism. Most, but not all, neurotransmitters are released by calcium-mediated *exocytosis* (the movement of material out of a cell using a sac or vesicle) after an action potential at the axon terminal.

The sequence of neurotransmission is quite similar to hormonal communication. Neurotransmission differs, however, in that neurons actually contact other specific neurons — or muscles or gland cells — directly at *synapses,* where information flows from one neuron to another across the synaptic cleft, the gap between a pre- and post-synaptic cell. The neurotransmitter released usually activates only receptors directly across the synaptic cleft in a single postsynaptic cell. This allows for significantly more complex communication with neurons than is possible with hormones. However, some specialized cells that are directly driven by neurons in brain areas like the hypothalamus do secrete hormones that circulate in the bloodstream. (See Chapter 4 for details about synapses and synaptic function.)

In some cases, however, a single presynaptic terminal can activate more than one post-synaptic receptor region. *Extra-synaptic neurotransmission* also happens, where neurotransmitter molecules escape from the synaptic cleft and activate distal sites on the postsynaptic neuron, or even other neurons.

Setting Boundaries: Cell Membrane Lipids

Just as the walls of your house separate the inside from the outside, so the cell membrane separates its inside (called the *cytoplasm*) from what's outside the cell. The word *cytoplasm* (the inside of a cell) is derived from the Greek words *cyto,* meaning "cell," and *plasma,* meaning "anything molded or formed." The cell membrane is often called the *plasma membrane.*

All animal cell plasma membranes are made primarily of molecules called *phospholipids.* Plant cells also have phospholipid membranes, but plants also have *cell walls* made of more rigid molecules such as cellulose, which gives them their stiffness. These phospholipid membranes in cells are everywhere, so if you think they're fundamental to life, you're almost certainly right! Although we don't know the details of how single cells evolved from the non-living soup of organic molecules in ancient waters billions of years ago, the formation of stable phospholipid "bags" of organic molecules probably preceded the evolution of DNA that now controls the activity and reproduction of cells.

Why are phospholipid membranes so essential to life? Phospholipids are molecules that spontaneously form membranes in salt solutions such as seawater, which is where life probably evolved. They do this because they're *polarized,* with different chemical properties at the two ends of the molecule (the next section explains this in more detail). The important thing about phospholipid membranes is that they're very stable in salt solutions and almost totally impervious to the movement of water or ions through them. Phospholipid membranes keep the inside of the cell in and the outside of the cell out.

Focusing on phospholipid chemistry

What are phospholipids and how do they form membranes? First, consider the common phospholipid molecule, as shown in Figure 2-1. To understand the membrane function, remember that phospholipid molecules have a *hydrophilic* (meaning, "water liking") "head" and two hydrophobic (meaning "water fearing") "tails." Molecules with this property are called *amphipathic*.

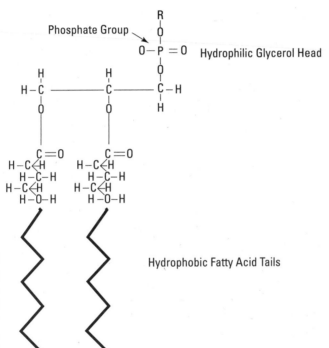

Figure 2-1: Phospho-lipid molecular structure.

 Why is a molecule hydrophilic? Water molecules (H_2O) are polarized because most of their electrons are concentrated around the oxygen atom, leaving the two hydrogen atoms with a deficiency of electric charge. So, the two hydrogen ends of the water molecule are slightly positive, with a slightly negative charge around the oxygen in the middle. Although water molecules move freely in the liquid state, most of the time adjacent water molecules have the hydrogen atoms in one water molecule near the oxygen atoms in adjacent ones.

 Common table salt (NaCl) dissolves in water because the positively charged sodium atom (Na^+) is attracted to the negative oxygen region of the water molecules and "lets go" of the chloride (Cl^-) to which it is bonded. The chloride, in turn, tends to stick to the hydrogen ends of the water molecule.

So, how does the hydrophilic water molecule relate to phospholipid membranes? When phospholipid molecules are floating around in water, the polar heads are attracted to and bind water molecules. But the hydrophobic tails don't bind water; instead, they're more likely to interact with each other. The most stable way for these molecules to arrange themselves, then, is for the hydrophobic tails to bind together, with the heads protruding outward from a bilayer and contacting water. The schematic structure of the molecule viewed this way is shown in Figure 2-2, and the stable bilayer (molecular layer two molecules thick) is shown in Figure 2-3.

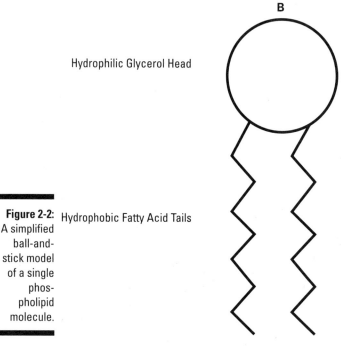

Hydrophilic Glycerol Head

Figure 2-2: Hydrophobic Fatty Acid Tails
A simplified
ball-and-
stick model
of a single
phos-
pholipid
molecule.

The last piece of this puzzle is that, unlike what might be implied in Figure 2-3, phospholipid bilayers won't form infinitely large sheets in aqueous environments. Instead, the only stable configuration is for the bilayer to close on itself and form a sphere. The size of this sphere is a function of the water forces and the chemistry of the phospholipid.

It's interesting that the extracellular fluid around cells in animals resembles the seawater in which cells originally evolved. If you think this wasn't an accident, you're right!

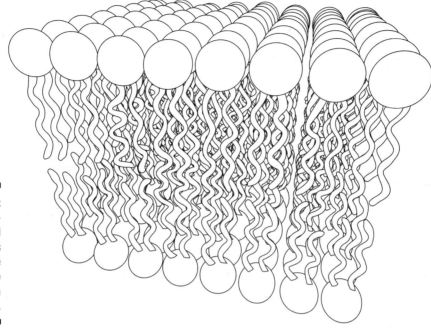

Figure 2-3:
Phospho-
lipid
molecules
assemble
to form the
plasma
membrane.

Seeing cells' differences

All of the cells in your body have the same lipid bilayer structure for their plasma membrane, but all cells are not the same. What makes a kidney cell or neuron or skin cell all different from each other? Two major differences apply to all the hundreds of distinct cell types in your body:

- ✔ **Different biochemical reaction sequences:** These sequences are particular to specific cell types controlled by selective expression of a subset of the total genes in each cell (although each cell has identical DNA).

- ✔ **Different protein structures in the plasma membranes:** These structures control the flow of ions and other substances through the cell's membrane.

These two differences are not entirely separate from each other. One of the major functions of the different biochemical reactions going on inside cells is generating and maintaining protein complexes for the cell membrane. All cells, of course, generate the phospholipids to maintain their plasma membranes.

Neurons differ from other cells in your body because they have a large number of specific types of ion channels made of protein complexes specified by a subset of the genes from the DNA in the cell nucleus. Not only do neurons have many more types of these channels than other cells, but many differences exist among neurons because of the hundreds of channel types they express, and the relative numbers of each.

Regulating Water and Cell Volume

The plasma membranes of neurons, as well as other cells in the body, are stable, but not rigid like the cell walls of plants. This means that neurons are flexible and can be deformed by mechanical pressure. Neurons exist within a matrix of glial cells and an extracellular matrix that holds the tissue together.

Although the extracellular matrix around cells is very effective in maintaining a supporting environment that prevents neurons from being damaged (to a limit, of course) by mechanical forces, neurons must actively resist another type of force — osmotic pressure.

Observing osmotic pressure

What is osmotic pressure, and why does it matter to cells? Well, you've probably heard the classic lines, "Water, water, everywhere; nor any drop to drink." Consider how people stranded in the middle of the ocean can't survive by drinking the seawater all around them. High concentrations of salts (primarily sodium chloride) are dissolved in seawater. If seawater is added to the already highly concentrated extracellular fluid around our cells, the result is that water will tend to move from the higher concentration inside our cells to the lower concentration (relative to the concentration of ions) outside. The plasma membranes of cells are not totally impermeable to water, because, among other reasons, membranes have water-permeable channels called *aquaporins.* This causes a net loss of water inside our cells so that they become hyperconcentrated with ions and die. Neurons, like other cells, have a variety of mechanisms for dealing with concentration balances between their cytoplasm and the extracellular fluid.

Responding to osmotic challenges

Osmotic imbalances are detected by a variety of sensors in cells, which respond in many ways such as with secretion, enzyme production, or changes in gene expression. Mechanosensitive channels in cell membranes respond to mechanical stress such as stretching of the membrane.

These channels open or close to allow bulk flow of ions through the membrane to balance between different concentrations inside versus outside. Protein pump molecules may selectively bring in or expel soluble ions in response to different total ionic concentrations inside versus outside the cell.

A recently discovered channel family termed TRPV (short for *transient receptor potential vanilloid*) responds to osmotic stress by allowing calcium influx. The increased calcium concentration inside the cell regulates volume by activating calcium-dependent potassium channels. Defective TRPV channels are associated with cystic fibrosis.

Moving water with aquaporins

Although phospholipid plasma membranes have some limited permeability to water, we know that in many neurons water channels called *aquaporins* control much of this movement. Aquaporin channels in the membrane tend to equilibrate water between the cytoplasm and extracellular fluid. In addition, aquaporin channels can be up or down regulated over longer time scales. Aquaporin channel deficiencies are involved in some types of diabetes.

Knowing the Neuron: Not Just Another Cell

At the most fundamental level, neurons differ from other cells because they express different portions of the DNA sequence, leading to the production of different proteins. These proteins result in two major types of differences between neurons and other cells:

- Structure
- Membrane receptors and ion channels

Noticing neuron anatomy

The most obvious feature of most neurons is their extensive dendritic branching patterns. Most neurons have several primary dendritic branches that leave the cell body. These typically divide numerous times (out to the tenth order or more) forming a tree-like structure often called the *dendritic tree* or *dendritic arborization*. Figure 2-4 shows two cells from a rabbit retina with very different arborizations.

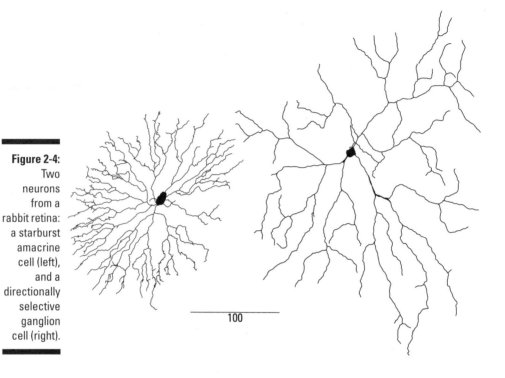

Figure 2-4:
Two
neurons
from a
rabbit retina:
a starburst
amacrine
cell (left),
and a
directionally
selective
ganglion
cell (right).

The dendritic arborization is where neurons receive most of their synaptic input — typically hundreds or thousands of synapses. These synapses are almost always a mixture of excitatory and inhibitory inputs. In many cases, the excitatory inputs are on *dendritic spines,* which are little mushroom-like appendages on the dendrites.

In any region of the nervous system are usually a finite number of distinct dendritic neuronal forms, between 10 and 30. Neurons are anatomically classified by the types of branching patterns using parameters such as total size, branching density, and the location of branches relative to other neurons. If you use a microscope to look at unstained tissue sections, these branching structures are usually not evident. Stains are necessary to reveal the structure of individual neurons.

The location of the dendritic branches with respect to nearby neurons determines some of what inputs may synapse on the neuron. The form of the branching structure determines how those inputs interact. Picture thousands of excitatory and inhibitory inputs going on and off in complicated patterns, producing a complex pattern of excitation and inhibition in the postsynaptic neuron, which is constantly changing. This neuron may itself synapse on hundreds of other neurons. Multiply this by 80 to 100 billion neurons and you have a circuit more complicated than any computer we have today!

Neurons also have an axon, their typical output structure. Usually a single process leaves the cell body and branches before forming synapses with other neurons. The axon conducts *action potentials,* millisecond-long electrical pulses that move from the cell body to the synaptic terminals of the axon, where they cause neurotransmitter to be released onto postsynaptic neurons.

Understanding what neurons do

Neurons enable sensation, communication, and movement in animals. They do this using their membrane receptors, ion channels, and exocytosis mechanisms. Reception and exocytosis themselves are both mediated by gated ion channels.

Taking in information: Receptors

Different types of receptors detect various kinds of energy from the environment. Here are a few examples:

- **Photoreceptors** capture photons of light.
- **Auditory hair cells** respond to acoustic energy, or sounds.
- **Mechanoreceptors** are located in the skin and respond to touch.
- **Olfactory and taste receptors** respond to molecules interacting with receptors in our noses and tongues.

Neurons also respond to each other via receptors for various neurotransmitters. Some neurons respond to hormones circulating in the extracellular space or bloodstream. Also, specific neural responses to extracellular ion concentrations can occur.

Transforming information: Interneurons

After neurons receive information from either the environment or other neurons, they process that information using electrotonic potentials and ion concentrations that interact within the neuron. Neurons then transmit information to other neurons or to muscles or glands.

A neuron's dendritic tree may have thousands of excitatory and inhibitory synaptic inputs, each of which may be modulated in a complex pattern over time. The way different inputs to the neuron interact also depends on their locations in the dendritic tree. Inputs that are near to each other may interact in a nonlinear way, exhibiting thresholds, saturation, multiplicative interactions, and other complex interactions.

In most neurons, all the inputs and their interactions result in a net flow of current into the cell body, or *soma,* and the initial segment of the axon. If the voltage produced by this current is below threshold, it doesn't produce any spikes. Above this threshold, the rate of action potentials, or spikes, is generally proportional to the net excitatory (depolarizing) current. The spikes are sent down the axon where, at the axon terminals, neurotransmitter is released. Neurons may release neurotransmitter on neurons a few tens of micrometers away or a meter or more away.

Moving our limbs: Motor neurons

Besides going to other neurons, the information that neurons transmit can also go to our muscles. All vertebrate neuromuscular transmission in vertebrates uses the neurotransmitter acetylcholine. The evolution of the nervous system is closely tied to the ability to move — animals have neurons, but plants don't. The nervous system allows us to move based on the environment (sensation) and on previous experience (learning). The nervous system also enables muscles in different parts of the body to work in a coordinated way to perform complex behaviors. For example, putting one foot in front of the other and walking — which most people do every day — is actually a highly complex behavior. Think of all the muscles that need to work together just so you can take a few steps!

When Things Go Wrong: Genetics and Neurological Illness

Genetics is absolutely amazing: A random shuffle of genes from two parents get thrown together, producing a working nervous system from the proteins encoded. This nervous system is produced with 80 to 100 billion cells and at least 100 trillion synapses. Of course, the process doesn't always have perfect results, and sometimes things go wrong. This section discusses some of these cases.

Nervous system disorders include some fairly well-understood sensory problems such as blindness, deafness, and motor disorders like myasthenia gravis (see Chapter 16), whose causes (but not necessarily cures) we know at the cellular level. Problems that affect mental functions are more complex, such as learning disabilities, schizophrenia, depression, bipolar disorder, and obsessive-compulsive disorder.

Neurological illnesses are among the most challenging and expensive health problems in the United States. This is particularly true for degenerative disorders such as Alzheimer's and Parkinson's diseases, which strike our increasingly elderly population.

Mutations and transcriptional errors

We know that many nervous system disorders are genetically based, even though we may not always know the genetic origin. So, how do genetic disorders happen?

Genetic *mutations* — which you probably know something about if you've ever read a comic book — are one cause of these disorders. Reproduction starts with *germ cells* (egg or sperm cells) being generated during meiosis. In this process, alternating partial segments from the parents' double-stranded DNA produce the offspring's unique DNA.

In the complex process of assembling a single chromosome of DNA from the two parental chromosomes, errors happen. These errors are one kind of mutation. Here are the three most common single chromosome mutations:

✔ **Deletion:** In deletion, a piece of a chromosome or sequence of DNA is missing. A partial sequence from neither parent ends up in the single chromosome of the egg or sperm, making that DNA shorter and missing the gene altogether.

✔ **Duplication:** In duplication, a partial sequence of DNA from one parent is inserted twice.

✔ **Inversion:** When inversion happens, a partial DNA sequence from one parent is inserted upside down in the offspring. As we discuss earlier in this chapter, DNA is always transcribed from the same direction, so when a partial sequence is inserted upside-down, the protein coded is completely different when it's transcribed.

Here are a few well-known examples of genetic disorders:

✔ **Down syndrome:** The most well-known example of a disorder with a known genetic cause is Down syndrome, which is caused by an extra chromosome 21 (trisomy 21). Down syndrome occurs in about 1 in 1,000 births.

✔ **Fragile X syndrome:** This disorder is the most common inherited cause of intellectual disability. It results from an X chromosome mutation. The features of Fragile X syndrome are mental retardation and a number of noted physical, emotional, and behavioral issues.

✔ **Rett syndrome:** Another inherited developmental brain disorder, Rett syndrome is characterized by abnormal neuronal morphology and reduced levels of neurotransmitters norepinephrine and dopamine.

✔ **Schizophrenia:** Rather than being due to a single mutation, schizophrenia has many genetic causes. It is a serious mental disorder that is characterized by severely impaired thinking, along with emotional and behavioral issues.

✔ **Autism:** This neurological disorder also has multiple genetic causes. As such, individuals with different mutations have somewhat different disorders of varying severity.

Autism is called a "spectrum" disorder because its multiple genetic causes create a range of phenotypic characteristics, depending on the person. Characteristics range from severe retardation to slight social ineptitude.

✔ **Asperger's syndrome:** Typically, Asperger's is included in the autism spectrum as autism without significant language delay or dysfunction. Like autism, Asperger's appears to arise from multiple mutation locations, and correspondingly very different types and severities of symptoms.

Modifying genes: Fixing or Frankenstein?

What can be done about genetically based neurological disorders? Can we fix broken genes?

Animal research

A huge research endeavor is going on, involving *transgenic animals* (animals whose genome has been changed by transferring genes from another species or breed, or by eliminating these genes altogether). The genetic compositions of these animals are different from so-called "wild type" animals. Many animal lines with these different genetic compositions originally arose from random mutations in offspring. They were then selectively bred as "models" for human diseases.

Today "knock-out" and "knock-in" transgenic animals exist. In these animals, scientists deliberately modify the genome by changing the DNA codons for single amino acids, multiple amino acids, or even entire genes.

Gene therapy

Human genetic manipulation may require both silencing a gene that produces a harmful protein and/or adding a gene to produce a needed one. This involves introducing exogenous DNA into the person's cells. This DNA may come from another organism or be synthesized in a lab.

The general term for genetic manipulation in humans for medical reasons is *gene therapy*. Gene therapy can be done in developed organisms rather than germ lines in several ways. One is to physically restrict the injection of the introduced DNA, such as in the eye to treat blindness, so that the gene can't get into any other body cells. Another way is using a tissue or cell type-specific promoter with the DNA so that it's only expressed in particular tissues.

Typically, the introduced DNA is packaged within a *vector* that is used to get the DNA inside cells within the body. One common vector is a virus, because viruses normally function by binding the cell membrane and inserting their DNA or RNA into the cell. The contents of a virus can be modified to produce a human gene. Also, exogenous DNA may be introduced that encodes a thera-peutic protein that works like a drug rather than the DNA corresponding to any actual human gene.

Chapter 3

Gating the Membrane: Ion Channels and Membrane Potentials

*I*f I told you that your brain is full of batteries, you'd probably wonder if I was insulting your intelligence or just plain crazy. But after you read this chapter, you'll see that neither is the case! Your brain's neurons are cells that specialize in rapid and precise electrical communication, integration, and processing of information. In order for neurons to perform these wonderfully complex tasks, they require a number of different cells and other components, such as membrane channels, gates, receptors, transporters, and more. In this chapter, I explore what neurons need in order to be able to detect and respond to other neurons, substances in the environment, and energy.

Looking at Membrane Channels

Neurons interact with other neurons (and the rest of the world) through membrane *protein complexes* (multiple proteins bound together in a structure such as a channel). (Refer to Chapter 2 for more about DNA.) After the proteins are produced, they're assembled into membrane complexes.

Talking about transporters

Cells contain *ions,* which are molecules that carry an electric charge. Many neurons contain *transporters* that have the task of pumping ions into and out of the cell.

All this transportation of ions creates a permanent imbalance between the ions inside the neuron and outside it. Different concentrations of ions exist on either side of the membrane.

You'll get a charge out of what happens next: These ionic imbalances turn neurons into batteries, capable of producing electrical currents that flow through discrete pathways for conduction through the membrane; the biophysical term for conduction is *permeability.* The conduction path is made up of ion channels, which have gates that open to allow ions like sodium, potassium, or chloride to move through the membrane.

Checking out channels

The things neurons do — such as receiving, processing, and transmitting information — all require membrane channels that form the following:

- ✔ **Ion-selective channels:** Membrane channels typically allow only certain ions, or groups of ions, to pass through the membrane. These channels may lack gates and, therefore, run continuously, or have gates dependent on the membrane potential or neurotransmitter binding.

- ✔ **Secretory mechanisms:** Membrane structures that use energy or concentration gradients to release substances outside the cell, such as neurotransmitters being released into the space between the pre- and postsynaptic neurons (the *synaptic cleft*) in a manner similar to how hormones are released into the bloodstream.

- ✔ **Membrane receptors:** Membrane channels called *ionotropic receptors* can bind neurotransmitters (called *ligands*) that allow the flow of ions through the membrane. Some receptors, called *metabotropic receptors* (discussed in more detail in Chapter 4) have the reception and channel functions located in separate protein complexes in the membrane.

Ion-selective channels

Ion-selective channels, as their name implies, control the movement of certain ions through plasma membranes. These channels are typically composed of four or more individual proteins (called *subunits*) that combine in the membrane to form a molecular pore. Most ion channels are selective — they only allow certain ions to pass and, often, only in one direction.

Ion channels can be un-gated or gated:

- **Constitutively open channels:** These are sometimes called *leakage channels* and are just like your reliable corner store because they're always open. Their *permeability* (ability to pass ions) is not modulated. However, the number of these channels in the plasma membrane (and, thus, the total membrane permeability) is controlled by DNA expression. This way, total permeability may be modified.

- **Gated channels:** These channels can be open or closed. Controlling ion movements through gated channels is fundamental to how neurons receive, process, and transfer information. *Sensory receptors* activate channels by receiving energy such as light or sound, or by external substances such as odors. Neurons communicate with other neurons through two types of gated channels:

  - **Ligand-gated channels** are channels that are opened as a result of a molecule (typically a neurotransmitter) outside the cell binding to a complementary receptor structure inside the channel complex. (The word *ligand* is from a Latin word meaning "to bind.") In *ionotropic receptors* (see Chapter 4 for more), the ligand binding site and gated pore are part of the same membrane protein complex. In *metabotropic receptors,* after binding a ligand, the receptor protein complex in the membrane activates a second messenger transmitter inside the cell whose actions may open or close other channels.

  - **Voltage-gated channels** open in response to changes in *membrane potential,* which is the voltage difference between the inside and outside of the cell. Typically, voltage-gated channels are closed when the neuron is not excited (at the "resting potential") and open when the cell is excited. When the neuron is excited (or stimulated), the membrane potential is depolarized (or more positive).

Secretory mechanisms

Neurons release neurotransmitters at their presynaptic terminals. In most neurons this happens by a process called *vesicular release* and works in a way that is similar to secretion. During vesicular release, calcium enters the presynaptic terminal through voltage-dependent calcium channels. (Chapter 4 discusses this process in more detail.)

Membrane receptors

Some membrane receptors act as sensors; they respond to energy or substances in the environment. To give just two examples, photoreceptors capture photons of light, and channels located in specialized hairlike structures on auditory hair cells open in response to sound waves that bend these hairlike structures.

Getting a Charge Out of Neurons

Neurons use electricity to communicate between different parts of the same neuron and between neurons. How this works is one of the most fascinating stories in all science.

The story starts with transporter pumps (refer to "Talking about transporters," earlier in this chapter) in the membrane that create ionic imbalances between the inside and outside of the cell. Not all ions get to move through the membrane, and the ligand-gated and voltage-gated channels act as the membrane's "bouncers," allowing only specific ions to move through. Then, voltage-gated channels amplify the effects caused by ligand binding so that distant parts of the cell's dendritic tree communicate these events to the cell's soma. The cell's soma then communicates the dendritic events to the axon terminal, which releases neurotransmitters that affect other neurons, and the symphony of brain activity plays on.

Believe it or not, every neuron in your body is actually a little battery that can make electric current flow. Think of the regular batteries you use every day. In these manmade batteries, chemical reactions in an *electrolyte* (salt solution) cause electrons to flow in an external circuit between two different electrodes that are immersed in the electrolyte.

 You can think of neurons in the same way. In neurons, ions in solution such as sodium, potassium, or chloride move through specific channels in the membrane when these channels are opened by ligands or electric fields (voltage). The reasons for ions moving through membrane channels are *diffusion* (concentration differences between inside and outside) and voltage differences between the inside and outside. The continuous running of the transporter pumps maintains these concentration differences — or ionic imbalances.

Pumping Ions for Information

One of the most important kinds of molecular pumps are *ion transporter pumps.* These pumps use energy derived from adenosine triphosphate (ATP) to move specific ions through the membrane.

Sodium-potassium pump

One transporter pump is the *sodium-potassium ATPase transporter.* It creates a large imbalance between — you guessed it — the concentrations of sodium and potassium inside and outside the cell. It also causes the inside of neurons to be negatively charged inside versus outside, which is necessary for neurons to work.

The sodium-potassium ion pump or transporter is sometimes called an *ion exchanger,* because it works with two different ions.

The sodium-potassium pump pushes sodium ions outside the cell and potassium ions inside. The exchange ratio is three sodium ions pumped out for every two potassium ions pumped in. These pumps are ubiquitously expressed in neurons and run constantly. By always running, they create a disequilibrium or imbalance in sodium/potassium concentrations across the membrane, as you can see in Figure 3-1.

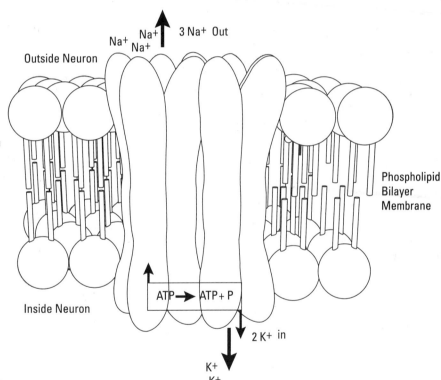

Na/K Transporter

Outside Neuron

Na+ Na+ Na+ Na+   3 Na+ Out

Inside Neuron

ATP → ATP + P

2 K+ in

K+ K+

Phospholipid Bilayer Membrane

Figure 3-1: The sodium-potassium pump creates a disequi-librium between sodium and potassium concentra-tions inside versus outside the cell.

Here are two important facts about the sodium/potassium imbalance:

✔ Compared to the extracellular fluid, which has high sodium and low potassium concentrations, the cell's cytoplasm has almost the opposite: very low sodium and high potassium.

✔ Because the sodium exit to potassium entry ratio is 3:2, a net loss of positive charge occurs inside the cell compared to outside. That is, neurons are negatively charged inside.

Because the negative potential inside neurons is based on the total difference in ionic concentrations between the inside and outside, if the transporter pumps stopped working and all other ion channels closed (in the *impermeable* state) a neuron's resting potential (when nothing is passing through) would still exist for a long time. Scientists have done experiments to verify this, using poisons to kill the pumps and channel blockers to close all the ion channels.

Other important pumps

Besides the sodium-potassium ion pump, other transporters exist that are also essential for different aspects of neural function. One is the *sodium-calcium exchanger.* The main function of the sodium-calcium exchanger is to remove calcium from the cytoplasm. (Calcium levels inside cells are usually held to levels of a few hundred nanomolar.) The sodium-calcium exchanger is found not only in the plasma membranes, but also in mitochondria and the endoplasmic reticulum of neurons. The sodium-calcium exchanger works by using the energy stored in the electrochemical gradient of sodium instead of chemical energy from ATP. The energy derived from three sodium ions flowing down this gradient brings in one calcium ion.

Another important class of transporters is the group of *cation chloride co-transporters* (sometimes called CCCs). Variants of these exchangers may bring in or push out chloride in exchange for potassium or potassium and sodium. Membrane transporters also exist for neurotransmitters such as glutamate, dopamine, serotonin, and norepinephrine. These transporters are involved in limiting synaptic transmission by scavenging neurotransmitters from the synaptic cleft, thereby recycling the neurotransmitter molecules. (Chapter 4 gets into the processes involved in neurotransmitter release.) In some special cases, transporters can also release neurotransmitters.

Discovering Diffusion and Voltage

Ask any neurobiologist, and she'll tell you that a big challenge in understanding the flow of currents through neural membranes is having to account for the two forces of imbalances: diffusion and voltage. Diffusion causes ions to move from regions of higher to lower concentration. As for voltage, the electrostatic force causes ions to move away from a like charge toward an opposite charge. Neurons have a net negative charge inside with respect to outside, and different concentrations of ions like sodium and potassium inside compared to outside. The following sections explore these ideas in more detail.

The upcoming sections look at how diffusion and electrostatic forces affect ion movement. Let's look at the forces influencing sodium ions as an example. The sodium concentration is very low inside compared to outside the cell. The inside of the cell is also negatively charged. So, when membrane ion channels that are permeable to sodium open, the concentration gradient pushes sodium from its high concentration outside into the cell. Similarly, the electrostatic force (voltage) will also draw the positively charged sodium from outside to the negatively charged inside. Opening sodium channels will cause a large sodium inrush from both diffusion and the electrostatic force.

What about potassium? Potassium has a higher concentration inside than out, so diffusion tends to move it outside if potassium channels are opened. On the other hand, the negative charge inside the cell attracts positively charged potassium, just like it does sodium.

The Nernst equation

So, which way will potassium ions move if potassium channels are opened? The *Nernst equation* — developed from basic thermodynamic principles by the 19th-century German chemist Walter Nernst — gives us the answer. It gives the "balance point" (called the *equilibrium potential*) between the diffusion and voltage forces, expressed in terms of voltage. This equilibrium potential (sometimes called the *Nernst potential,* for obvious reasons) is the voltage (inside the cell versus outside) that would exactly balance the tendency of ions to diffuse down their concentration gradient. In other words, if the inside of the neuron is at the Nernst potential for an ion, no net movement of that ion will occur when the relevant channels are open.

A separate Nernst equation is written for each ion. The Nernst equation giving the equilibrium potential for sodium, E_{Na}, would be written as follows:

$$E_{Na} = 59.8 \text{ mV } \log_{10} ([Na^+]_{outside}/[Na^+]_{inside})$$

The constant 59.8 mV comes from the evaluation of several other constants (RT/zF), where R = the universal gas constant, T = temperature in degrees Kelvin, F = Faraday's constant, and z = the ion valence (for Na^+ z = 1).

For a typical neuron frequently studied, like the squid axon, Na_{inside} might equal 50 mM (millimolar), whereas $Na_{outside}$ is typically 440 mM.

This gives

$$E_{Na} = 59.8 \text{ mV } \log_{10} (440/50) = 56.5 \text{ mV}$$

What this means is that the potential inside the neuron would have to be raised from its –60 millivolt (mV) resting potential to +56.5 mV to balance the tendency of sodium ions to rush into the neuron by diffusion due to the much higher concentration outside than inside.

For potassium, where the concentrations are about 400 mM inside versus 20 mM outside, E_K = 59.8 mV $\log_{10}$ ([K^+]$_{outside}$/[K^+]$_{inside}$) = 59.8 mV $\log_{10}$ (20/400) = –77.8 mV.

This means that the potential inside the cell would have to be made more negative than –77.8 mV to keep potassium from going outside the cell through a membrane permeable to potassium due to the much larger concentration of potassium inside the cell than outside.

For chloride, E_{Cl} = 59.8 mV $\log_{10}$ ([Cl^-]$_{outside}$/[Cl^-]$_{inside}$) = –59.8 mV $\log_{10}$ (560/52) = –61.7 mV.

Note that a minus sign (–) appears in front of the 59.8 constant because the valence, z, of chloride is negative (–1). The reversal potential for chloride is often near the resting potential because chloride leak channels (channels without gates) exist in most neurons. These channels are always open and allow chloride to move through the membrane until its equilibrium potential is reached.

The concentration of chloride ions is much higher outside the cell than inside for the equilibrium potential of about –60 mV, close to the resting potential of many cells. The negative charge inside the cell compared to outside repels negative chloride ions. Also, many organic ions exist inside a cell that are negatively charged.

Chloride channels may be inhibitory even if the reversal potential for chloride is slightly above the resting potential. That's because opening chloride channels will oppose depolarization by opening nearby sodium channels. Moreover, the open chloride channels reduce the membrane resistance, and by Ohm's law (V = I · R), reduce the depolarizing voltage produced by sodium currents.

The Goldman–Hodgkin–Katz equation

The Nernst equation (refer to the previous section) tells you what the reversal potential would be for a single ion. But multiple ionic concentration differences exist across the neural membrane, and the most important are sodium, potassium, and chloride. But another question is, given the concentration differences of these different ions, what is the actual membrane potential for a given set of permeabilities to the different ions?

The *Goldman–Hodgkin–Katz equation* determines the voltage that results from ionic currents across the membrane. It expands on the Nernst equation by taking into account multiple ions and their individual permeabilities (that is, if you eliminate all but one ion from the Goldman equation, you get the Nernst equation). What the Goldman equation shows is that, for a given set of ionic concentration gradients across the membrane, the voltage inside the cell (across the membrane) will be driven toward the Nernst equilibrium potential of the most permeable ion.

The Goldman–Hodgkin–Katz equation is as follows:

$$V_m = \frac{RT}{zF} \ln \frac{P_K\left[K_0\right] + P_{Na}\left[Na_0\right] + P_{Cl}\left[Cl_i\right]}{P_K\left[K_i\right] + P_{Na}\left[Na_i\right] + P_{Cl}\left[Cl_0\right]}$$

The chloride versus terms are reversed in the numerator and denominator of the Goldman-Hodgkin-Katz equation. This takes into account that z for chloride is –1, while it is +1 for sodium and potassium.

The Goldman–Hodgkin–Katz equation was derived from the Nernst equation but takes into account the important fact that the membrane potential tends to move toward the reversal potential of the ion to which the membrane is most permeable. Note that, if you set the permeabilities of two of the ions to zero, the Goldman–Hodgkin–Katz equation reduces to the Nernst equation for the remaining ion that has some finite permeability.

The neuron is at its resting potential when it isn't being stimulated, or excited. The permeability for chloride tends to be high in the resting state of neurons, so the chloride current contribution is relatively dominant then.

The potassium current also pulls the membrane potential toward the potassium reversal potential because the resting membrane permeability is much higher to potassium than sodium. The reversal potential for potassium is generally more negative than the resting potential (–75 mV versus –65 mV).

During an action potential, however, the sodium permeability becomes much higher than the potassium permeability, so the intracellular potential is driven toward the positive sodium equilibrium potential. In the next section, I show you what happens when the membrane permeability for sodium and potassium ions are regulated by voltage-gated ion channels.

Signaling with Electricity in Neurons

The sodium-potassium pump (refer to the section "Pumping Ions for Information," earlier in this chapter) creates large concentration imbalances between the neuron's cytoplasm and the extracellular fluid, and a net negative charge inside the neuron of about –65 mV (that is, the resting potential). How the neuron uses these concentration and charge imbalances for information processing is fundamental to what they do. Gated ion channels (refer to the "Ion selective channels" section, earlier in this chapter) change the neuron's permeability to particular ions. These permeability changes lead to ionic current flow and corresponding changes in the membrane potential. Membrane potential changes control voltage-gated channels and neurotransmitter release.

In the following sections, we discuss what happens when the ionic permeability changes, specifically in the action potential.

Exploring potential

The *resting potential* is the voltage across the membrane when the neuron is not strongly driven by excitatory inputs. It's established by ionic gradients and charge imbalances that occur because the sodium-potassium transporter pumps are constantly working. At this resting potential in most neurons, some leakage current flows through open chloride channels and a small conductance of potassium channels.

If we use the Goldman–Hodgkin–Katz equation (refer to the "Goldman–Hodgkin–Katz equation" section, earlier in this chapter) to solve for the voltage across the membrane given the sodium, potassium, and chloride permeabilities, we get a resting potential of about –65 mV. (In most cells, this value varies somewhat across neurons.) Because chloride passively distributes its concentration across the membrane — due to diffusion and electric field forces created by sodium-potassium pumps — we find that the resting membrane potential is due mostly to the resting potassium conductance. Opening sodium channels that *depolarize* the inside of the neuron change all this drastically.

Controlling ion permeability: Gated channels

Earlier in this chapter, I explain that ion channels can be gated either by ligands (neurotransmitters) or voltage. Gating changes the channel's state from closed to open, or vice versa. Gated channels are at the core of how neurons integrate and process inputs, and how they communicate with other neurons (or, as neurobiologists always say, "No neuron is an island").

Neurons receive messages in the form of neurotransmitters through ligand-gated channels on their dendrites, soma, and, in some cases, axon. These inputs are excitatory if the receptors flux sodium ions, inhibitory if they flux potassium or chloride.

Opening channels changes the voltage across the neurons membrane by the flow of ions. We use the Goldman–Hodgkin–Katz equation to calculate the membrane potential that results. If the neuronal membrane potential becomes sufficiently less negative (depolarized), the effect may be to open voltage-gated ion channels. Two of the most important voltage-gated ion channels are those of the sodium and potassium channels that lead to the action potential, an all-or-nothing spike of voltage that serves as the basic unit of electrical signaling in neurons.

Making Spikes with Sodium and Potassium Channels

Imagine a neuron at its resting potential of about –65 mV. Some other neuron that is presynaptic to this one releases glutamate, which binds to the first neuron's excitatory glutamate receptors. This process opens a glutamate receptor, which passes a (mostly) sodium current. Sodium rushes into the cytoplasm from outside the neuron and depolarizes it, reducing potential across the membrane from –65 mV to around –20 mV. This is above the threshold for voltage-gated sodium channels in the first neuron's membrane, which are now open.

Getting back to resting potential

Opening voltage-gated sodium channels, which increase the flow of sodium into the cell, further depolarizes the cell. This opens any other nearby voltage-dependent sodium channels. The situation is one of typical *positive feedback* in which the neuron is increasingly being driven toward the sodium equilibrium potential (approximately +55 mV, depending on the cell, from the Nernst equation). This amplification causes the neuron to remain stuck in this depolarized condition, unless something happens to get it back to its resting potential. Two things can work to do this:

- ✔ Sodium channels close themselves.
- ✔ Voltage-dependent potassium channels open.

In this chapter, I cover voltage-dependent sodium channels as though they only exist in two states — open or closed — but that isn't quite right. A third state exists: When the neuron is in the resting state, the voltage-dependent sodium channels are in a state that is *closed, but capable of opening* (meaning they can be opened by voltage). When the membrane potential crosses the threshold, the channels transition to the *open* state. The third state occurs in less than one millisecond after the channels open. A mechanism within the channel causes the voltage-dependent channels to close themselves and transition to a state that is *closed, but not immediately capable of reopening.* That is, even though the membrane voltage may continue to remain above their opening threshold, they won't open again. This process is called *inactivation.* The transition to this third, closed state causes the neuron to *repolarize* (meaning return to the resting potential), along with potassium channel activity, which we discuss in the next section. Milliseconds after the neuron repolarizes, the voltage-dependent sodium channels transition from the inactivated state back to the original closed state. Then the cycle can begin again.

Voltage-dependent channels

The sudden opening and then closing of many voltage-dependent sodium channels produces an *action potential,* or *spike* — sharp voltage change across the cell's membrane.

If you do a computer simulation of the action of voltage-dependent sodium channels using their known kinetics, the simulated action potential lasts longer than actual spikes in most real neurons. The reason is that *voltage-dependent potassium channels* also exist, and they're almost always near voltage-dependent sodium channels. (They also open when the neuron is depolarized, but more slowly than the sodium channels.) When these voltage-dependent potassium channels open, potassium flows out of the cell, which drives the membrane potential toward the potassium equilibrium potential around –75 mV. This shortens the duration of the action potential because opening potassium channels repolarizes the cell more rapidly than closing the voltage-dependent sodium channels.

Reaching action potential

The voltage-dependent potassium channels also close on their own after opening, but much more slowly than the sodium channels. A lingering potassium current remains after each action potential that makes firing another action potential more difficult, because a subsequent depolarizing input must fight this hyperpolarizing potassium current.

The period immediately following an action potential when it's more difficult or impossible to elicit a second action potential is called the *refractory period*. It has two phases:

- ✔ **Absolute refractory period:** The absolute refractory period is when the sodium channels are in the inactivated state. In this state no additional action potential can be elicited, no matter how strong the depolarizing input.

- ✔ **Relative refractory period:** The relative refractory period is when the potassium channels are still open, but the sodium channels have transition from closed, inactivatable, to closed, activatable. Another spike is hard — but not impossible — to produce because of the relative refractory period after the sodium channel transitions (from the inactivated to the closed state) and potassium currents are lingering.

See how these events play out in Figure 3-2.

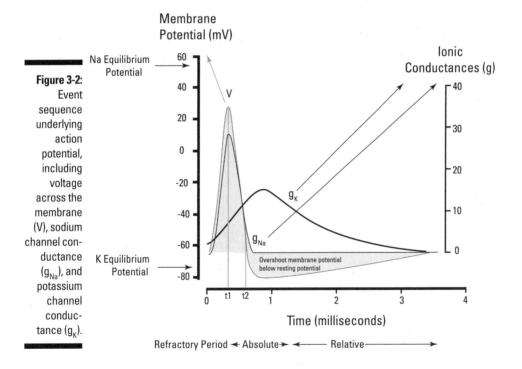

Figure 3-2: Event sequence underlying action potential, including voltage across the membrane (V), sodium channel conductance (g_{Na}), and potassium channel conductance (g_K).

The trace in Figure 3-2 labeled "V" is the membrane potential, and the scale for this trace is on the left. At the start of the plot, the membrane potential is at the resting level, or about –65 mV. As sodium channels open, the potential moves toward the sodium equilibrium potential (although it may not actually reach this 55 mV level). The membrane potential then declines to a level below the resting potential, and then finally returns to the resting potential.

The other two traces in Figure 3-2 show the sodium and potassium permeabilities that control this membrane potential. The action potential (voltage, membrane potential trace) is caused by any input that depolarizes the cell enough to open the voltage-dependent sodium channels. The permeability (a biophysical term corresponding to electrical conductance) of the sodium channels is given by the g_{Na} trace, whose values (conductance) correspond to the axis on the right. This conductance is nearly zero at the resting potential, rises to a maximum near the membrane potential peak, and then returns to zero through the transition from the open to the inactivated state (refer to "Getting back to resting potential" earlier in this chapter).

The opening and closing of the voltage-dependent potassium channels, whose conductance is g_K, happens more slowly than the sodium channels. They tend to drive the membrane potential toward the potassium reversal potential, usually near –75 mV. The depolarizing phase of the action potential tends to be stopped by the closing of the sodium channels (which the voltage-dependent sodium channels do on their own) and the opening of potassium channels.

The absolute refractory period is the time during which the sodium channels are in the inactivated state, before they transition to the closed state. The relative refractory period occurs after the action potential when potassium channels remain open and sodium channels have partially recovered from inactivation. The lingering potassium current drives the membrane potential below the resting potential, and makes it harder to elicit a spike than was the case in Figure 3-2 when the cell was at the resting potential at the beginning of the plot.

The sodium-potassium transporter pump runs all the time, causing the imbalance in ionic concentrations between the inside and outside of the neuron. A single action potential creates a temporary current through the membrane, which changes the voltage across the membrane, but it has little effect on the total ion concentrations within the entire cell. Even if all the sodium-transporter pumps shut down (refer to the "Sodium-potassium pump" section, earlier in this chapter), up to millions of action potentials can occur before the cell starts to lose its concentration difference with respect to the cell exterior.

Refractory periods and spike rate coding

Neurobiologists generally model synaptic inputs to neurons as currents injected into the dendritic tree (refer to Chapter 2) that are transformed into a train of spikes at the cell soma or axon initial segment. If the firing rate were exactly proportional to total synaptic current (above threshold), the relationship between synaptic current and spike rate would be called *linear.* However, in reality, this relationship is not linear for two main reasons:

✔ Leakage currents through the membrane tend to shunt away synaptic current more for low, slowly changing current levels than for rapidly changing ones.

✔ At high spike rates, the refractory period requires disproportionally more synaptic current to increase the spike rate. In fact, as the absolute refractory period is approached, no amount of increased synaptic input current can increase the spike rate.

One interesting result of this second factor is that the relationship between synaptic input current and spike rate in most neurons is more like a logarithmic function than a linear function. Psychophysical laws such as Weber's and Fechner's laws have long demonstrated that our perception of magnitude in senses such as sight, sound, and touch also follow a logarithmic relationship, where doubling the stimulus magnitude produces less than a doubling of the sensory perceptual magnitude. Direct experimental comparisons between perception of magnitude and neural firing rates have shown that the logarithmic spike compression underlies the logarithmic perception — that is, the perceptual magnitude follows the neural firing rate, which itself is logarithmically related to the magnitude of the stimulus.

Cable properties of neurons: One reason for action potentials

Neurobiologists continue to unveil new complexities about neurons, while continuously proving that we have much more to learn. Creating an accurate model of the activity of just one neuron — the complex, time-varying changes in its thousands of synapses and millions of voltage-dependent membrane ion channels — can take 100 percent of the processing power of a quite large computer.

A major reason why the interactions among inputs to a neuron can be so complicated is that neural dendrites have what are called *cable properties* for transmitting signals. This means that the way synaptic signals on different points on a dendrite interact depends on the structure of the dendritic tree between the two points. This includes whether the inputs are on the same or different dendritic branches. The reason the dendritic branch structure makes so much difference is that electrical parameters of the dendrites — such as membrane resistance, membrane capacitance, and dendritic axial resistance—(which we discuss in a moment) are distributed along the dendrite or dendritic tree. Understanding how synaptic inputs interact within the dendritic tree is modeled using *cable theory,* which was originally developed for transoceanic submarine telegraph cables. The application of this theory to neurons was championed by Wilfred Rall, who made influential contributions to our undertanding of dendritic integration.

Synaptic input current is typically divided into *passive* versus *active conduction properties.* Passive properties are those in the absence of voltage-dependent ion channels that themselves cause currents to flow through the membrane in response to synaptic input currents (and other voltage-dependent channels). Active properties involve voltage-dependent ion channels such as the voltage-gated sodium channel that can act to amplify signals.

Passive electrotonic conduction

A dendrite can be modeled (electrically) as an insulating membrane that separates an inner conductive core from the outer, extracellular fluid (which is also conductive). The membrane has resistance, which is normally very high except where ion channels and capacitance exist.

Capacitance occurs when a thin insulator separates two conductors, such as the neural membrane separating the conductive fluids inside and outside the cell. Normally, no current will flow across an insulator between two conductors. But, if the insulator is thin, and its area is large, transient current can flow due to a redistribution of charges as positive charge on one side of the insulator attract to negative charges on the other side (or vice versa).

To understand what membrane resistance means to spreading synaptic current, think of a water pipe. Suppose a water pipe is standing straight up and connected to a faucet at the bottom that is turned off. If you suddenly turn on the faucet, water will gush out of the top of the pipe almost immediately. The same idea applies to a neuron for a synaptic input on a dendrite with very high membrane resistance (no leakage) and no membrane capacitance between the synapse and another location on the dendrite. Now suppose the pipe has many small holes all along its length. When the faucet is turned on, some water will exit the end of the pipe almost immediately. But a lot of water will escape through the holes along the way, so the force won't be as strong when the water gushes out of the top. In other words, the holes, like low membrane resistance, will weaken the "signal" reaching the top of the pipe from the opened faucet at the bottom.

The water pipe idea can also help us to understand membrane capacitance. Suppose the pipe is not a stiff metal one, but a very stretchy rubber hose. If you suddenly turn on the faucet, the water flow creates a bulge at the end of the hose near the faucet. The water travels down and creates another bulge, and so on, until water finally begins to leave the open end of the hose.

Eventually, the flow out the end of the pipe will be equal to the flow into the pipe at the faucet. Membrane capacitance works in the same way, by delaying and soothing sharp inputs at one point on a dendrite while they're on their way to other dendritic locations.

The highly stretchable hose is like membrane capacitance. Even if the end of the hose — which you can think of as the energy storage mechanism — farthest from the faucet were closed, opening the faucet would allow some water flow until the force stretching the hose was exactly equal to the force where the water enters the faucet. This flow is always transient, however, just like the flow of current through a capacitor, which has a low resistance to changing voltage but blocks constant voltage.

The combination of low membrane resistance (holes in the pipe) and high membrane capacitance (stretchable pipe) means that synaptic input currents in one dendritic location may be severely weakened, delayed, and smoothed when they arrive at some other location. Figure 3-3 is a model that represents both continuous membrane resistance (due mostly to ion channels) and membrane capacitance.

An axonal or dendritic process has continuous axial resistance (r_a), membrane resistance (r_m), and membrane capacitance (c_m).

Figure 3-3: Electrical model of the distributed membrane resistance and capacitance in a neural process such as a dendrite or axon. In thin processes, the axial resistance r_a can become significant.

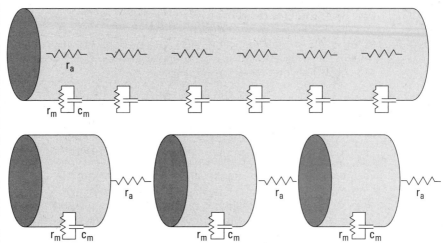

The process may be approximated in simulations by a finite number of small or unit cylinders having discrete values of r_a, r_m and c_m.

In real neurons, synaptic signals are so reduced over distances larger than about 200 micrometers that they become ineffective (low amplitude and slow time course). To communicate synaptic inputs over larger distances, neurons require *active propagation,* which I discuss in the next section.

Active propagation of depolarization

Most neurons have dendritic trees with diameters of less than a few hundred micrometers. This is the limit for passive signal propagation from the most distal dendrites to the soma. Larger neurons need to overcome the problems of weakened signals and signal smoothing if they are to communicate over distances larger than a few dendritic trees.

In the earlier section titled "Cable properties," I mention that the analysis of dendritic signal propagation uses *cable theory,* derived from undersea telegraph cable technology. An undersea telegraph cable is a conductor such as a copper wire, insulated, and surrounded by seawater, which itself is conductive. This is like a neural process such as a dendrite immersed in conductive extracellular fluid (which, by the way, is somewhat similar in ionic composition to seawater).

When testing began for the first undersea telegraph cables, it was found that signals (telegraph pulses) applied at one end were lost through the insulating layer and smeared out and delayed over time (due to the capacitance of the cable) when they were received some distance from the source. The solution for telegraph cables was placing repeaters along their length that boosted the signal back to its original strength before it was lost.

Just like telegraph cables, neurons also use repeaters. Neuronal repeaters are the voltage-dependent sodium channels (we discuss them earlier in this chapter) working with the action potential. Voltage dependent-sodium channels cause further depolarization, which amplifies the depolarization signal in the membrane. This amplification in axons allows neurons to send pulses over arbitrarily long distances, exceeding meters.

The first long-distance neural signal amplification system to evolve was continuous in unmyelinated axons, with voltage-dependent sodium channels placed continuously.

Neuroscience research is full of surprises. One from the last two decades is that neurons use signal amplification not only in their long axons, but also in their dendritic trees. This signal amplification can be done with either voltage-dependent sodium channels or voltage-dependent calcium channels, often located at branch points in the dendritic tree. These channels not only amplify, but also participate in the computing that takes place in the neuron's dendritic tree. This is because the dendrite can use amplification to control the flow of information throughout the dendritic tree. The neuron's dendritic tree can be divided into many subunits that interact and make complex processes — such as recognizing a particular pattern of action potentials on the dendritic tree — happen.

Insulating with Glial Cells

Many student neuroscientists are surprised when they learn that the most numerous cells in the nervous system are not neurons, but *glia,* which make up the nervous system's connective tissues. In fact, glia outnumber neurons by about 10:1. Many types of glial cells with different functions exist (see Figure 3-4):

✔ *Astrocytes* are glial cells that form part of the blood-brain barrier and regulate ionic concentrations of extracellular fluid.

✔ *Microglia* scavenge for and clean up extracellular debris from dead cells and injury.

✔ *Schwann cells* and *oligodendrocytes* wrap axons to enhance signal propagation. (See the next paragraph for more.)

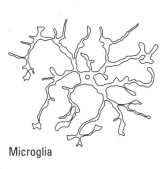

Microglia

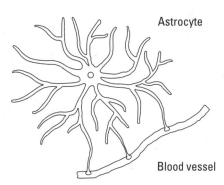

Astrocyte

Blood vessel

Figure 3-4:
Types of glia cells (microglia, astrocytes, and myelin-producing Schwann cells and oligodendrocytes).

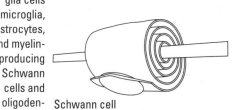

Schwann cell

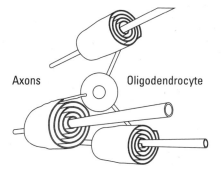

Axons

Oligodendrocyte

As the previous list shows, an important function of glial cells is that they wrap axonal membranes to enhance signal propagation. The glial cells that do this are *Schwann cells* in the peripheral nervous system and *oligodendrocytes* in the central nervous system. These cells produce *myelin*, which is the fatty tissue made of lipids and lipoproteins that encloses certain axons and nerve fibers.

Both types of glial cells form a spiral, multilayered wrapping on a portion of an axon. This wrapping has two main effects:

✔ It greatly increases the membrane resistance (lowering leakage).

✔ It reduces membrane capacitance (refer to "Passive electrotonic conduction") by increasing the distance between the fluid inside the axon and the fluid outside. The increase in membrane resistance prevents the signal from weakening, and the reduction in capacitance decreases the time smearing of the signal.

However, neither of these effects is enough to conduct action potentials for more than a few hundred micrometers without amplification, which is where repeaters come in. In glial-wrapped, or myelinated, axons, the glial wrapping contain breaks or gaps, approximately every millimeter. Located at these breaks, called *nodes of Ranvier,* is a high concentration of voltage-dependent sodium channels. The action potential jumps at high speed from node to node in a process called *salutatory conduction.* This conduction speed is about ten times faster than it is in unmyelinated fibers.

Chapter 4

Sending Signals: Chemical Release and Electrical Activation

In This Chapter

▶ Signaling with chemical and electrical synapses

▶ Being open to receptors for neurotransmitters

▶ Pooling resources with interneurons and circuits

*N*eurons have three main functions: detecting inputs at their membranes; putting all this information together; and communicating the results to other neurons, muscles, or glands. This chapter discusses how neurons accomplish the third function, communication, using neurotransmitters that bind to different types of membrane receptors.

So, why is all this communication necessary, anyway? A big job for your nervous system is communicating with muscles to produce and control behavior. In vertebrates, neuromuscular transmission involves activating receptors on muscle cells, which causes them to contract. Most of the time multiple receptors activate multiple muscle cells through a coordinating network of neurons. Everything works together, so you can walk, breathe, and turn the pages of this book. This chapter covers how this happens.

Looking at Synaptic Transmission

Synaptic transmission is a specialized type of cell-to-cell (neuron-to-neuron) communication that occurs at synapses. *Synapses* are small contact areas between cells that mediate this communication. Two major types of synapses exist, each using different mechanisms for communicating with other neurons:

▶ **Chemical synapses:** Most chemical synapses use a secretion mechanism. The presynaptic neuron releases small packets (called *vesicles*) of neurotransmitter molecules that cross the gap (called the *synaptic cleft*) between the pre- and postsynaptic neuron. These neurotransmitter molecules bind *receptors* (protein complexes in the postsynaptic membrane). These receptors either open ion channels directly (*ionotropic receptors*) or open or close ion channels indirectly (*metabotropic receptors*). If the ion channel is selectively *permeable* to sodium (that is, it allows sodium ions to pass), it's an *excitatory* receptor. If the channel is permeable to potassium or chloride, it is typically an *inhibitory* receptor. (Refer to Chapter 3 for more about receptors and ion channels.) The next section goes into chemical synapses in more detail.

✓ **Electrical synapse:** The other major type of synapse is called an *electrical synapse.* In electrical synapse, a channel on the presynaptic cell lines up with and binds to a similar channel on the postsynaptic cell. This is called a *gap junction.* A pore then exists that connects the cytoplasm of the presynaptic cell directly with the cytoplasm of the postsynaptic one that allows not only can ions like sodium, potassium, and chloride pass, but small dissolved organic molecules up to atomic weights of several hundred Daltons.

Checking out chemical synapses and neurotransmitter release

In chemical synapses, a specialized ending of the presynaptic cell (traditionally called an *axon terminal* or *bouton*) releases neurotransmitters. Neurotransmitters can be released in several ways. The most common method is when vesicles of neurotransmitter fuse with the plasma membrane. This causes neurotransmitter molecules to get dumped into the synaptic cleft, where they diffuse to the postsynaptic receptors. The arrival of an action potential (refer to Chapter 3) at the axon terminal usually triggers this process.

Other mechanisms of neurotransmitter release are based on transporters. *Transporters* are pumps that move ions or small charged molecules — such as neurotransmitters — through the cell membrane. Transporters involved in synaptic transmission are typically those where membrane potential (refer to Chapter 3) controls ion movement.

Sometimes pairs of ions work together to co-transport ions, such as the sodium-potassium ATP co-transporter I discuss in Chapter 3.

Synthesis of neurotransmitters

How neurotransmitters are *synthesized* (made from precursor molecules) depends on where they're synthesized and how they're released:

✓ **In neurotransmitter terminals:** Some neurotransmitters, such as acetylcholine, are synthesized in the neurotransmitter terminals from choline that has been reabsorbed and recycled from a previous release.

✔ **In the nucleus:** Neuromodulator transmitters, such as neuropeptides like enkephalins and neuropeptide Y, are typically synthesized in the rough endoplasmic reticulum and packaged in vesicles like secretory proteins. These vesicles are transported down the axon by the cytoskeleton to the synaptic terminal. Neuromodulators usually have slower and more diffuse effects than neurotransmitters.

Presynaptic nerve terminals and neurotransmitter release

For most small-molecule neurotransmitters, an action potential arrives causing neurotransmitters to be released at the axon terminal. The axon terminal contains *synaptic vesicles* (small membrane-bound organelles filled with neurotransmitter molecules). Figure 4-1 shows this "classic" mechanism for chemical neurotransmitter release, which I describe next.

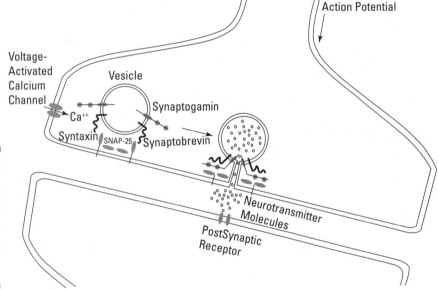

Figure 4-1: Structure, molecules, and sequence for neurotransmitter release.

This sequence of events for releasing neurotransmitter takes only a few tenths of a millisecond:

1. **An action potential travels down the axon and reaches the synapse.**

2. **This action potential depolarizes the presynaptic terminal membrane.**

3. **The depolarized terminal causes voltage-dependent calcium channels to open.**

   Refer to Chapter 3 for a description of voltage-dependent channels.

4. **Calcium ions enter the presynaptic membrane, rapidly increasing the calcium concentration.**

5. **The elevated calcium concentration activates proteins (such as synaptotagmin and synaptobrevin) on some of the neurotransmitter-filled synaptic vesicles that are docked onto the synaptic membrane.**

6. **The changes in vesicle proteins cause these proteins to bind to several other proteins (syntaxin and SNAP-25) at the presynaptic membrane.**

7. **The vesicle fuses with the membrane.**

8. **This fusion causes the vesicle contents — including the neurotransmitter molecules — to be dumped into the synaptic cleft between the membranes of the pre- and postsynaptic neurons.**

Neurotransmitter release at some synapses involves transporters. In many chemical synapses, transporters in the postsynaptic membrane remove neurotransmitters from the synaptic cleft to prevent excitation of the postsynaptic cell. (See the next section for more about excitatory neurotransmitters.) However, some transport mechanisms work in reverse, releasing the neurotransmitters into the synapse in a process called *nonvesicular release*.

There are approximately 15 small molecules that function as neurotransmitters in neural communication, and on the order of 50 neuroactive peptides. Several hundred distinct receptor types exist for these neurotransmitters.

Excitatory neurotransmitters

Neurotransmitters can be divided into groups in various ways. One important distinction is between those that tend to act on rapidly responding ionotropic (channel-containing) receptors and those that act on metabotropic (indirect receptors).

Most rapid action in the nervous system is controlled by small molecule neurotransmitters that act on ionotropic receptors. These can be divided into excitatory and inhibitory neurotransmitters. Just remember that it's actually what happens at the receptor that determines the neurotransmitter action.

Excitatory neurotransmitters promote the opening of ion channels that are permeable primarily to sodium. The main small-molecule excitatory neurotransmitters in the nervous system that cause rapid neural responses are glutamate and acetylcholine. Although both of these neurotransmitters are generally associated with fast synaptic transmission, both glutamate and acetylcholine can activate certain classes of metabotropic receptors and in some areas of the nervous system even lead to inhibition.

Embracing your inhibitions

Neurobiology students often find inhibitory receptors puzzling. Why are they necessary? One answer is that many behaviors that are triggered by sensory input must, under some circumstances, be inhibited. For example, if you're holding a hot stick over a campfire and it starts to burn your hand, you have a reflex to drop the stick and withdraw your hand. But if you're using that stick to cook your last hot dog over that fire, you may be willing to endure the brief pain and hold on to the stick a bit longer if you're hungry.

Another reason is computational. Neural circuits, like electronic circuits, tend to work better if inhibition can modulate excitation so it doesn't get out of control. One thing that happens in the brain when inhibition doesn't properly modulate excitation is epileptic seizures.

Inhibitory neurotransmitters

Inhibitory neurotransmitters open channels for potassium or chloride. The main small-molecule neurotransmitters that mediate fast inhibitory synaptic transmission are GABA (for gamma-Aminobutyric acid) and glycine. Receptors called $GABA_A$ are ligand-gated chloride channels, whereas $GABA_B$ receptors are metabotropic receptors that open potassium channels indirectly via G-proteins.

Neuromodulators and neuropeptides

Neurons also use about 50 to 100 short-chain proteins, called *peptides,* as neurotransmitters or neuromodulators. *Neuropeptides* are related to peptide hormones, and in fact, some neuropeptides are also hormones. However, neuropeptides are released by neurons at synapses and not into the bloodstream like hormones. Many neuropeptides are involved in motivational aspects of brain function, such as reward, reproduction, and social behavior.

Neuropeptides typically act at what are called *metabotropic g-protein-coupled receptors* (see the "Meeting metabotropic receptors and second messenger systems" section, later in this chapter). This allows neuropeptides to have long-term, diverse effects, such as altering gene expression or *synaptogenesis* (the process of forming synapses). Neuropeptides are often released by the same neurons that release conventional small-molecule neurotransmitters such as glutamate or GABA.

Neurons release neuropeptides through vesicular release like conventional neurotransmitters (we explain conventional neurotransmitter release earlier in this chapter), but with some important differences. Neuropeptides are released from *dense-core vesicles* (so-called because of their appearance in the electron microscope), whereas small-molecule neurotransmitters are released from smaller synaptic vesicles that do not have a dense core. (The term *dense-core vesicle* comes from the way these vesicles look under the electron microscope, which I cover later in this chapter.) The properties of synaptic release for dense-core vesicles are very different than for conventional synaptic vesicles.

Neurotransmitters are structurally classified into amino acids, peptides, monoamines, and miscellaneous (but important) others:

- ✔ **Amino acid neurotransmitters:** These include glutamate (which accounts for over 90 percent of brain synapses), GABA (which accounts for over 90 percent of inhibitory synapses), glycine, aspartate, and D-serine.

- ✔ **Monoamines and other biogenic amines:** These include dopamine (the drugs cocaine and amphetamine affect dopamine transmission), epinephrine (formerly, adrenaline), norepinephrine (formerly, noradrenaline), histamine, and serotonin (5-HT).

- ✔ **Neuropeptides:** Among the more than 50 neuropeptides are somatostatin, substance P, neuropeptide Y and several opioid peptides such as β-endorphin.

- ✔ **Other important neurotransmitters:** These include acetylcholine and adenosine, and even gases such as nitric oxide and carbon monoxide.

Eyeing electrical synapses at gap junctions

A very ancient type of synapse between neurons is the *gap junction*. Gap junctions exist not only between neurons, but also between other cells, such as secretory cells. Gap junctions are made when the pre- and postsynaptic neurons each form from hemichannels whose exterior sides bind to produce a continuous pore that links the cytoplasm of one cell to the cytoplasm of the other. Figure 4-2 shows how gap junctions (visible using electron microscopy, which we tell you about later in this chapter) would appear at high magnification.

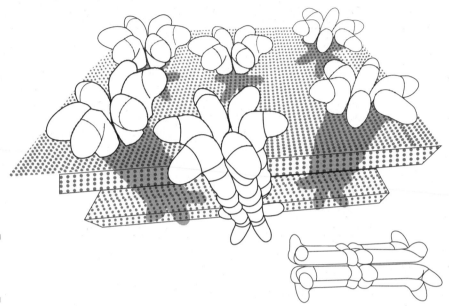

Figure 4-2:
Gap junction
synapses.

The pore in the gap junction is much larger than the channel in a typical ion channel. Because the pore is larger, it allows not only most dissolved atomic ions — such as sodium, potassium, and chloride — to pass through, but also allows small dissolved organic molecules up to several hundred Daltons in atomic weight. Hundreds or thousands of gap junction channels may be packed together in a small region of membrane.

Electrical currents pass through the connecting gap junctions from one cell to the other. These currents make the postsynaptic cell respond in a manner similar to the presynaptic cell. The advantages of this type of synapse are speed and synchronicity because the post-synaptic cell(s) follow the presynaptic cell(s) in lockstep.

Gap junction neurotransmission does have its limits. The following two limits help to explain why large-brained animals such as mammals have such a dominance of chemical over electrical synapses (as I explain in the previous section about chemical synapses):

 ✔ **Classic inhibition is not possible.** Because the postsynaptic cell does exactly what the presynaptic cell does, classical inhibition (refer to the sidebar "Embracing your inhibitions") is not possible.

✔ **Effects are limited.** The current generated by the presynaptic cell crosses more membrane, reducing the voltage across the total membrane of the two cells compared to the presynaptic cell alone. This means that a presynaptic cell can only drive a few postsynaptic cells and must be much bigger than the postsynaptic targets to have much effect on them.

Neurobiologists say gap junction synapses are *sign-conserving* because the postsynaptic cell follows the potential generated by the presynaptic cell. Normally this means that these synapses are excitatory only. However, in some cases, *gap junction coupling* occurs — shunting away excitatory current from the presynaptic cell reduces the excitatory current received by other parts of the presynaptic cell. This reduces the influence of the excitatory neurotransmitter.

Gap junction synapses are common in invertebrates, but they make up only a small minority of the synapses in vertebrates, especially mammals. In fact, scientists used to believe that the neocortex of mammals had almost no gap junctions at all. However, recently scientists are seeing that inhibitory networks in the cortex use gap junction synaptic coupling.

Being Receptive to Neurotransmitter Receptors

The effect of a neurotransmitter on the postsynaptic cell depends on what receptor is activated. Although receptors are highly specific for single neurotransmitters, many different types of receptors exist for each neurotransmitter. Some receptors act more rapidly than others, and some have longer lasting effects.

Two major classes of neurotransmitter receptors exist, distinguished by whether the receptor itself gates an ion channel (ionotropic) or whether the receptor's activation has indirect effects (metabotropic). These receptors are the topic of the next two sections.

After neurotransmitter release, the neurotransmitter molecules must be removed so the cycle of synaptic transmission can continue. Three main mechanisms remove the neurotransmitter molecules:

✔ **Simple diffusion:** The neurotransmitter may diffuse away from the synaptic cleft. In some cases, the neurotransmitter may activate other receptors in a process called *extra-synaptic transmission*.

- **Destruction or inactivation:** Enzymes within the synaptic cleft or neural membranes may destroy or inactivate the neurotransmitter. One prominent example of this process is the destruction of acetylcholine by the enzyme acetyl cholinesterase within the synaptic cleft.

- **Reuptake:** Transporters may reuptake the neurotransmitter — or one of the products left over after enzymes destroy the neurotransmitter, as in the previous bullet — back into the presynaptic axon terminal. Afterward, the neurotransmitter or its components may be reprocessed and released again.

Introducing ionotropic receptors

In ionotropic receptors, when the neurotransmitter is bound, the receptor proteins refold in such a way that a pore opens, allowing particular ions to pass through it. This pore is usually ion selective and allows sodium, potassium, chloride, or calcium to pass (although many receptors allow a minority flow of a second ion). The receptor many also be *rectifying,* allowing the selected ion to flow (or flux) in one direction (into or out of the cell).

Most fast excitatory and inhibitory receptors involved in the immediate control of the brain and behavior are ionotropic, using the neurotransmitters glutamate and GABA. Some ionotropic receptors have multiple neurotransmitter binding sites. However, having multiple binding sites may include — in addition to one for a particularly fast neurotransmitter — sites for neuromodulatory neurotransmitters. These are often metabotropic, activating slower second messenger systems. The most important ions in neuronal excitability are sodium, potassium, and chloride; *ionotropic receptors* (receptors with integral, ligand-gated channels) exist for all three of these ions.

Although it is common (including in this book) to refer to "excitatory" and "inhibitory" neurotransmitters, the effect of the transmitter on the postsynaptic cell depends primarily on which ions are permeable through the receptor channel that opens after binding the neurotransmitter. So, dividing excitatory and inhibitory receptors into three main groups is actually more correct:

- **Excitatory receptors whose channels flux primarily sodium:** An influx of sodium into neurons causes *depolarization* (positive movement away from the negative resting potential) and is excitatory.

- **Inhibitory receptors whose channels flux primarily chloride:** The chloride equilibrium potential for most neurons is just below the resting potential. Ligand-gated opening of chloride channels *hyperpolarizes* the cell (makes the cytoplasm more negative) and is inhibitory. In addition, opening chloride channels resists the depolarization that is caused by opening other excitatory sodium channels, even if the chloride equilibrium potential is close to the cell's resting potential. This is sometimes called "silent" or "shunting" inhibition.

The most important excitatory ionotropic receptors are those for the neurotransmitters glutamate and acetylcholine. Glutamate receptors are by far the most numerous and important excitatory receptors in the central nervous system, whereas virtually all vertebrate *neuromuscular transmission* (the activation of muscles by neurons) is via acetylcholine.

Most inhibitory ionotropic receptors chloride. The most important inhibitory neurotransmitters in the nervous system are GABA and glycine (an amino acid). The most important GABA chloride receptor type is called a $GABA_A$ channel (there is a similar, but much rarer, $GABA_C$ receptor type). Most glycine-activated ionotropic channels are inhibitory chloride permeable channels. For GABA, metabotropic potassium channel receptors also exist.

Neuromuscular activation occurs by ionotropic acetylcholine receptors, called *nicotinic receptors* (because they can be activated by nicotine).

Meeting metabotropic receptors and second messenger systems

In contrast with ionotropic receptors, metabotropic receptors have no ion channel. Instead, when they bind the neurotransmitter molecule on the extracellular side of the membrane, a change in structure occurs in the receptor that activates an enzyme (directly or indirectly). This activated enzyme (called the *primary effector*) converts a substrate *within the cytoplasm* into what's called a *second messenger.* This second messenger may open or close ion channels by binding at a channel site on the *inside of the membrane.*

Second messenger cascades can cause multiple actions. They may open several nearby channel pores from the inside or change the expression of DNA in the nucleus. These types of effects tend to be much slower but longer lasting compared to those in ionotropic receptors. (An exception is the NMDA receptor that fluxes both sodium and calcium.)

The second messenger system for most metabotropic channels involves what are called *g proteins,* so these receptors are sometimes referred to as g protein-coupled receptors.

Dale's law

In the mid 20th century, neuroscience students were taught a principle called Dale's law:

> The same chemical transmitter is released from all the synaptic terminals of a neuron.

Modern biochemical techniques have shown, however, that this law, at least as stated in this form, is not universally correct. The most common "violation" of Dale's law is the coexistence of the release of a fast, ionotropic neurotransmitter such as glutamate, with a slower, metabotropic transmitter peptide such as somatostatin. Often, the effect of the peptide is regulatory, because

strong, prolonged release of the ionotropic excitatory transmitter that may overstimulate the postsynaptic cell also down-regulates the receiving cell's response to the excitatory transmitter. This process is a kind of homeostasis.

You can find some even more extreme violations of Dale's law. Starburst amacrince cells in the retina release acetylcholine at their dendritic terminal regions but GABA all along their dendrites. Both of these are fast, ionotropic transmitters, but one is excitatory and the other inhibitory.

Over a hundred of types of metabotropic receptors exist, but they use only a limited number of second messenger pathways:

- ✔ Cyclic adenosine monophosphate (AMP) pathway
- ✔ Inositol triphosphate/diacylglycerol (IP3/DAG) pathway
- ✔ Arachidonic acid pathway

The cyclic AMP pathway is the most important in neuronal communication. When the metabotropic receptor is bound by the ligand, membrane-bound enzyme adenylyl cyclase is activated, which is the primary effector. This, in turn, converts adenosine triphosphate (ATP) in the cytoplasm into the second messenger cyclic-AMP (cAMP), which diffuses within the cytoplasm to activate the secondary effector, protein kinase A (PKA). Protein kinases are capable of adding phosphate groups (*phosphorylating proteins*) to regulate channel gates or protein translation.

Many neurotransmitters activate ionotropic receptors in some neural circuits, and metabotropic receptors in others. Metabotropic receptors for glutamate and GABA exist, for example. Some metabotropic glutamate receptors are inhibitory because they open potassium channels. $GABA_B$ receptors are metabotropic and inhibitory because they open potassium channels. Metabotropic receptors are typically the targets of neurotransmitters such as dopamine, epinephrine, norepinephrine, histamine, and many neuropeptides.

Making connections with the neuromuscular junction

Neurons synapse mostly on other neurons, but the ultimate outcome of neural computation is usually activating muscles to do something.

Muscles are groups of muscle cells. Muscles contract because the muscle cells contract along their length parallel to the long axis of the muscle. Your body has two main types of muscle:

- ✔ **Smooth muscle:** Found in blood vessel linings, the digestive and urinary tracts, the uterus, and other places where they mediate internal, homeostatic functions. You don't control these functions; your autonomic nervous system does. (I cover muscles and muscle control in more detail in Chapter 6.)

- ✔ **Striated muscle:** Used for making voluntary actions. The nervous system controls these muscles. Muscle cells are excitable cells, like neurons, that can produce action potentials. In voluntary muscles, action potentials are produced when presynaptic motor neuron terminals release the neurotransmitter acetylcholine, which binds to a postsynaptic receptor on the muscle cell. This is an ionotropic receptor. The *end-plate* is the postsynaptic region of the muscle fiber where motor neuron axon terminals synapse. (Cardiac muscle is a different kind of striated muscle.)

The major steps in neuromuscular transmission are as follows:

1. **The motor neuron presynaptic terminal releases acetylcholine.**

   The acetylcholine crosses the synaptic cleft and binds to the postsynaptic receptor on the muscle cell end plate. Typically one motor neuron axon terminal exists per muscle cell, although a single motor neuron axon can branch and innervate many muscle cells.

2. **The acetylcholine binds a nicotinic acetylcholine receptor.**

   Nicotinic acetylcholine receptors are ionotropic receptors that are primarily selective for sodium but also pass some potassium.

3. **The ion flux through the receptor channel produces the muscle end-plate potential.**

   This is similar to the excitatory post-synaptic potential produced by excitatory synapses on neurons that open sodium channels.

4. **The end-plate potential causes a muscle action potential.**

   This action potential has an ionic basis that is similar to the neural action potential, except that it's much longer lasting (5 to 10 milliseconds).

5. **The action potential activates voltage-dependent calcium channels (L-type)in the muscle cell membrane.**

    Gating voltage-dependent calcium channels causes the an internal organelle called the sarcoplasmic reticulum within the muscle cell to release calcium, transiently increasing the free calcium concentration in the muscle cell cytoplasm.

6. **The increase in calcium within the muscle cell causes the actin and myosin myofilaments to slide over each other. These myofilaments run the length of the muscle cell and are responsible for muscle's ability to contract.**

    This causes the muscle cell to contract along its length. This process uses ATP as an energy source.

Acetylcholine only binds for a short time on the receptor. After the acetylcholine molecule comes off the receptor, degradation molecules (called *cholinesterases*) in the synaptic cleft destroy the acetylcholine molecule so that it can't bind again.

The choline product of the degradation of acetylcholine is taken back up (reuptake) by the presynaptic terminal, reconverted into acetylcholine, and repackaged into vesicles for later release.

The muscle cell end-plate receptor is called *nicotinic* because nicotine (yes, from tobacco) is an effective agonist for this receptor. An *agonist* is an substance that is not normally released onto the muscle receptor, but that is effective in producing the same effects as the normal neurotransmitter.

Dividing and Conquering: Interneurons and Circuits

Understanding the function of a neural circuit or brain area can be difficult for neurobiologists because most neurons in the middle of the brain are still quite a mystery. We don't know exactly what their input is, where their output goes, or what their output does.

One instructive way to analyze the function question was proposed by David Marr and Tomaso Poggio of the MIT Artificial Intelligence Laboratory. They suggested that function in the nervous system could be approached at three levels:

✔ **Computational level:** What is the overall task of the system? For example, the autopilot in an airplane has the task of keeping the plane on the correct heading at the right altitude, among other things.

✔ **Algorithmic/representational level:** How does the system operate? For the autopilot, algorithms compute how much elevator change in degrees should be made for a particular altitude error.

✔ **Physical implementation level:** What's the actual hardware? Autopilots can be digital or analog, controlling the plane with wires, hydraulics, or electric motors.

We investigate nervous system function at all three of these levels. This is typically easiest to do for parts of the nervous system close to sensory input or motor output, where you can observe the correlation between the circuit and its result. For example, you can shine light on a photoreceptor and observe its electrical response. In the upcoming sections, we apply each of these three levels to look at different nervous system functions.

Recent technical progress in physiological measurement and neural response manipulation has expanded our understanding into the middle of the brain — where the greatest mysteries remain.

Pooling sensory input

One place in the nervous system where considerable work has been done at the circuit level is the retina. On the computational level, the retina's job is to allow us to see. On the algorithmic level, the retina allows us to see using five major cell types arranged in two synaptic layers that extract and transmit specific aspects of the visual world to the brain. On the physical implementation level, the information sent to the brain goes over the axons of about 20 different ganglion cell classes, each of which has a representative at almost every point in the retina.

Neural convergence occurs when the inputs from many sources are pooled and transmitted in the output of fewer neurons. For example, the retinas of animals that are at least partially nocturnal have photoreceptors called *rods.* These rods can operate in light levels where only a few photons per second are available to be captured. The rods have multiple photopigment molecules that capture photons, and multiple rods that connect to a single ganglion cell. Pooling inputs reduces the total number of neurons and complexity of the system, with some sacrifice in preserving information about exactly where the photon was absorbed. Pooling always occurs to some degree in sensory system relays to the brain, and commonly that deals with sensitivity-efficiency trade-offs.

Coordinating motor output

Walking or swimming to get somewhere (computational) requires multiple muscles in multiple limbs to coordinate with each other in time and space. This coordination involves neural sensors that report limb position and forces, and neural integrating circuits that coordinate and sequence limb movements (algorithmic). A hierarchy of controllers work together to coordinate these sequences, starting with simple reflex controllers in the spinal cord, to spinal cord cyclic pattern generators, to error generation in the cerebellum that interact with the thalamus, basal ganglia, and motor cortex (implementation).

 The superior colliculus is a good example of a controlled motor output for which we know the neural basis. This midbrain structure receives a large input from the retina, so it has cells in its superficial layers that respond to visual input. But the function (computational) of the superior colliculus appears to be to code eye movements — *saccades* — for orienting our attention (algorithmic). This happens by a projection from the superior colliculus to the pulvinar and frontal lobe areas of the brains, so that shocking a given area on the colliculus produces an eye movement toward whatever we're seeing that is drawing our attention (implementation).

Comparing brains to computers

One of the hottest topics in neuroscience is comparing the computational power of the brain with that of computers. But how do we compare the two? We know that human and animal brains can do things — such as recognize complex patterns — that are extremely difficult to program computers to do. Of course, computers can do things like calculate the value of π to thousands of decimal places in a few milliseconds, which humans cannot do.

 Brains and computers compute in fundamentally different ways, even when doing the same task (same computation, probably different algorithms, and certainly different implementations). Only our brains use neurons. Given what we know about how neurons work, how do they do computations and what sort of computations do they do?

If you think of a very simple case where a neuron has two inputs, each of which by itself is above the threshold (more properly, the voltage at the soma due to the net synaptic current produced by those inputs is above the threshold), then the neuron is like an *OR gate* (it fires if either one or the other input is active).

But if the somatic response to each of the two input neurons (inputs A and B) is a bit more than half as much as the threshold, the neuron becomes an *AND gate*. That is, the output neuron is active only if both A and B inputs are active.

Because the output of neurons can also be inhibitory, they can function as inverters, or *NOT gates*. The combination of OR, AND, and NOT is more than sufficient for the nervous system to implement the same logical power as present in digital computer circuits.

However, in trying to compare the computing power of brains to computers, several problems remain. Most digital computers are serial devices, executing one instruction at a time. The brain is massively parallel, however, potentially executing billion of actions simultaneously. Individual synapses in neurons can also execute complex analog computations such as multiplication, division, and logarithmic transforms that make them more like analog than digital computers. We clearly need to know more about how neurons actually work in neural circuits. (The appendix at the end of this book explores how we study neurons and the nervous system.)

Part II
Neuroanatomy: Organizing the Nervous System

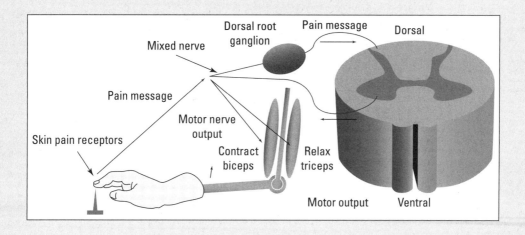

Find out more about consciousness in an article at www.dummies.com/extras/neurobiology.

In this part . . .

- ✔ Find out how your brain commands movement, and how your muscles accomplish it.

- ✔ See how your brain works through the spinal cord to control movement and regulate your organs.

- ✔ Discover what the oldest parts of your brain have in common with the brains of animals.

- ✔ See how behavior is generated by a hierarchical control system running from the neocortex to the brainstem.

- ✔ Discover how the neocortex — the newest and most powerful part of the brain — works with the older parts of the brain we inherited from our mammalian ancestors.

Chapter 5

Movement Basics: Muscles and Motor Neurons

. . . .

In This Chapter

▶ Dealing with distinct muscle types and functions

▶ Checking out how muscle cells contract

▶ Manipulating muscle contraction

▶ Locating your limbs

▶ Reacting to reflexes

▶ Considering the factors of exercise, aging, and sex

. . . .

*E*ven when you're sitting quietly — perhaps as you are right now, reading this book — your body is always moving. You consciously control some of the movements your body makes, while other types of movement happen without your even being aware.

Our bodies have distinct muscle types that produce involuntary, cardiac, and voluntary movement, all of which this chapter explores. Then I discuss how muscles are able to move because muscle cells contract to produce movement. Our bodies have different neural circuits that control these contractions. Speaking of circuits, this chapter tells you about sensory feedback circuits, which allow muscle reflexes to occur quickly and automatically, and take care of all the details of movement so you don't have to concentrate on every step you take.

The final sections of this chapter discuss what exercise does to our muscles, gaining and losing muscle mass as we age, and the difference in muscle composition between men and women. So, don't move a muscle, and read on!

Making a Move: Muscle Types and What They Do

The body produces very different kinds of movement — from intestinal contractions to heartbeats to voluntary bending (flexion) and stretching (extension) of limbs. Different kinds of neural circuits control these movements, and mediate reflexes, rhythmic motor patterns, and voluntary movement sequences that we consciously control. The two major types of muscle in the body are smooth and striated.

Processing with smooth muscle

Smooth muscle controls involuntary movements that you're generally not aware of, such as stomach and intestinal contractions. The autonomic nervous system (see Chapter 6) regulates these involuntary movements using the smooth muscles. The body's smooth muscles are located in a variety of places such as the walls of blood vessels, the iris of the eye, the bladder, and, for women, the uterus.

Smooth muscle types include single-unit and multiunit smooth muscle. In single-unit smooth muscle, the autonomic nervous system generates an action potential in one cell that is spread to other muscle cells through gap junctions (refer to Chapter 3). The result is that the entire muscle — which is made of many cells — contracts as a unit. In contrast, in multiunit smooth muscles, different motor neuron terminals contact, or *innervate,* individual cells. This allows for graded responses and finer neural control.

Smooth muscle differs significantly in structure and function from striated muscles, such as cardiac and skeletal muscle. It typically has greater elasticity and can contract even when already extended, which is an important function in organs like the intestines and bladder.

Striated muscle for hearts and limbs

Striated muscle enables voluntary movements of which you're fully conscious — movements typically controlled by high-level brain activity. It gets its name because of its striped appearance. Because muscles can only pull, and not push, *antagonistic* (or opposite) muscle pairs control most limbs; one muscle is a flexor, and the other is an extensor. (See "Pulling Your Weight: How Muscle Cells Contract," later in this chapter.)

The two major types of striated muscle are cardiac muscle and skeletal muscle. Cardiac muscle produces *heartbeats* (contractions of the heart muscle for pumping blood). Striated skeletal muscles are attached to bones through tendons to produce movement of the body.

A specialized type of striated muscle causes your heart to beat with a force like that of voluntary muscle. But the force and rate of your heartbeat is not under conscious control.

Skeletal muscle

Skeletal muscles consist of long, thin cells called *muscle fibers.* These muscle fibers typically extend the entire length of the muscle and are up to 30 centimeters long, but less than 0.1 millimeter wide. (Very few cells, besides neural axons, are centimeters long.)

Muscle cell membranes are similar to those of neurons. Their membranes have nicotinic receptors for the neurotransmitter acetylcholine (ACh) in a structure called the muscle *end plate* (refer to Chapter 4). Acetylcholine binds to these receptors and causes sodium channels to open. This depolarizes the cell and triggers a muscle cell action potential by activating voltage-dependent sodium channels. Each action potential produces a contraction of the muscle fiber, called a *twitch.*

Muscle contraction is based on the movement of myosin and actin fibers (which I discuss in a moment). The two major types of muscle filaments are Type I (slow-twitch) fibers and Type II (fast-twitch) fibers, both of which exist in skeletal muscle. The characteristics of both types are as follows:

- **Type I, slow-twitch fibers:** Type I, slow-twitch muscle is dense with mitochondria and myoglobin, which gives this type of muscle tissue its characteristic dark red color. Myoglobin is an iron-containing, oxygen-binding protein found in vertebrate muscle tissue, related to hemoglobin. Slow-twitch fibers can contract for long periods of time, but with less force than fast-twitch. They use fats and carbohydrates as fuel.

- **Type II, fast-twitch fibers:** Type II, fast-twitch fibers contract powerfully and rapidly. However, they also fatigue quickly, and after a short burst of activity their contraction starts becoming painful. They're the main fiber type that contributes to the total force a muscle can exert. Weight-bearing exercise increases mass primarily in this fiber type.

  Two kinds of Type II fast-twitch fibers exist:

  - **Type IIb fibers,** the speed champions, are able to contract up to ten times faster than Type I fibers. Because the Type IIb fibers are anaerobic, they look like "white meat" because they have less mitochondria and myoglobin.

- **Type IIa fibers,** the medium speed fibers, contract at a speed that is somewhere between that of Type I and Type IIb.

Type I slow-twitch fibers use aerobic metabolism (they require oxygen), whereas fast-twitch fibers use anaerobic metabolism (they do not require oxygen). Performing endurance activities such as marathon running depends mostly on aerobic slow-twitch fibers. Short-duration power movements, such as sprinting, use anaerobic fast-twitch fibers. This results in an energy/oxygen debt that the body must pay back over time by eating and consuming glucose (but a necessary and worthwhile one when escaping a predator, for example).

Cardiac muscle

Cardiac muscle is an involuntary striated muscle found in the heart. Cardiac muscle cells are called *myocardiocytes* or *cardiomyocytes.* Cardiac muscle is very resistant to fatigue, having a high density of mitochondria. Just like voluntary, striated skeletal muscle, cardiac muscle relies on the proteins actin and myosin for contraction, and has a striated appearance because of alternating segments of thin and thick protein filaments. Like smooth muscle, however, it's controlled by the autonomic nervous system.

Twitching fast and slow: Muscle composition

The ratio of fast- and slow-twitch muscle fibers is varied in major muscles such as quadriceps (thigh muscle) in humans. People with a smaller percentage of fast-twitch fibers may be better marathon runners; those with a larger percentage, better sprinters. One effect of weight-bearing exercise is that increases the percentage of fast-twitch fiber mass in the muscle, which increases strength.

Pulling Your Weight: How Muscle Cells Contract

Muscles can only pull, not push. Antagonistic muscle pairs control our limbs — the *flexor* flexes (bends) the limb and the *extensor* extends (straightens) the limb. Figure 5-1 shows the antagonistic pair that moves the lower leg. The quadriceps is the extensor that straightens the leg and supports you in an upright position. The hamstring is the flexor that bends the limb when you walk.

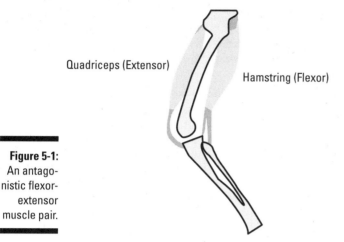

Quadriceps (Extensor)

Hamstring (Flexor)

Figure 5-1:
An antago-
nistic flexor-
extensor
muscle pair.

Muscle cells are excitable cells like neurons, in that they can produce action potentials. Voluntary striated muscles contract in a sequence of events. It starts with the presynaptic motor neuron terminal releasing the neurotransmitter acetylcholine, and ends with actin and myosin filaments sliding over each other in a contraction. I outline the events in the next section.

Releasing acetylcholine

Motor neurons are neurons that control muscles. Most skeletal muscles are controlled by alpha motor neurons (which I discuss further in the "Alpha motor neurons" section, later in this chapter) whose cell bodies are in the spinal cord. Virtually all striated muscle neurotransmission in vertebrates is controlled by acetylcholine released by motor neurons. Read on to find out how it all works.

Patterning muscle contractions

Muscles can be activated by reflexes, rhythmic motor patterns, or consciously controlled voluntary movement sequences. For typical skeletal muscles such as those that move the arms and legs, the alpha motor neuron is the final common pathway for these three possible activations:

✔ **Reflexes:** A reflex involves the activation of a sensory receptor, such as a pain receptor, in the limb that may fire action potentials when you touch something sharp (see Figure 5-4, later in this chapter). The axon of this receptor projects to the spinal cord through the dorsal root, and excites, in a reflex arc, an alpha motor neuron that causes the body to withdraw the limb (usually using a flexor muscle).

- ✔ **Rhythmic motor patterns:** Circuits in the spinal cord that are spread along the spine to control rhythmic motor patterns. These circuits control sequences, such as the alternating movement of the two legs for walking and the alternating movement of the arms working in anti-phase with the legs.

- ✔ **Consciously controlled muscle movement sequences:** Originating in a complex neural circuit, these sequences involve the frontal lobe, basal ganglia, thalamus, and cerebellum. The neural circuit projects to motor neurons in the primary motor areas of the frontal lobe, located just before the central sulcus. These motor neurons project down the spinal cord and synapse on the last neurons in the chain, the alpha motor neurons.

Alpha motor neurons

Alpha motor neurons are located in the spinal cord and brainstem. Their cell bodies are in the spinal cord gray area, which is part of the central nervous system. However, because their axons leave the central nervous system to project to muscles, they're considered part of the peripheral nervous system. Either the brain or the spinal cord circuits can activate alpha motor neurons.

Another motor neuron type that leaves the spinal cord is the *gamma motor neuron.* It innervates the intrafusal muscle fibers (which contain sensory neurons) of muscle *spindles* (which are sensory receptors) and is involved in sensory feedback from the muscle. (See "Knowing Where Your Limb Is Located," later in this chapter, for more about gamma motor neurons.)

The motor unit

One alpha motor neuron together with the many muscle fibers it innervates is called a *motor unit.* Several motor units are typically involved in producing the contractions of a single muscle (group of muscle fibers). A *motor pool* is the set of all the motor units within a muscle.

A given alpha motor neuron innervates only muscle fibers of the same type (fast- or slow-twitch). The alpha motor neuron action potential causes all the fibers to which it projects to contract. The force of the muscle contraction is controlled according to the number of motor units that are activated and their rate of firing.

A great deal of variation exists within one muscle and across many muscles in the number of muscle fibers that are innervated by a single alpha motor neuron. Typically, motor units that innervate muscles that control large body parts — like the legs — may contact up to 1,000 muscle fibers, whereas motor units that innervate small muscles may only contact 10 muscle fibers. To achieve fine motor control, the body varies the activity of a larger number of alpha motor neurons to have a graded activation of muscle fibers.

A condition called *post-polio syndrome* results from the polio disease killing large numbers of alpha motor neurons. Rehabilitation from polio happens, in part, by a training process causing the smaller number of remaining alpha motor neurons to innervate more muscle fibers and restore some muscle force. But, as people age, they lose some of these remaining alpha motor neurons. In post-polio syndrome, so few alpha motor neurons are left that they can't effectively innervate all the cells in the muscle, and a person can regress to a pre-rehab state.

Sliding filaments: Actin and myosin

Typically, one motor neuron axon terminal exists per muscle cell, although a single motor neuron axon can branch and innervate many muscle cells. Thousands of acetylcholine receptors exist across from each alpha motor neuron presynaptic terminal.

Calcium

The muscle cell action potential activates voltage-dependent calcium channels in the muscle cell membrane (called L-type calcium channels), causing the sarcoplasmic reticulum within the muscle cell to release calcium. This increase in calcium in the muscle cell causes actin and myosin myofilaments to slide over each other to shorten their overlap (see Figure 5-2) and the muscle cell contracts along its length. The process of muscle contraction uses adenosine triphosphate (ATP) as an energy source.

Muscle cells are long and thin, and organized lengthwise into muscle fibers. A muscle consists of many fibers. The more muscle fibers contract, the shorter the muscle gets. This, in turn, is controlled by the number of muscle cells activated (the number of active alpha motor neurons) and their rate of activation (the motor neuron firing rate). The force of the contraction is also proportional to the number of parallel muscle fibers. Therefore, the number of motor neurons activated and their rate of activation can very precisely control muscle force to produce finely graded contraction forces.

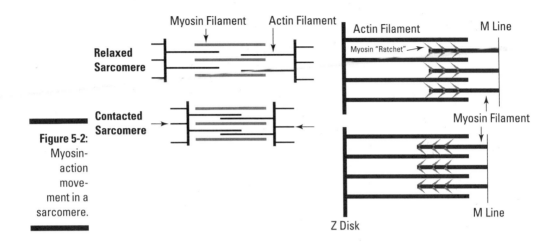

Figure 5-2:
Myosin-
action
move-
ment in a
sarcomere.

Troponin

Calcium entering the muscle cell controls its effects using a protein called troponin. When the muscle fiber is not contracted, troponin is bound to the actin molecules, preventing them from interacting with myosin. Calcium released from internal organelles within the muscle fiber during the muscle cell action potential binds to troponin. This causes troponin to partially release from actin, which then allows the actin to bind with myosin.

Muscle cells are composed of many actin and myosin filaments in series. Myosin interacts with actin like a molecular ratchet. The myosin binds, rotates, and rebinds along an actin filament so that it slides along it using ATP as an energy source. The myosin ratchet draws one actin filament to which it is attached along the myosin it is ratcheting along, shortening the *sarcomere* (sarcomeres have microscopically visible structures called Z lines). This shortens the entire muscle fiber and contracts the muscle.

Figure 5-2 shows how the muscle shortens, moving the Z lines closer together on the left. On the right is a detail of how the myosin filament ratchets move the myosin fiber along the actin.

Controlling Muscle Contraction

Muscles can exert small or large forces. This enables a person to cradle an egg with the same hand that can break a board in martial arts. Force is controlled in two main ways: One is by varying the firing rate of motor neurons, which determines how much contraction occurs in the muscle fibers they innervate. The other is by varying the number (and types) of muscle fibers activated.

Modulating firing rate

One factor that determines muscle force is the frequency with which the muscle fibers are stimulated by their innervating alpha motor neurons, called the *motor unit firing rate*. This varies from single action potentials that produce a single-twitch contraction, to firing rates of hundreds of spikes per second that can produce a the maximal contraction, called a *fused tetanic contraction*. In general, the firing of many alpha motor neurons increases gradually (in spite of recruitment — see the next section) as muscle force is increased. This provides a nearly continuous ability to increase force as the muscle load demands.

Receiving inputs

Inputs from cortical motor neurons, sensory receptors in the muscle and tendons, and interneurons in the spinal cord control the firing of alpha motor neurons. Alpha motor neurons project not only to muscles but also to extrafusal muscle fibers (see "Knowing Where Your Limb Is Located," later in this chapter). Extrafusal fibers are involved in sensory feedback to the spinal cord for well-controlled muscle activity.

Moving through action potentials

Alpha motor neuron axons have large diameters and are heavily myelinated by both oligodendrocytes and Schwann cells (refer to Chapter 3). These features increase the speed of their action potentials, shortening the time between a central command or sensory reflex input, and the action. Oligodendrocytes *myelinate* (cover) the segment of the alpha motor neuron axon that is in the spinal cord. As alpha motor neuron axons leave the spinal cord from the ventral root, they're wrapped by Schwann cells, which typically myelinate axons in the peripheral nervous system.

Figure 5-3 shows an alpha motor neuron axon branching into several terminals on the left; on the right, you see a magnified view of the end-plate synapse. The curve shows the long duration muscle end-plate potential.

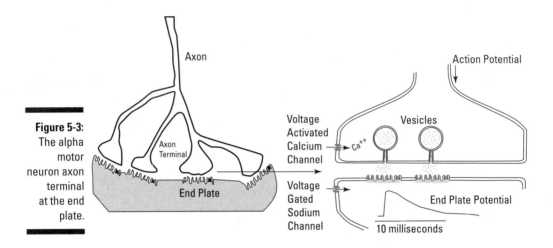

Figure 5-3:
The alpha motor neuron axon terminal at the end plate.

Recruiting motor neurons

In stimulating muscles, the central nervous system recruits motor neurons, in order, from smallest to largest, to increase the force being exerted from weak to strong. The smaller diameter axon motor neurons tend to innervate Type I slow-twitch, fatigue-resistant muscle fibers. For higher forces, larger axon diameter Type II alpha motor neurons are activated that innervate fast-twitch, stronger, but more quickly fatigued muscle fibers (refer to the "Skeletal muscle" section, earlier in this chapter).

Alpha motor neuron axons are classified by size. Different sizes have different functions:

✔ **Type Aα axons:** Large-diameter, well-myelinated fibers that conduct action potentials rapidly. These large-diameter alpha motor neurons typically innervate muscle fibers that produce the highest contraction forces.

✔ **Type Aγ axons:** Conduct less rapidly, and innervate muscle spindles to keep the spindle taught and able to sustain the contraction as the whole muscle contracts.

Knowing Where Your Limb Is Located

Knowing where you are helps you get where you're going. To move your limbs, you have to know something about where they are when you start the movement, and then be able to keep tabs on where they are as the movement progresses.

Muscle spindle and gamma motor neurons

An important type of motor neuron doesn't directly cause the muscle to contract at all. *Gamma motor neurons* project to sensory receptors within the muscle called muscle spindles. Within these structures, there are sensory neurons called *Ia sensory fibers* that signal the degree of contraction of the muscle. The gamma motor neuron input keeps the intrafusal fibers taut so they can signal when the overall muscle is contracted or relaxed. Gamma motor neurons are typically activated simultaneously with alpha motor neurons.

Golgi tendon organs

Sensory receptors within the muscle tendons are called *Golgi tendon organs*. They give feedback about muscle tension, the force of muscle contraction. Golgi tendon organs are located at the junction between the muscle and the tendon that attaches to a bone. Golgi tendon organs are innervated by *Ib sensory fibers*. These are smaller than the larger Ia fibers (refer to the previous section) that innervate the muscle spindles.

Ib fibers from the Golgi tendon organs form a feedback loop by entering the spinal cord and synapsing on alpha motor neurons. The kneejerk reflex is a classic example of this feedback. When a doctor taps the rubber hammer on your patellar tendon, that tap causes the tendon to stretch, as it would if your knee buckled while you were standing. The stretching tendon activates the quadriceps extensor muscle to compensate. Of course, in the exam room, your lower leg just swings forward.

Joint receptors for position

Sensory receptors called *mechanoreceptors* in the joints and the tissues around joints send information to the spinal cord about joint position and movement. Some information about joint position comes from receptors in the skin near joints, because this skin is stretched or relaxed as the joint moves. Free nerve endings report painful, extreme joint positions. In other words, they let you know when you just don't bend that way!

Reflexing without Reflecting

Reflexes are one of the most fundamental brain circuits. In a reflex, receptor activation produces a motor response through a very short synaptic pathway.

Withdrawing a limb

A classic example is the limb withdrawal reflex. Touching something sharp can elicit this reflex (see Figure 5-4). The neural circuit for this reflex exists at the level of the spinal cord, and normally happens without our conscious control — although we can override it centrally if we know in advance what is going to occur.

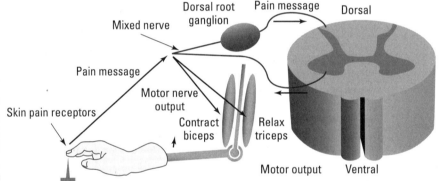

Figure 5-4: A spinal reflex neural circuit.

The purpose of the withdrawal reflex is to protect us from damaging stimuli so we don't get hurt. It typically begins by activating pain receptors that indicate tissue damage. These receptors, called *nociceptors,* project to the spinal cord and activate — through a polysynaptic reflex circuit — flexor muscles that withdraw the limb.

Staying put

Although most of the time we think of reflexes as producing movement in response to some stimulus, some reflexes exist to keep us in the same place. If you were unloading a truck, for example, and someone tossed you a box and you caught it, your new weight and the load on your legs would suddenly change. The alpha motor neuron firing rate that a second ago was just right to hold you upright is now inadequate. Feedback mechanisms through the spinal cord allow the brain to command the *position* of your limb. The spinal circuit works out the muscle contraction *force* necessary to keep you in the standing position.

Seeing the spinal flexor reflex

Figure 5-4 shows the components of a spinal flexor reflex. Touching a sharp point activates pain receptors that project to the spinal cord through the dorsal root. Pain receptors may make a monosynaptic contact with alpha motor neurons that activate the flexor muscle (biceps) to move the hand away from the sharp point. Or pain receptors may also participate in poly-synaptic reflexive reduction in the tension of the triceps, the extensor. (Refer to "Monosynaptic and polysynaptic reflexes," earlier in this chapter, for more on these terms.) Projections to other spinal cord segments allow us to balance and compensate for the rapid hand movement. This fast reflex happens at the spinal level before the pain signal even reaches your brain!

Keeping the spinal cord in the loop

Sensory receptors in the muscles, joints, and tendons work in feedback loops that allow your brain to tell your limbs to move. Fast neural circuits in your spinal cord take care of the details, adjusting for different loads and conditions.

What your brain does for limb position is like setting a thermostat to keep your home at a certain temperature. The thermostat has a sensor that turns the furnace on if the temperature goes below a set point, or off if the temperature goes above that point. This works regardless of the outside temperature (load), or changes in the furnace's capacity (such as the air filter being dirty and clogged).

Monosynaptic and polysynaptic reflexes

Spinal cord feedback loops adjust muscle force in either monosynaptic or polysynaptic reflex loops:

- **Monosynaptic reflexes:** Earlier in this chapter, I discuss the kneejerk reflex — more properly called the *patellar tendon reflex.* This involves tapping the tendon attached to the quadriceps muscle of the leg, which stretches it. This produces a monosynaptic reflex, where Ia sensory fibers in the muscle spindles (the sensory receptors) directly contact alpha motor neurons that innervate the quadriceps, causing it to contract, and your knee jerks.

Monosynaptic reflexes are often embedded in more complex, polysynaptic reflexes.

✔ **Polysynaptic reflexes:** One of the most common polysynaptic reflexes is the reciprocal inhibition of one set of muscles that happens when the other member of its antagonistic pair is activated. (Refer to the earlier section "Pulling Your Weight: How Muscle Cells Contract.") In the patellar tendon reflex, for example, as the quadriceps extensor is activated, the hamstring flexor is inhibited. This happens because the Ia sensory fibers that directly activated the alpha motor neuron for the quadriceps also activate an inhibitory interneuron in the spinal cord. The inhibitory interneuron reduces the firing of the alpha motor neurons that drive the hamstring flexor muscles.

If you touch something hot, a monsynaptic connection occurs from the nociceptive sensory fiber to the extensor alpha motor neurons. At the same time, the sensory neurons contact inhibitory interneurons that reduce the drive to flexor muscles, allowing you to withdraw your hand very quickly.

Also, we do not actually totally relax one muscle of an antagonistic pair when activating the other. Fine, steady control may require partial activation of both muscles simultaneously. The fine motor control happens by descending control from the brain acting on spinal interneurons. Other interneurons may project to other spinal cord segments, adjusting muscle contractions in your legs to balance you when you move your arms.

Overriding a reflex

Although local spinal cord neural circuits carry out the details of cortical brain commands, sometimes cortical, high-level commands override the local reflex circuits. You can hold on to a hot cup of coffee despite your reflex to let go.

Alpha motor neurons and spinal interneurons receive inputs from a variety of cortical and subcortical areas. These include the primary motor cortex, and projections through the corticonuclear, corticospinal, and rubrospinal tracts. Commands from the primary motor cortex are modulated by activity in the cerebellum, which receives sensory information from some of the same sensory receptors as spinal reflexes.

Exercise and Aging

Exercise builds muscle mass and strength. Muscles get bigger and stronger in response to damage to the muscle fibers from the exercise. The muscle growth involves the production of more actin and myosin filament proteins.

Lack of activity causes the opposite to happen: loss of muscle mass due to the breakdown of muscle proteins. One example of how we lose muscle mass is when astronauts spend months in the low gravity of space. Without the force of gravity to make muscles work, astronauts have been known to lose nearly one-quarter of their muscle mass in a few months.

Use it or lose it: The effects of exercise

Exercise increases the mass of fast-twitch muscle. Endurance training, such as long-distance running, can allow people to gain more of the slower Type IIa fibers versus the faster Type IIb fibers. (Refer to "Skeletal muscle" earlier in this chapter.)

After a person is paralyzed, the ration of fast-twitch Type II muscle fibers to slow-twitch Type I fibers does seem to increase. Slow-twitch Type I fibers may be lost because of the lack of neural innervation that is necessary to maintain muscle.

Slowing down with age

Without some change in lifestyle, such as taking up weightlifting, most people start losing muscle mass around age 25. By the age of 75, people are down to about half the muscle mass they had before age 25.

Changes also occur in the alpha motor neurons that control muscles. These neurons fire fewer action potentials per second in older versus younger people. Declines in both the muscle and neural innervations result in weaker muscles that act more slowly.

Muscle mass in men and women

Developing muscle mass is easier for males because of male hormones (androgens). Even in preschoolers, boys have significantly more muscle mass than girls of the same age.

The lower forces that women's muscles generate may lead to increased joint instability in athletics, making injuries more likely. For example, damage to the anterior cruciate ligament, in the knee, is common in female athletes such those who play soccer. Some differences in skeletal composition also put females at a disadvantage compared to males in athletics. Women's wider pelvises put more stress on their knees. Although androgen hormones help males add muscle mass, female hormones such as estrogen have little effect on it. Women do have advantages in some types of muscle endurance, however.

Chapter 6

The Spinal Cord and the Autonomic Nervous System

*A*lthough the brain usually gets the credit for being the smart one, the spinal cord is pretty intelligent, too. The brain is like the architect, while the spine is the contractor. The brain, using its vision and memory, decides where you want to go, like an architect decides the design of the building. But the spinal cord, the contractor, is certainly no slouch — it executes the plans, taking into account a ton of variables. For example, the brain decides that you're going to take a walk. But when you walk, the spine helps to keep you on track if you step in holes, trip over branches, carry loads, and move your arms in complex ways that require a constant, complex balancing act to remain on path.

This chapter explores how the spinal cord is a complex computer that can function quite well with little brain input. I look at how the different spinal segments communicate with each other and with sensory receptors in the muscles, tendons, and joints to move the limbs, and how the spine processes sensory information from outside the body. I also look at the central pattern generator that controls locomotion, as well as how the spinal cord is the seat of the autonomic nervous system — is the "brain" that controls body functions such as heart rate, intestinal movement, and bladder function.

Segmenting the Spine

The spine starts at the bottom of the brain at a brainstem structure called the *medulla*. It begins with a segment called *cervical 1* (C1). The spine runs from cervical to thoracic to lumbar to sacral. Although the spine is outside the brain, it and the brain (including the retina) comprise the central nervous system.

The spinal cord is embedded in and protected by *vertebrae* — a series of small bones that form the spine. Figure 6-1 shows how this is arranged. What we casually call the "backbone" is a set of spinal vertebrae that run from the neck to the "tail bone," which is actually a remnant of our pre-ape lineage. The spinal cord runs between the main vertebra bodies and the bones of the back that you can feel through your skin. Between the vertebra bodies are *spinal disks*, which are rubbery pads that cushion and separate the vertebra bodies. A herniated disk is a common back injury.

At every spinal cord segment, pairs of spinal nerves project to the left and right side of the body, at about the level of each disk. The bulges in these nerves (see Figure 6-1) are the *dorsal root ganglia*. The dorsal root ganglia contain the cell bodies of sensory receptors whose axons project to the periphery and into the interior of the spinal cord.

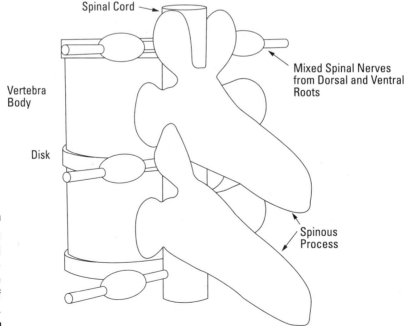

Spinal Cord

Mixed Spinal Nerves from Dorsal and Ventral Roots

Vertebra Body

Disk

Spinous Process

Figure 6-1: The spinal cord in relation to the vertebrae of the back.

Output motor neurons from the *ventral root* (the nerve exits on each side of the ventral surface) of the spinal cord join the sensory axons at the dorsal root ganglia. This forms a mixed nerve distal to the dorsal root ganglia. The interior of the spinal cord is part of the central nervous system, but the axons projecting outside the spinal cord are part of the peripheral nervous system. (I discuss the central and peripheral nervous systems later in this chapter.) All the spinal nerves distal to the dorsal root ganglia consist of both sensory and motor fibers, so they're called "mixed" nerves.

Sensory nerves have their cell bodies in the dorsal root ganglia. They participate both in local reflexes and in sending sensory information to the brain. The motor output of the spinal cord is from the cell body through the ventral root. The cell bodies that form ventral root axons, called *alpha motor neurons* (refer to Chapter 5), are located in the spinal gray area.

The human spinal cord has 31 spinal cord nerve segments (different from the number of vertebrae). These include 8 cervical segments, 12 thoracic, 5 lumbar, 5 sacral, and 1 coccygeal segments (several coccygeal segments are joined into a single segment to form one pair of coccygeal nerves). Figure 6-2 shows you where these segments are located along the spine, as well as their functions. Nerves exiting the spinal cord form a *plexus,* which is a network of nerves. The spine is associated with five plexi: cervical, brachial, lumbar, sacral, and coccygeal. (The thoracic nerves are not associated with a plexus.) Earlier, in Figure 6-1, you can see how the spinal nerves exit directly from the spinal cord in the upper segments of the vertebral column. In the lower vertebrae, the nerves tend to travel a segment or two down the column before exiting.

Cervical nerves

The top of the spinal cord starts where the medulla ends. The first seven vertebra segments are called *cervical.* From these seven segments, eight pairs of cervical nerves (C1 to C8) exit on the left and right sides of the spinal cord to innervate the periphery with sensory and motor neurons.

The nerves leaving the various segments of the spine are, in many cases, similar to nerves leaving the core areas of the brain (such as the brainstem), where they're called *cranial nerves.*

Note that the spine has eight cervical spinal nerves, but only seven cervical spinal segments. Nerves C1 to C7 exit the spinal cord from just above their corresponding vertebra. However, starting at the C7–T1 (for thoracic 1) junction, the spinal nerve roots exit below their corresponding vertebra. The spinal nerve emanating from between C7 and T1 is called C8.

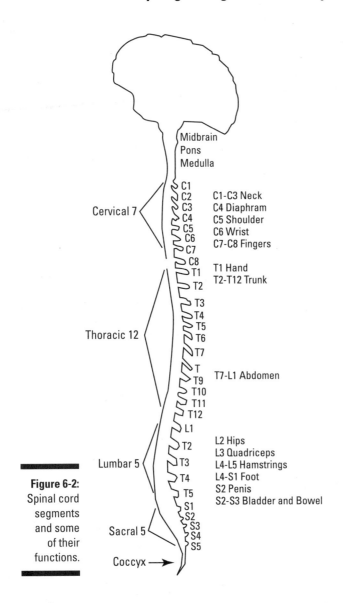

Midbrain
Pons
Medulla

Cervical 7

C1
C2
C3
C4
C5
C6
C7
C8
T1
T2

C1-C3 Neck
C4 Diaphram
C5 Shoulder
C6 Wrist
C7-C8 Fingers

T1 Hand
T2-T12 Trunk

Thoracic 12

T3
T4
T5
T6
T7
T
T9
T10
T11
T12

T7-L1 Abdomen

L1
T2
T3
T4
T5
S1
S2
S3
S4
S5

L2 Hips
L3 Quadriceps
L4-L5 Hamstrings
L4-S1 Foot
S2 Penis
S2-S3 Bladder and Bowel

Lumbar 5

Sacral 5

Coccyx →

Figure 6-2:
Spinal cord
segments
and some
of their
functions.

Cervical nerves collect sensory information from and project motor commands to several specific parts of the body:

✔ Nerves C1 and C2 control the head via neck muscles.

✔ Nerves C3 and C4 control the diaphragm for respiration.

✔ Nerve C5 innervates upper-body muscles, such as the biceps and deltoids.

✔ Nerve C6 goes to the wrist and provides a partial innervation of the biceps.

✔ Nerve C7 projects to the triceps.

✔ Nerve C8 controls and receives inputs from the hands.

Injury to the cervical spine often results in severe disability or death from respiratory failure. Disabilities include quadriplegia, paralysis, and loss of feeling in both the arms and the legs.

Thoracic nerves

The thoracic nerves (T1 to T12) are the 12 spinal nerves that exit from the 12 thoracic vertebrae. They're organized as follows:

✔ T1 projects into the brachial plexus, which includes nerves that innervate the arms and upper back.

✔ T2 to T6 project to the *intercostal* (between the ribs) chest muscles and receive sensory information from the skin of the chest and upper back.

✔ T7 to T11 innervate the skin and intercostal muscles of the abdomen and lower back.

✔ T12 projects with another nerve called the *iliohypogastric nerve* (a branch of L1, the first lumbar nerve) to innervate the gluteus muscles and skin of the buttocks.

Lumbar nerves

The five lumbar vertebrae comprise the lower back. From these five vertebrae emerge five pairs of lumbar spinal nerves. All the lumbar nerves emerge from just below the corresponding vertebra. These nerves innervate the lower abdomen, back, and buttocks. L1 through L4 innervate the thigh muscles, such as the quadratus lumborum and iliopsoas for flexion. L2 through L5 mediate thigh adduction.

Sacral nerves

The sacral spinal nerves (S1 to S5) start below L5 and emerge from the spinal cord through openings called *foramen* in the fused sacral vertebrae. After emerging from the spinal cord the nerves join either the sacral or lumbosacral plexus (refer to "Segmenting the Spine," earlier in this chapter, for more on plexi). Sacral nerve functions include innervation of the skin and muscles of the thighs, buttocks, legs, and feet. S2, S3, and S4 also send parasympathetic fibers (see the section "Fighting or Fleeing: The Autonomic Nervous System," later in this chapter) that innervate the colon, rectum, bladder, and genital organs.

The functions of the sacral nerves (S1 to S5) include the following:

- S1 is involved in flexion of the leg and foot and extension of the toes.
- S2 is involved in flexion of the foot and toes, as well as control of the urethral sphincter.
- S3 is important in control of the bladder.
- S4 controls reproductive organs, such as the testes and uterus.
- S5 supplies the coccygeus muscle, which controls muscle tension in the pelvis.

Below the spinal cord are three to five additional fused vertebra called *coccygeal segments,* which are not associated with spinal nerves.

Spinal membranes

The *spinal cord* (the neural part of the spine) is covered and protected by the same three membranes that protect the other part of the central nervous system, the brain. These membranes, sometimes called *meninges,* are the dura, arachnoid, and pia mater. The outermost membrane is the dura, which is fibrous and protects the spinal cord. Next is the arachnoid, consisting of filaments that resemble a web, that are connected to the underlying pia. The space underneath the arachnoid (subarachnoid space) is filled with cerebrospinal fluid. Underneath the arachnoid is the pia, which is highly vascular.

Spying on the Spinal Cord

The central nervous system consists of the brain and spinal cord. The brain is a concentrated cluster of billions of neurons. Among mammals, the size of the brain varies greatly. But the spine, extending from the bottom of the brain at the medulla to the base of the tail (or vestigial tail), varies much less among mammals.

The spinal cord is an extended brain whose different segments (with some overlap) control the four limbs (and other body parts) to act in unison. However, the spinal cord lacks vision, hearing, smell, taste, and balance senses. These senses are concentrated in the head, which, in four-legged and swimming animals, is first to encounter stimuli during movement. The brain has an elaborate structure for processing sensory information and coordinating it with bodily movement.

The spinal cord consists of three types of neural circuitry:

✔ Sensory-motor "arcs" that function mostly within one segment of the spine

✔ Sensory and motor projections that coordinate multiple segments of the spine

✔ Sensory projections to the brain, and motor commands from the brain, in specific spinal tracts

The following portions of this chapter discuss sensory-motor integration in local circuits in the spine and brain.

Dorsal inputs, ventral outputs

Looking into the spinal cord reveals that it consists of a central gray matter area that contains neural cell bodies, surrounded by white matter composed almost exclusively of axon tracts. The gray matter in the center of the cord is shaped like a butterfly and consists of cell bodies of interneurons and motor neurons (as well as their dendrites and axons). The tips of the wing-like gray areas in the spinal cord are called *horns*. Figure 6-3 shows a schematic section of the spinal cord, so you can see the central gray-matter and peripheral white-matter areas. The white-matter axon tracts carry information up and down the spinal cord to other segments and the brain.

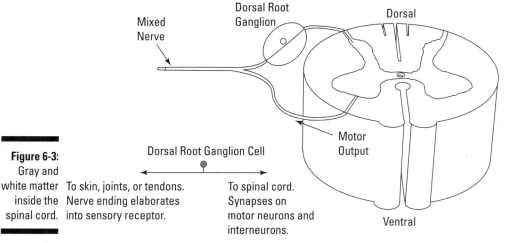

Figure 6-3:
Gray and white matter inside the spinal cord.

Mixed Nerve

Dorsal Root Ganglion

Dorsal

Dorsal Root Ganglion Cell

To skin, joints, or tendons. Nerve ending elaborates into sensory receptor.

To spinal cord. Synapses on motor neurons and interneurons.

Motor Output

Ventral

In the center of the gray area is a canal that contains *cerebrospinal* (brain and spine) fluid. The fluid is continuous with the brain. It merges with the ventricles of the brain by extending through the brainstem and opening up into the fourth ventricle in the medulla. Cerebrospinal fluid has several complex functions in the central nervous system. These include regulating chemical concentrations (such as by buffering), providing mechanical protection (such as by functioning as a shock absorber). Because of the continuity between the spinal and brain cerebrospinal fluid, anesthetics can be injected below the cauda equina between L3 and L5 into the spinal cord and will, through circulation of the fluid, reach the brain.

The way the spinal cord is organized, motor axon output from the spinal cord always exits from the ventral side (the side toward the front of our bodies), whereas sensory input always comes into the spinal cord through the dorsal (back) side. The motor output is carried by alpha motor neurons (refer to Chapter 5) whose cell bodies are in the ventral gray area and whose axons project to motor end-plate regions on muscles.

The sensory neurons have a structure that is rather unusual compared to that of the classic neurons. Typically, neurons have dendrites that receive inputs and an axon that sends outputs to other neurons. The sensory neurons of the spinal cord have their cell bodies in a neuron cluster (called a *ganglion*) of neurons just outside the cord — the dorsal root ganglion. Neurons of the dorsal root ganglion have no dendrites.

Coming in the back

As Figure 6-3 shows, a single axon emanates from the sensory neural cell body in a dorsal root ganglion and then *bifurcates* (splits itself into two, like a fork in a road) within the ganglion. One end of the axon goes to the periphery — such as the skin, a joint, a tendon, or an organ — and *becomes the sensory receptor*. Sensory input (such as mechanical stimulation) produces action potentials in the axon terminal. These action potentials travel what would normally be considered a retrograde path back toward the bifurcation point. The action potentials continue past this bifurcation, now in an orthograde (normal) direction away from the soma to their terminals in the spinal cord gray area. Here, the action potentials make conventional synapses, releasing the neurotransmitter glutamate. Dorsal root ganglion sensory neurons participate in monosynaptic and polysynaptic reflexes (refer to Chapter 5). They also send sensory information to the brain about the body through the white-matter tracts of the spinal cord.

Going out the front

Motor neuron axons leave the ventral spinal cord and join the same nerve as the sensory input that is distal to the dorsal root ganglion. The distal side of the dorsal root ganglion is a mixed nerve that contains both sensory and motor nerve axons. Within this mixed nerve, the sensory nerves that go toward the spinal cord are called *afferents* (the name for nerves going toward the central nervous system). The motor nerves that are carrying signals toward the muscles away from the spinal cord are called *efferents*.

Dorsal and ventral axons leave the spinal cord in each segment through several "rootlets" that join up in the dorsal root ganglion.

Reflecting on what hit you: The basic spinal reflex

In Chapter 5, I explain that a reflex is the basic unit of sensory motor integration — a stimulus (such as to a pain receptor on the finger) leads to a direct movement (such as withdrawing the finger). Other simple reflexes, however, are not so automatic; instead, they're mediated by the brain. For example the breath-holding reflex occurs when your face goes under water.

One thing spinal reflexes have in common with other reflexes is that they occur before your brain knows what's going on. That's because the time for the neural signals to go from the sensory receptor to the spinal cord and back to activate the muscles is faster than the time signals take to go up the spinal cord to your brain.

Defining reflexive action

A withdrawal reflex can begin with your finger touching something hot, like the handle of a pot on the stove. The pain receptors for heat send their retrograde action potentials along their axons up the arm to the shoulder and then to the dorsal root ganglion of the second thoracic segment (T2) that receives pain information from the finger.

These pain-produced action potentials continue past the axonal bifurcation in the dorsal root ganglion into the spinal gray area. (Refer to the "Dorsal inputs, ventral outputs" section, earlier in this chapter.) There the axon terminals release the neurotransmitter glutamate onto alpha motor neurons (monosynaptic reflex) and onto spinal cord interneurons (polysynaptic reflex).

Spinal interneurons are so called because their inputs and outputs are entirely within one spinal cord segment.

Opposing forces: Flexor-extensor muscle pairs

Antagonistic flexor-extensor muscle pairs control almost all joints in the body (although, for most joints, other muscles also produce or control rotation). The spinal interneurons modulate the firing of alpha motor neurons that project to both the biceps and the triceps — a flexor-extensor pair. For flexion, spinal interneurons increase the activation of the biceps *flexor* muscle (monosynaptic) and decrease the activation of the triceps *extensor* muscle (polysynaptic) so the biceps relax.

Mechanics: Monosynaptic reflex pathway

The monosynaptic pathway (refer to Chapter 5) consists of what's called a *reflex arc* from a sensory neuron to an alpha motor neuron. The two neurons meet at a synapse in the spinal cord ventral gray zone. A typical reflex involves a *nociceptive* (pain) sensory neuron projecting to an alpha motor neuron that activates a flexor muscle. Flexors move limbs toward the body, away from the point of sensory activation.

Modulating reflexes

Most reflexes involve more than activating a single flexor muscle. Almost always the antagonistic extensor muscle must be simultaneously deactivated to allow the flexor muscle to move the limb. (Think of the biceps-triceps I discuss earlier in this chapter.) In a strong reflex generated at the fingertip, finger flexors, arm flexors, and shoulder flexors may all be activated for fast, strong withdrawal.

Moving a limb also requires that other body parts move for counterbalance. This is all coordinated by projections of interneurons that send the pain signal to other spinal segments. Sending the pain signal to other spinal segments helps to coordinate the withdrawal of the limb, which involves not only your arm, but also other joint movements for balance, such as decreasing the extension force of the leg on the same side as the arm that is brought toward the body.

Overriding the reflex

The complete reflex circuit exists at the spinal level and is independent of the brain. It occurs before the sensory signal even reaches the brain. However, you can override spinal reflexes if you know in advance that they're about to occur.

For example, say you pick up a hot pan from the stove. Your reflex may be to drop it immediately. But your brain, not wanting to clean up the huge mess that you would make if you did simply let go of the pan, may override this reflex. Overriding the reflex allows you to keep holding on long enough to set the pan down safely.

At a more fundamental level, overriding reflexes is essential to locomotion. You can think of walking as a process of falling forward and catching yourself again and again. In the falling forward phase, you override your balance reflexes until the point where you swing a leg forward. If you do this in a pattern, alternating the legs, you're walking.

Spinal pattern generators

Early in the 20th century, it was shown that animals could walk and run on treadmills even if the spinal cord connections to their brains were severed. This means that the basic rhythmic patterns for locomotion can be produced by the spinal cord without the need for any descending commands from the cortex. The spinal cord neuronal circuits that produce these rhythmic patterns of neural activity are called *central pattern generators* (CPGs).

CPGs normally produce rhythmic patterned outputs in response to sensory feedback; however, sensory feedback isn't required for CPGs to produce these outputs. Sensory feedback helps coordinate efficient locomotion in the limbs, for instance. The brain normally initiates and controls the activity of spinal CPGs through descending axonal projections that make up high-level commands, such as changing your gait. For example, you start walking faster because you suddenly realize you're late for an appointment.

Locomoting with alternate limb movement

Walking and other forms of locomotion involve moving all four limbs. CPGs are distributed throughout the lower thoracic and lumbar spinal cord. These circuits generate motor neuron firing patterns that synchronize rhythmic contractions of flexor-extensor muscles of the arms and legs. As the legs move in antiphase with each other, the arms move in the opposite antiphase — so your left arm goes forward at the same time as your right leg.

Balance is mediated by having lumbar pattern generators affect pattern generators in cervical segments. It's also subject to top-down control from inputs from the visual and *vestibular* (your sense of balance) systems. Your visual system generates commands to keep you from running into trees. Your vestibular system prevents you from falling if you step in a hole, and makes sure your body is in the right posture for the conditions around you, such as if you're running on a slope.

CPGs require neural circuits that interact in such a way that half of the circuit increases in activity while the other half decreases. Scientists believe this alternating phase activity is based on what are called *half-center scillators*. These are circuits of neurons that are mutually inhibitory. Consider two neurons, each of which by itself has no rhythmic activity, but the coupling between the two causes each to oppose (inhibit) the firing of the other. After one neuron has reached its maximum firing rate for some time, a feedback process causes it to reduce firing on its own. This decreases the inhibition of the other neuron, which increases its firing and further inhibits the first neuron.

Changing pace, walking, and running

Our immediate needs for balance and central commands to change gaits — such as from walking to running — modulate CPGs. Virtually all gaits involve alternating lower limbs, and simultaneously alternating upper limbs in antiphase. A gait is normally established by a command from the brain to begin the gait by setting parameters for the CPGs, followed by a hierarchical set of reflex circuits. These circuits move the limbs and make many adjustments according to the ground surface and muscle fatigue during the movement.

Feeling and Acting: The Peripheral Nervous System

The nerves and ganglia outside the spinal cord (and brain) constitute the *peripheral nervous system* (PNS). The PNS connects the central nervous system (brain and spinal cord) to the limbs and organs. The peripheral nervous system is divided into the somatic nervous system and the autonomic nervous system. (I discuss the autonomic part of the PNS later in this chapter.) Sensory neurons of the dorsal root ganglia and axons of the motor neurons leaving the ventral root are part of the somatic PNS.

Most of the cranial nerves (see Chapters 7 and 8) are also part of the PNS.

Besides its function in feedback control of limb position and movement (called *proprioception* and *kinesthesis*), the peripheral nervous system mediates the senses of touch, including temperature and various kinds of pain.

Getting stimulated by neural sensors

The skin consists of an outer layer of dead cells, called the *epidermis,* and an inner layer of living cells called the *dermis* (see Chapter 11 for more detail on this). Cells in the dermis are continuously dividing, migrating to the epidermis, and dying, allowing you to scrape the surface of your skin in normal activity without damaging the living cell layer.

Within the dermis are skin receptors. These include touch receptors *(mechanoreceptors),* hot and cold temperature receptors *(thermoreceptors),* and pain receptors *(nociceptors).* Like the neural sensors for limb position and muscle tension, these sensory neurons have their cell bodies in the dorsal root ganglia. Much of their output, however, goes to the thalamus *(ventral posterior nucleus)* through two major spinal cord white matter tracts (see Figure 6-4):

   ✔ **Medial lemniscal pathway:** This tract has large fibers that carry not only the various kinds of touch sense (pressure, flutter, vibration) but also information relayed from joint position *(proprioception).*

   ✔ **Spinothalamic:** The smaller fibers of the spinothalamic pathway carry mostly pain and temperature information.

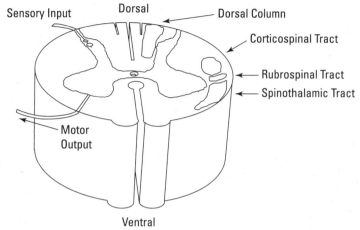

Sensory Input
Dorsal
Dorsal Column
Corticospinal Tract
Rubrospinal Tract
Spinothalamic Tract
Motor Output
Ventral

Figure 6-4:
Spinal cord
tracts.

Moving around: Neural effectors

The cell bodies of alpha motor neurons (among other cells) are located in the ventral horns of the spinal cord gray matter (refer to "Dorsal inputs, ventral outputs" earlier in this chapter). Alpha motor neurons drive the muscles and receive three kinds of inputs:

- ✔ **Direct commands from the primary motor cortex in the frontal lobe:** Primary cortex motor neurons project to alpha motor neurons mainly via the corticonuclear, corticospinal, and rubrospinal tracts.

- ✔ **Monosynaptic activation by sensory receptors:** This activation occurs in reflex arcs involving peripheral sensory neurons (in the dorsal root ganglia) such as muscle spindles, Golgi tendon organs, mechanoreceptors, and thermoreceptors. Pain-withdrawal and kneejerk reflexes both involve monosynaptic connections from the sensory to the motor units.

- ✔ **Polysynaptic activation in multi-muscle coordination:** Alpha motor neurons receive most of their input from local interneurons. These interneuron circuits are involved in locomotion and complex, multi-muscle coordination and reflexes.

The following section discusses the basic elements of muscle activation from the spinal cord. For more detail, refer to Chapter 5.

Zeroing in on motor neurons-effectors

Alpha motor neurons typically innervate muscles on the same side of the body on which they exit the spinal cord. One alpha motor neuron and all the muscle fibers it projects to are called a *motor unit*. The set of all the alpha motor neurons that project to a single muscle is called the *motor neuron pool*.

Fine muscle control is generally achieved by having a large number of alpha motor neurons, each having fewer muscle outputs, compared to having a small number of alpha motor neurons innervate hundreds of muscle fibers.

Alpha motor neurons are located in what's called *lamina IX* in the middle of the ventral horn of the spinal cord's gray matter. Alpha motor neurons that innervate more distal muscles are located more laterally in the gray matter than those that innervate proximal muscles. Also, alpha motor neurons that innervate extensors tend to be located more ventrally than those that innervate flexors.

Some alpha motor neuron axon collaterals synapse on a specific type of spinal cord interneuron called a *Renshaw cell*. Renshaw cells are inhibitory interneurons. They feed back onto the alpha motor neuron to suppress excess activity that may cause muscle damage. Gamma motor neurons also exit the ventral root and innervate muscle spindle intrafusal muscle fibers, which are involved in sensory feedback from muscles (refer to Chapter 5).

Doing the heavy lifting: Muscle cells

Calcium entering into the muscle cell mediates its effects by acting on a protein called *troponin*. When the muscle fiber is not contracted, troponin binds to actin molecules, preventing them from interacting with myosin. Increased calcium concentrations during the muscle cell action potential cause calcium to bind to troponin, releasing actin to bind to myosin.

Myosin interacts with actin like a molecular ratchet in a cycle: It binds, rotates, and rebinds along the adjacent actin filament so that it slides along the filament. This process used ATP as an energy source. The result is that the muscle fiber shortens.

Correcting Errors: The Cerebellum

The *cerebellum* (Latin for "little brain") is a part of the brain that plays an important role in motor coordination, precision, and timing. It's capable of learning motor sequences and generating error signals when body movement doesn't match the brain's commands. The cerebellum receives inputs from sensory neurons of the spinal cord and integrates these inputs with other parts of the brain to fine-tune motor activity.

The cerebellum juts out from the back of the brainstem. It sits just below the posterior part of the cortex (see Figure 6-5). The cerebellum is an ancient, highly complex brain structure. Like the newer neocortex, the cerebellum is a thin, large neural layer that is folded up to fit in a small space. The cerebellum also is necessary for several types of motor learning (see the upcoming section "Stepping in holes, and what to do about it"). Most notably, it adjusts relationships between sense and motor functions for coordination.

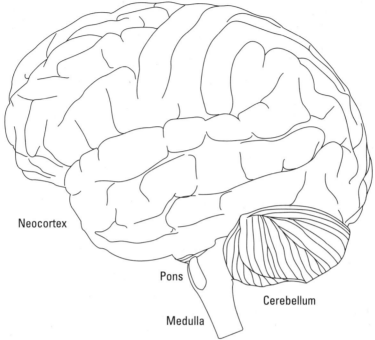

Figure 6-5:
The
cerebellum.

The cerebellum is evolutionarily old. It has a similar form in both mammals and non-mammalian vertebrates such as fish and amphibians. It's also complex and may contain as many neurons as the rest of the central nervous system (80 to 100 billion neurons). Cerebellar lesions result in decreased muscle tone, clumsy and abnormal movements, and loss of balance.

Cerebellar structure

The cerebellum's appearance doesn't tell us much about its internal structure or organization. The cerebellum receives information from the entire body (*somatosensory* information) via the spinal cord, plus vestibular and visual information from the brain. These inputs synapse in the outer superficial layers of the cerebellum, called the *cerebellar cortex*. After processing in the cerebellar cortex, neurons there project to deep cerebellar nuclei that are the output of the cerebellum. The control output of the cerebellum is *ipsilateral* (on the same side of the body) because they cross the midline twice.

The cerebellum has three main divisions, which you can see in Figure 6-6:

- **The neocerebellum:** The neocerebellum is the most lateral part of the cerebellum. Its inputs are proprioceptive signals from the cerebral cortex, and it projects to the red nucleus and the ventro-lateral thalamus, which in turn projects to premotor areas of the brain such as the supplementary motor cortex and premotor cortex. These are the brain areas that provide general commands for movement. The cerebellum uses its previous knowledge of similar movement sequences to refine these plans. For example, if you're about to throw a bowling ball, your cerebellum has stored success/failure information about the entire sequence of movements you need to perform, from the first steps you take in preparation to the time you release the ball.

- **Spinocerebellum:** The spinocerebellum is in the center of the structure, comprising the vermis and paravermis. It receives proprioceptive and auditory inputs, and projects to deep cerebellar nuclei called the the fastigeal and interposed nuclei, which in turn project to the brainstem and primary motor cortex to control alpha motor neurons. This is a lower level of control than that mediated by the neocerebellum and is more concerned with finer details of movement.

- **Vestibulocerebellum:** The vestibulocerebellum receives inputs from the vestibular nuclei, semicircular canals, superior colliculus, and visual cortex. It projects into the oculomotor system to adjust eye movements and into vestibular recipient zones for correction of balance mechanisms.

Stepping in holes and what to do about it

The cerebellum compares what the brain commands the body to do with what the body does. It receives commands from the motor and premotor cortex about where the body is supposed to be, and uses sensory feedback to recognize where the body actually is. It uses an internal "model" of movement sequences to compare commands with execution. Using this model, the cerebellum recognizes any errors and sends programming information back to the cortex through the thalamus to change the command sequence in response to the errors.

The spinocerebellum and neocerebellum generate different kinds of responses to errors. At the lower level, the spinocerebellum may adjust your body posture and immediate stride when you're running on uneven ground with bumps and holes. At a higher level, the neocerebellum may cause you to change your gait and slow down if you're heading for a tree.

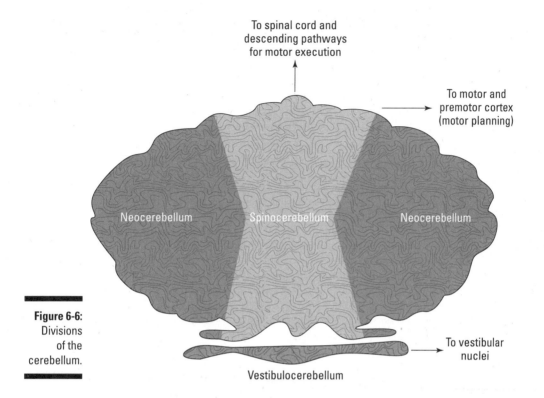

To spinal cord and
descending pathways
for motor execution

To motor and
premotor cortex
(motor planning)

Neocerebellum   Spinocerebellum   Neocerebellum

To vestibular
nuclei

Vestibulocerebellum

Figure 6-6:
Divisions
of the
cerebellum.

One reason that you get better at doing things — like hitting a tennis ball — with practice is that your cerebellum learns which motor sequences work and which don't. This type of learning is called *motor learning.* You aren't conscious of motor learning, but it's essential for doing all skilled action. The cerebellum has a set of powerful learning circuits that carry out this adaptive behavior. Damage to the cerebellum doesn't cause paralysis because your basic motor command and execution structure is intact. However, it does result in disorders in fine movement, posture equilibrium, and, of course, future motor learning.

Carrying the load: Feed-forward force calibration

In short-distance circuits, like those involved in spinal reflexes, feedback control is fast enough to do what it's supposed to do. In feedback control, a neural comparator constantly evaluates the difference between the command position and the actual position, and sends error-correcting commands to the appropriate muscles to reduce the error to zero. But in long, complex circuits, like from the brain to the extremities, feedback circuits may be too slow to work efficiently.

For these command circuits to work properly, timing is very important. For example, adjusting the extensor force in a leg won't do any good if the gait has already shifted the weight to the other leg. Or consider a simple act like throwing a baseball: It involves a *learned* preparation phase of positioning the legs, rotating the shoulders, and holding the ball out and away from the body. Then the throw itself consists of a sequence of rapidly executed plans for moving the leg, rotating the shoulder, moving both the upper and lower arm in synchrony, and releasing the grip on the ball at the right moment. Timing is everything if you're going to throw a strike. And timing has to be programmed *in advance.*

The cerebellum acts as a feed-forward control system, in contrast (and complementary) to the spinal cord feedback system. In the *cerebellar feed-forward system,* the cerebellum receives sensory information during movement with which it produces a model that can generate an optimal sequence of output commands *in the future.* Feed-forward systems learn (by practice) the correct sequence of commands to program a task — like throwing a ball — without having to rely on long feedback loops to correct for errors.

Imagine a thermostat. Suppose it's controlling the temperature in a nuclear power plant, which takes a long time to heat up or cool down. When the thermostat trips at the desired temperature, the plant will still keep running for some time and overheat. But in a feed-forward system, the controller (cerebellum) would learn how long it takes to shut down the plant, and program the thermostat to turn off at the exact right time before the temperature could reach its set point.

Cerebellar circuits

During movement, motor command and sensory status information come into the outer layers of the cerebellum. In the outer layers, a highly regular set of neural circuits — that include several prominent cell types, such as Purkinje and granule cells — process the information. The folded cerebellar cortex provides considerable area for all these circuits. After processing, these circuits project to a set of deep cerebellar nuclei, which are the cerebellar output.

In the cerebellar cortex, each cerebellar Purkinje cell receives inputs from thousands of what are called *parallel fibers,* which are the axons of granule cells, but only from one climbing fiber, which is one of the external inputs. The other external input is via what are called *mossy fibers.* Both Purkinje cells and mossy fibers project to the deep cerebellar nuclei, the output of the cerebellum.

The parallel fibers can be regarded as a matrix of different timings of one muscle's action during a sequence. The single climbing fiber is the "teaching signal" that induces a long-lasting change in the strength of the appropriate parallel fiber inputs. In other words, if you throw the ball too low, the next time the cerebellum will program for you to release the ball slightly earlier (or program some other adjustment to raise the ball's trajectory).

Recent imaging studies show that motor learning in the cerebellum underlies some cognitive activities that were thought to be quite abstract, such as playing chess. When experienced chess players are contemplating game moves, their cerebellums are activated, suggesting that movement sequences in chess are represented in the cerebellum. The cerebellum may also be involved in higher cognitive functions such as language.

Fighting or Fleeing: The Autonomic Nervous System

Your body does many things of which you're not directly conscious, such as regulating body temperature, blood flow, respiration, and *circadian rhythms* (your body's internal clock). Your *autonomic nervous system,* a part of the peripheral nervous system, regulates all these functions.

The body's tendency to regulate its internal physiological processes — such as body temperature — and keep them stable and constant is called *homeostasis.* These homeostatic functions are necessary for life. Homeostatic functions of the nervous system evolved before all the brain's higher cognitive abilities. Even invertebrates, like worms and insects, maintain internal regulation.

The two main subdivisions of the autonomic nervous system

The autonomic nervous system itself has two main subdivisions — sympathetic and parasympathetic — which are, in a large sense, antagonistic to each other:

- ✔ **The sympathetic system:** This "fight or flight" system regulates your body for fast and enduring physical action by, for example, by diverting blood supply from digestion to the muscles.

- ✔ **The parasympathetic system:** The parasympathetic system does the opposite of the sympathetic system. It reduces voluntary muscle blood supply and enables digestion, immune responses, wound healing, and other types of body maintenance.

See Figure 6-7 for some of the functions of these two different branches of the autonomic nervous system.

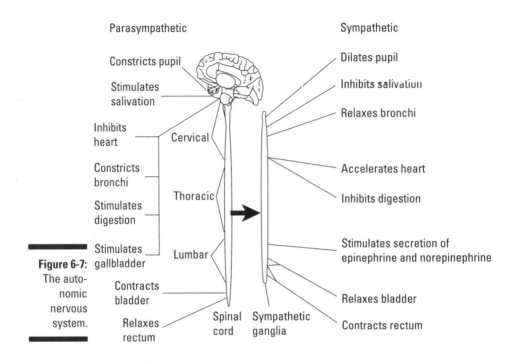

Parasympathetic — Constricts pupil — Stimulates salivation — Inhibits heart — Cervical — Constricts bronchi — Thoracic — Stimulates digestion — Stimulates gallbladder — Lumbar — Contracts bladder — Relaxes rectum — Spinal cord

Sympathetic — Dilates pupil — Inhibits salivation — Relaxes bronchi — Accelerates heart — Inhibits digestion — Stimulates secretion of epinephrine and norepinephrine — Relaxes bladder — Contracts rectum — Sympathetic ganglia

Figure 6-7: The autonomic nervous system.

REMEMBER

Why does the autonomic nervous system have this dual, antagonistic structure? Your ancestors once had to chase down their meals before they could eat. The sympathetic, "fight or flight" system increased their heart rate and respiration for high activity, diverting blood flow away from the digestive system to the skeletal muscles. After they captured their meal, their parasympathetic systems slowed down their overall metabolism and directed blood flow to their digestive systems, allowing the extraction of nutrients. All vertebrate animals have this dual system.

Both the sympathetic and the parasympathetic subsystems involve neurons in spinal segments and cranial nerves that use acetylcholine as the initial neurotransmitter. But in the sympathetic nervous system, neurons project to an external ganglion whose relays cells release noradrenaline (norepinephrine) that acts on adrenergic receptors at the target organs.

Getting ready for action: The sympathetic system

The need to engage in strenuous, immediate, and enduring activity activates the sympathetic division of the autonomic nervous system. This system originates with *cholinergic* (cells in which acetylcholine is the neurotransmitter) neurons located in the thoracic and lumbar segments (T1 to L2) of the spinal cord. These neurons synapse (releasing acetylcholine) on neurons in *sympathetic ganglia,* a system of neurons outside the spinal cord running roughly parallel to it (refer to Figure 6-7). Neurons in the sympathetic ganglia synapse on target organs such as the heart, lungs, blood vessels, and digestive tract. These second-order neurons use norepinephrine (noradrenaline) as a neurotransmitter.

Sympathetic neurons also project to the *adrenal medulla* (part of the adrenal glands on the top of the kidneys) where post-synaptic neurons release epinephrine and norepinephrine into the bloodstream.

Taking care of yourself: The parasympathetic system

Neurons of the parasympathetic nervous system are located primarily in the sacral spinal cord and brainstem (cranial nerves III, VII, IX, X). Parasympathetic nerves also use acetylcholine as a neurotransmitter, but instead of relaying through a spinal cord ganglion, these neurons synapse directly on neurons in a diffuse system of various smaller ganglia near the target organs, such as the heart. The target organ receptors for these parasympathetic ganglia have muscarinic receptors, a metabotropic receptor type for acetylcholine (refer to Chapter 4).

The autonomic nervous system input and output

The autonomic nervous system senses conditions within the body. It has inputs from sense organs and brainstem nuclei such as the nucleus of the solitary tract, and outputs to major organs such as the heart and glands that secrete hormones.

Sensory projections to the nucleus of the solitary tract

The autonomic system has sensory neurons that detect levels of metabolites, gases, and other conditions important for body function, including oxygen, carbon dioxide, sugar, and arterial pressure. Blood oxygen and carbon dioxide are detected by receptors called *baroreceptors,* which are located in the carotid body where the carotid artery *bifurcates* (forks off into two segments). Baroreceptors send blood pressure signals via the vagus nerve (the tenth cranial nerve, which controls the viscera and conveys visera sensory information back to the central nervous system), and via the nucleus of the solitary tract in the medulla of the brainstem. The nucleus of the solitary tract projects to the nucleus ambiguus (a nucleus dorsal to the inferior olivary nucleus that receives motor neuron innervation through the corticobulbar tract) and vagal nucleus (dorsal motor nucleus of the vagus), which release acetylcholine as part of the parasympathetic system to slow down the heart.

To regulate body temperature, thermoreceptors in the *hypothalamus* (a set of nuclei that lie below the thalamus) send signals to autonomic motor neurons and the pituitary to produce responses such as shivering or sweating. Many other autonomic sensory receptors also project to the medulla of the brainstem in the nucleus of the solitary tract, an integrator of visceral information.

The hypothalamus is an important controller of the autonomic nervous system. The hypothalamus is involved in controlling thirst, hunger, body temperature, fatigue, and circadian rhythms. The hypothalamus is activated by inputs from the ventrolateral medulla that carry information from the stomach and heart, and from pacemaker cells that control respiratory rhythms. The hypothalamus is comprised of a number of nuclei, some of which exert their effects by acting on the pituitary gland.

Control of the endocrine system

The *endocrine system* is the system of glands that secrete hormones directly into the bloodstream to maintain homeostasis. Groups of glands that signal each other are called an *axis,* such as the hypothalamic-pituitary-adrenal axis.

Two examples of autonomic control of the endocrine system are the pancreas and adrenal medulla. Sympathetic activation decreases insulin release from the pancreas, while parasympathetic activation increases it. Sympathetic activation increases both epinephrine and norepinephrine secretion from the adrenal medulla.

The autonomic nervous system influences the hypothalamus, and the hypothalamus secretes *neurohormones* (hypothalamic-releasing hormones) that act on the pituitary gland at the base of the brain to release specific pituitary hormones.

The following are some of the numerous hormones the hypothalamus secretes:

- **Vasopressin:** A peptide hormone that regulates the kidneys to help reabsorb and conserve needed substances in the blood. It also constricts the peripheral vasculature, increasing blood pressure in the arteries.

- **Somatostatin:** Somatostatin peptides act on the anterior lobe of the pituitary to inhibit the release of thyroid-stimulating and growth hormones. Somatostatin also suppresses the release of pancreatic hormones and reduces smooth-muscle contractions in the intestines.

- **Oxytocin:** Oxytocin is essential for female reproduction, triggering distension of the cervix and uterus and stimulating breastfeeding. Synthetic oxytocin (Pitocin) is often administered during labor to accelerate the birth process. Circulating oxytocin levels enhance maternal behaviors such as social recognition and pair bonding.

- **Growth-regulating hormones:** The hypothalamus also controls the release of several growth-regulating hormones such as somatotropin (growth hormone) that produces growth factors and increases protein synthesis.

Chapter 7

The Busy Brain: Brainstem, Limbic System, Hypothalamus, and Reticular Formation

*W*hen it comes to the human brain, it's fair to say "You've come a long way, baby!" Our human brains evolved from those of primates, which evolved from those of mammals, which, in turn, evolved from brains of lower vertebrates like amphibians and reptiles.

The brain and its parts have many, many complex functions, besides allowing you to think deep thoughts. The brain integrates spinal cord control with sensory information from the eyes and ears, allowing you to keep your balance. It creates and retains short- and long-term memories, and controls the motivations behind our behaviors. As if that weren't enough, the brain is always working behind the scenes to control functions that are essential to life, like heart rate, blood pressure, and breathing. It also regulates the rhythms of the body's internal clock, telling you when to sleep and when to wake. This chapter explores all these functions and more.

The Brainstem: Medulla, Pons, Midbrain

The medulla, pons, and midbrain make the transition between the brain and spinal cord. These are old brain structures that have developed over millions of years — they probably evolved in primitive fish over 500 million years ago.

Together the medulla, pons, and midbrain are called the *brainstem*. These structures add the first non-skin sensory input (such as from the eyes, ears, and semicircular canals) to spinal cord control of basic behaviors such as locomotion coordination. They also control eye movements and (with the hypothalamus) homeostasis functions such as respiration, heart rate, and temperature (refer to Chapter 6).

All the cranial nerves (which I discuss more fully in the "Counting the Cranial Nerves" section, later in this chapter), except cranial nerves I and II, originate in the brainstem. Figure 7-1 shows the brainstem in relation to the rest of the brain and spinal cord. The medulla, pons, and midbrain have very different appearances and functions.

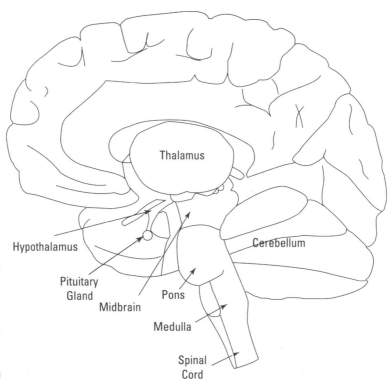

Figure 7-1:
The brain-
stem:
medulla,
pons, and
midbrain.

Meeting the medulla

The most ventral (bottommost) area of the brain is called the *medulla* (or *medulla oblongata*). The lower border of the medulla is the top of the spinal cord. The transition between the top of the spinal cord and the medulla occurs at a hole in the occipital bone at the base of the skull called the *foramen magnum*.

Carrying information

The medulla connects the brain to the spinal cord. Much of a cross section of the medulla consists of neural fiber tracts. These fiber tracts carry sensory information from the skin, muscles, and tendons up to the brain, and motor command information from primary motor cortex in the frontal lobe down to the spinal cord to control the body's muscles.

Two areas of cells in the medulla, called the *gracile* and *cuneate nuclei,* (dorsal column nuclei) are primarily involved with ascending tactile sensory proprioceptive information, and serve as a relay station in the dorsal column–medial lemniscus pathway.

Examining important functions

If you look at the medulla (refer to Figure 7-1), its appearance is not much different from the cervical spinal segments below it. However, instead of receiving sensory information from the skin of the arms, and joint and tendon signals from the arm muscles, the medulla receives information from taste receptors on the tongue, the skin of the head, the heart and lungs, major blood vessels, and the digestive system. Sensory fibers of the somatic and autonomic cranial nerves carry this information to the medulla.

Functions of the medulla include the following:

- The medulla's motor output goes to muscles of the tongue, the soft palate and larynx associated with producing speech, and to the glandular portions of these organs.
- The medulla helps regulate important body homeostasis functions such as respiration, heart rate, digestion processes, and blood vessel functions (refer to Chapter 6).
- The medulla controls "mouth reflexes" such as vomiting, coughing, sneezing, and swallowing.

Because the medulla controls so many body functions that are crucial to life — such as heart rate and respiration — any extensive damage to it is typically fatal.

Noting the nuclei

The medulla has several *nuclei* (collections of cell bodies whose axons project elsewhere). Figure 7-2 shows some of these nuclei. Keep in mind, however, that the medulla is longer than the cervical spinal cord segments below it, and not all the nuclei you see in Figure 7-2 would appear in every cross section.

Major Nuclei of the Medulla

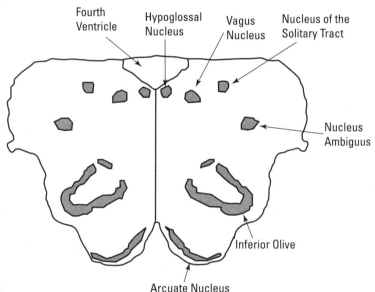

Figure 7-2:
Medulla
cross
section.

The nuclei of the medulla are as follows:

- ✔ **Nucleus of the solitary tract:** The nucleus of the solitary tract is notable because it receives taste inputs from the glossopharyngeal nerve, the IXth cranial nerve. Neurons that synapse in the nucleus of the solitary tract also mediate a number of reflexes, such as the gag and cough reflexes, respiratory reflexes, the carotid sinus, and aortic reflexes. Reflexes involving the *baroreceptors* (blood pressure) and gastrointestinal system also involve this nucleus. Taste sensation also arrives at this nucleus from the facial nerve.

- ✔ **Vagus nucleus:** Also called the dorsal nucleus of the vagus, this is cranial nerve X. Axons from this nucleus are preganglionic cholinergic sympathetic fibers that emanate from the brainstem near the inferior olive. This nucleus controls parasympathetic functions in the lungs, gastrointestinal tract, and abdomen.

✔ **Hypoglossal nucleus:** The hypoglossal nucleus gives rise to cranial nerve XII. This nerve innervates the muscles of the tongue that control chewing, swallowing, and speaking.

✔ **Nucleus ambiguous:** The inputs to this nucleus come from the corticobulbar tract, and its outputs are motor neurons that travel via the vagus nerve (cranial nerve X) to the pharynx, larynx, and esophagus.

✔ **Inferior olive:** The inferior olive within the medulla receives inputs from the dorsal column nuclei. Its outputs interact extensively with the cerebellum for motor coordination and learning. Inferior olive output axons, called *olivocerebellar fibers,* cross the midline on their way up to the contralateral cerebellum and enter it through a tract called the *inferior cerebellar peduncle.* Within the cerebellum, they become the climbing fibers that synapse on Purkinje cells. The climbing fibers generate error signals for learning by Purkinje cells, which are the major output of the cerebellum via the deep nuclei.

Tracts of ascending (from spinal sensory neurons) and descending (from motor cortex) axons that go through the medulla cross over to the opposite side of the centerline of the body at what's called the *decussation of the pyramids.* This crossover causes each of the two cerebral hemispheres to receive sensory input from, and control muscles on the opposite side of, the body. The place where sensory input traversing the medulla crosses the midline is called the sensory decussion.

Presenting the pons

Above the medulla lies the pons. You can see in Figure 7-1, earlier in this chapter, that the pons bulges out in front of the ventral surface of the medulla below it, and behind the pons is the cerebellum. Above the pons is the midbrain.

The pons contains nuclei that mediate several important functions:

✔ **Hearing:** One function of the pons is *sound localization* — identifying the origin of a sound and how far away it is. It does this with neural comparisons of the intensity and timing of the sound between the two ears (in cooperation with the inferior colliculus in the midbrain).

✔ **Keeping your balance:** Neural circuits for balance involve inputs to the medulla and several nuclei within the pons *(pontine nuclei)* from the vestibular system in the inner ear (the semicircular canals). Outputs from these nuclei project to the cerebellum and frontal lobes.

Damage to the pontine nuclei (as well as to the vestibular system) can produce chronic dizziness and extreme postural instability.

- ✔ **Looking around:** Pontine nuclei are involved in the control of eye movements.

- ✔ **Sleeping:** Pontine nuclei help to control sleep.

- ✔ **Making faces:** The pons receives sensory input from the face and sends motor neurons to facial muscles to control both voluntary and involuntary facial expressions.

- ✔ **Secreting:** The superior salivary nucleus in the pons helps to produce tears and secrete saliva.

- ✔ **Working with the medulla:** Neural circuits involving both the pons and medulla control respiration, swallowing, and bladder emptying.

Four cranial nerves (for more see the "Counting the Cranial Nerves" section, later in this chapter) emanate from pontine nuclei: the trigeminal nerve (V), the abducens (VI), the facial nerve (VII) and the cochlear nerve (VIII). These four nerves function in sensory processing of hearing, balance, and facial sensations such as touch, pain, and taste.

Mentioning the midbrain

The top level of the brainstem is called the midbrain (or mesencephalon). The midbrain works with the pons to control eye movements and help localize sound.

Moving the eyes

In mammals, the major visual area in the midbrain is called the *superior colliculus* (which is the equivalent of the optic tectum in non-mammalian vertebrates). In cold-blooded vertebrates, such as frogs, the midbrain is typically the highest-level brain structure, with the large optic tecti being the major visual processing centers that are crucial for visually guided behavior. Mammals analyze visual input in the visual cortex and use the superior colliculus to control rapid eye movements called *saccades*.

Localizing sound

The midbrain helps to localize sound through the following path: Auditory fibers from the *superior olive* (a group of brainstem nuclei involved in processing auditory inputs) project to a processing area below the superior colliculus called the *inferior colliculus* (see Figure 7-3). Neurons of the inferior colliculus project to neurons in the auditory part of the thalamus (called the *medial geniculate nucleus*). The medial geniculate nucleus projects to the auditory part of the neocortex on the top part of the temporal lobe. Neurons in the auditory pathway help localize the source of sound using *interaural time difference* (the difference in arrival time of the sound between the two ears) and *interaural intensity difference* (the difference in sound magnitude between the two ears).

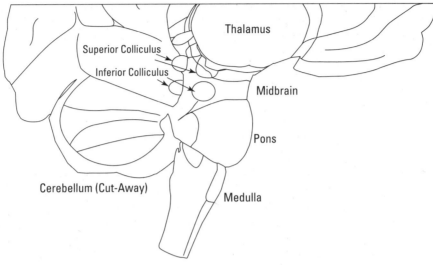

Other functions

The midbrain also includes a structure heavily connected with the basal ganglia, the substantia nigra (refer to Chapter 8). Other nuclei in the midbrain, such as the locus coeruleus and raphe, make extensive but diffuse modulatory projections throughout the neocortex. These projections are involved in setting basic brain states, such as what you're attending to, alertness, drives, and goals.

Recently, addiction researchers have focused considerable attention on the midbrain ventral tegmental area. This nucleus sends *dopaminergic axons* (axons that release the neurotransmitter dopamine) to a forebrain area called the nucleus accumbens, which in turn projects to the prefrontal cortex. This circuit has been shown to be important in reward and addiction.

Counting the Cranial Nerves

Like skin on the rest of the body, the skin of the face and head has sensory receptors and muscles that move the face to produce facial expressions. Some *cranial* (related to the cranium or skull) nerves that emanate from the brain are involved in peripheral sensation and muscle control, much like the nerves leaving the spinal cord (refer to Chapter 6).

But some organs are unique to the head. The eyes, ears, nose, and tongue have no counterpart in the spine, and some of the nerves serving those senses are quite different from anything in the spine. The body has 12 cranial nerves (each is assigned a number), 10 of which emerge from the brainstem. The cranial nerves are considered part of the peripheral nervous system, except for the optic nerve (II), because the retina, from which it originates, is part of the central nervous system even though it's outside the skull. (This is fortunate because seeing through your skull bone would be difficult!) Controlling eye position through the six eye muscles is distributed across several cranial nerves.

The body has two of each cranial nerve, and the nerves are generally bilaterally symmetrical about the midline. The 12 cranial nerves are as follows:

- **The olfactory nerve (I):** Transmits the sense of smell from the nose. It terminates in the anterior olfactory nucleus.

- **The optic nerve (II):** Carries messages from retinal ganglion cells to the lateral geniculate nucleus of the thalamus, the superior colliculus, and more than ten other retinal recipient zones.

- **The oculomotor nerve (III):** Is primarily a motor nerve for controlling eye movements and pupil dilation. The axons of this nerve originate primarily in the oculomotor nucleus and the Edinger–Westphal nucleus.

- **The trochlear nerve (IV):** Is a motor nerve that emanates from the dorsal midbrain trochlear nucleus and controls the superior oblique eye muscles.

- **The trigeminal nerve (V):** Has both sensory and motor axons. Sensory input comes from the face, and motor output controls chewing. It originates in the trigeminal nucleus of the pons, with help from the spinal trigeminal nucleus and mesencephalic trigeminal nucleus. A motor component involved in chewing comes from the trigeminal motor nucleus.

- **The abducens nerve (VI):** Is a motor nerve originating from the abducens nucleus. It synapses on the lateral rectus eye muscle.

- **The facial nerve (VII):** Has sensory and motor axons associated with the facial nucleus, nucleus of the solitary tract, and superior salivary nuclei. Facial expressions are controlled by motor innervation of this nerve. Taste information from the front of the tongue also reaches the brain by this nerve. Motor output includes some of the salivary glands and the lacrimal gland.

- **The acoustic (vestibulocochlear) nerve (VIII):** Is a sensory nerve that transmits auditory and vestibular information to the brain from the spiral ganglion and Scarpa's ganglion. Its axons originate in the cochlear and vestibular nuclei.

- **The glossopharyngeal nerve (IX):** Originates in the medulla, and has sensory and motor axons. It carries taste information from the back of the tongue. Axons in the nerve also come from the nucleus ambiguus and inferior salivary nucleus. Motor output controls the secretion of the parotid gland.

✓ **The vagus nerve (X):** Originates in the posterolateral sulcus of the medulla, the nucleus ambiguus, the dorsal vagal nucleus, and the solitary nucleus. Motor output controls laryngeal and pharyngeal muscles — the larynx and pharynx in the throat. This nerve also has a parasympathetic output to control mucous membranes in the thorax and abdomen. Taste sensory information from the epiglottis travels to the brain by the vagus. The vagus is also crucial for controlling the vocal cords.

✓ **The accessory nerve (XI):** Is a motor nerve originating mostly from the nucleus ambiguus and spinal accessory nucleus. This nerve innervates the sternocleidomastoid and trapezius muscles, which help to move the neck and turn the head.

✓ **The hypoglossal nerve (XII):** Is primarily motor and originates in the medulla hypoglossal nucleus. It controls the tongue and is important for speaking and swallowing.

Controlling Your Motives: The Limbic System

The term *limbic system* refers to a group of nuclei and tracts above the brainstem and below the neocortex originally postulated to control drives and instincts. It is phylogenetically very old, and exists in non-mammalian vertebrates, which perform complex behaviors with little or no neocortex. They use subcortical neural control in areas like the basal ganglia and limbic system.

Above the limbic system is the corpus callosum, then the cingulate gyrus, then neocortex. The vast majority of the cortex (outer surface and associated white matter) of the mammalian brain is neocortex. Evolution tried two other types of cortex before settling on building the brain mostly from neocortex. These are mesocortex and allocortex, shown in Figure 7-4. These evolutionarily older types of cortex are associated with the limbic system. The limbic system is a collection of structures from the midbrain, diencephalon, mesocortex, and allocortex.

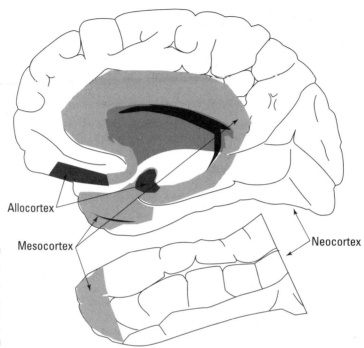

Figure 7-4:
Neocortex,
mesocortex,
and
allocortex.

Allocortex

Mesocortex

Neocortex

Emotional processing

Although science fiction often portrays emotionless characters such as Mr. Spock as superior beings, would we really be better off without emotions? Why would we have evolved emotions if they only get us into trouble? The answer is that emotions allow us to avoid trouble far more often than they cause it.

Remember: Emotions existed before reason. Feelings — the content of emotions — are the brain's way of telling us if something is good or bad, and whether it's important, without having

to go through a long and perhaps faulty chain of reasoning about the results of some action (or inaction). Emotions are the means by which the part of your brain that processes incoming sensory information communicates likely outcomes to the part of your brain that executes actions. This communication depends on a set of sub-neocortical structures called the *limbic system* that are in brain regions that are cortex, but not neocortex.

A look back on the limbic system

In his triune brain model, Paul D. MacLean, an American neuroscientist, hypothesized that the limbic system controlled emotion, instinctive behavior, motivation, memory, and sense of smell. The triune consisted of three major structures sequentially added during evolution: the reptilian complex (basal ganglia), the paleomammalian complex (limbic system), and the neomammalian complex (neocortex).

The reptilian complex basal ganglia were hypothesized to function in instinctual behaviors such as aggression. The paleomammalian brain (limbic system) supposedly arose later in evolution and mediated motivation and emotion for feeding, reproductive behaviors, and parenting. The neomammalian complex (neocortex) enabled language, abstract reasoning, and complex planning.

The limbic system was proposed to consist of the cingulate cortex, hippocampal complex, amygdala, septum, anterior thalamic nuclei, limbic cortex, and hypothalamus. The hippocampus is essential for transferring memory from short to long term, whether it has any emotional content or not. The result is that use of the term *limbic system* is controversial among neurobiologists. The idea of an evolutionarily old, subcortical processing system whose output is an emotional state that affects behavior still has considerable validity, but the group of brain structures lumped together as a limbic system or module is clearly not valid. I discuss several of these structures later in this chapter and book.

Mesocortex and allocortex versus neocortex

Mesocortex is a six-layered brain structure in what's called the paralimbic region between neocortex and allocortex. It includes the cingulate gyrus, insula, some of the orbitofrontal cortex, and the parahippocampal gyrus. Allocortex (or archicortex) is the oldest cortex, having one to four layers. It's the type of brain structure in the hippocampal complex and primary olfactory cortex (also sometimes called paleocortex). These structures predate the neocortex in evolution, and are crucial for brain function even in animals like humans who have very large neocortices.

Organizing thoughts and activities: The cingulate gyrus

One of the original limbic areas is the cingulate gyrus, a mesocortical area that lies mostly between the corpus callosum fiber tract and the neocortex (see Figure 7-5).

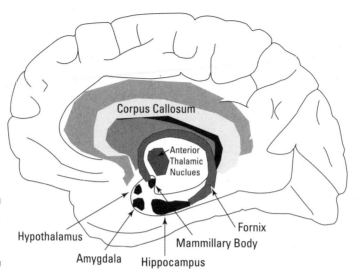

Figure 7-5:
The limbic
system.

The cingulate gyrus receives inputs from the thalamus and the neocortex, and projects to the entorhinal cortex around the hippocampus via the cingulum. One function proposed for the cingulate gyrus is to allocate processing among other cortical areas, making it a mediator of executive function.

The cingulate gyrus is typically divided into anterior and posterior regions, with the dividing line above the anterior thalamus:

✓ **Anterior cingulate cortex:** This area appears to be involved in motivation and the perception of pain, or even the expectation of pain. Imaging studies show that it's activated when we make mistakes and when we receive conflicting information.

✓ **Posterior cingulate cortex:** Less is known about this area, but it appears to be involved in awareness and the allocation of working memory along with the dorsolateral prefrontal cortex.

Making memories: The hippocampus

You can remember the phone number of a pizza takeout place for only about as long as it takes to dial it, but you never forget your Social Security number (unless you develop a form of dementia like Alzheimer's disease). The hippocampus controls the formation of long-term memories like your Social Security number.

Creating a memory

Short-term memory is disposable: You retain the memory for as long as you need it, and then discard it or forget it. Temporary short-term memory is held in what's also called *working memory,* in the lateral prefrontal cortex. The only information that passes from your short-term to long-term memory is information you rehearse or to which you're repeatedly exposed. Rehearsing or repeating engages a reciprocal circuit between the hippocampus and neocortex that converts the memory to long-term. So, when you're learning something by heart, you're really learning it by hippocampus.

Making associations

The hippocampus is an allocortex structure located (bilaterally, of course) at the medial aspect of the temporal lobe (refer to Figure 7-5). It receives inputs through the parahippocampal gyrus and entorhinal cortex from virtually the entire neocortex. Figure 7-6 illustrates the hippocampus.

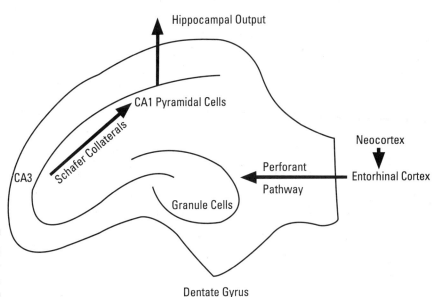

Figure 7-6:
The hippo-
campus.

The output of the hippocampus on each side of the brain is through a fiber tract called the *fimbria.* The axons from the hippocampi on each side of the brain merge at the midline where the tract is called the *fornix* (refer to Figure 7-5). The fornix divides at the anterior commissure at the most anterior and ventral end of the corpus callosum. The anterior axon tract is called the precommissural fornix. It projects to the nucleus accumbens (involved in reward, and implicated in addiction) and to septal nuclei. Some fornix axons form what is called the post-commissural fornix and project through the hypothalamus to the mammillary bodies. These in turn project to the anterior nuclei of the thalamus, which projects to the cingulate cortex.

The hippocampus is an association engine for memory. The representation of any event is distributed across the entire neocortex. For example, what you see is found in various parts of the visual system, and the meanings of words you hear and read are around language areas. All the information in the brain about what is going on now is projected and organized through the parahippocampal gyrus and entorhinal cortex to cells in the hippocampus that respond to coincidence, including previous partial memories of related events.

For example, say that yesterday you were driving your red car down Route 17 to meet Bob and Carol, and it was snowing. Particular cells in the hippocampus are activated by red, not green, and Route 17, not Route 101, and Bob and Carol, not Ted and Alice, and by snow as opposed to rain.

The synapses between these particular cells undergo synaptic strengthening in a process called *long-term potentiation*. With practice, and often during sleep, the hippocampus reciprocally fires back at the neocortex cells that generated the long-term potentiation, and produces a long-term memory by enabling the cells in the neocortex to form their own mutually excitatory memory circuit that can be activated by future input, independent of the hippocampus.

The amygdala

Just anterior to the hippocampus is another structure originally included in the limbic system: the amygdala (bilaterally, of course). Like the hippocampus, the *amygdala* is a memory structure that interacts with the neocortex. However, unlike the hippocampus, the amygdala seems be associated particularly with memories having high emotional salience, such as fear. Besides projecting back to the cortex (mostly the orbitofrontal cortex), the amygdala projects to the hypothalamus and other brain areas associated with emotional reactions to stimuli. The amygdalae are essential for the formation of memories associated with emotional events, such as in *fear conditioning*, where a context that predicts a painful outcome becomes associated with the outcome and itself induces fear.

Several well-documented clinical cases exist in which sociopaths were determined to have damage to their amygdalae. Like the hippocampus, the amygdala appears to be involved in forming long-term memories in the neocortex, primarily, the orbitofrontal cortex. The orbitofrontal cortex is involved in emotional responses to contexts, such as being nervous when betting a large sum of money. Lesions to the anterior temporal lobe that include the amygdala produce *hypo-emotionality* (a loss of emotional response), loss of fear, and *hypersexuality* (increased desire for sexual behavior) in experiments on nonhuman primates — called Klüver–Bucy syndrome. Some patients with severe amygdala damage cannot experience any fear at all.

Short- and long-term memory: The case of H.M.

The famous clinical case of the patient H.M. shows the importance of the hippocampus in learning. H.M. was an epileptic who suffered from seizures that appeared to originate in the temporal lobes. H.M. had both hippocampi removed to try to end the seizures.

After the surgery, H.M.'s previous long-term memories were still intact. He also appeared to function normally in any situation that lasted for only a few minutes. However, H.M. could form no new long-term memories. Doctors would have extended conversations with H.M., but when they left the room and returned, H.M. would have no recollection of ever having seen them.

The process of transferring information from short- to long-term memory requires, as the case of H.M. demonstrates, the action of the hippocampus. HM was studied extensively over many years. He lived the rest of his life in an eternal present and always thought that today's date was the date that he'd had his surgery. He never formed any new long-term memories.

Regulating the Autonomic Nervous System: The Hypothalamus

The *hypothalamus* is a collection of nuclei where the nervous system is linked to the endocrine system by the pituitary gland. It's located below the thalamus, and together with the thalamus, epithalamus, and the subthalamus makes up the diencephalon. The hypothalamus controls circadian rhythms, sleep, thirst, hunger, body temperature, and some parenting behaviors.

Sleeping and waking: Circadian rhythms

An important nucleus in the hypothalamus is the *suprachiasmatic nucleus* (SCN). This nucleus controls *circadian rhythms* (our sleep/wake cycle). In sleep, consciousness is absent or severely reduced, but in a different way than during hibernation or a coma. Even though almost all vertebrates sleep, scientists have no universally accepted theory for sleep's function.

Synchronizing our intrinsic clocks with external light involves a special class of retinal ganglion cells in our eyes called *intrinsically photosensitive ganglion cells,* which project to the SCN. These cells have their own visual pigment that allows them to directly respond to light.

Sleep cycles through several characteristic stages, each of which has unique properties. If you observe someone sleeping you can see periods in which his eyes are moving nearly continuously, whereas during other periods the eyes don't seem to move very much at all. This distinguishes rapid eye movement (REM) sleep from non-REM (NREM) sleep.

The predominant brain waves that can be detected with electroencephalography (EEG) also differ between sleep and wakefulness, and between different sleep phases. Figure 7-7 shows a typical night's sleep phase plot, which is called a *hypnogram*.

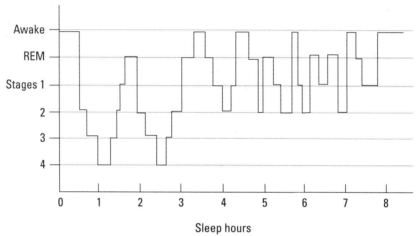

Figure 7-7: A hypnogram.

REM sleep

REM sleep is the e most like being awake. Most dreams occur in REM sleep. This sleep stage appears to be important because if humans are sleep deprived they spend proportionately more time in REM sleep. Infants not only sleep more than adults, but also have a larger proportion of REM sleep. No one is sure why we dream. One theory is that synapses that are activated during waking activities are pared back (in a process known as *normalization*) so that the brain is ready for renewed synapse growth during learning.

REM sleep is characterized by high frequencies in the EEG. These high frequencies are associated with motor activities that occur in dreams, such as running, that are associated with frontal-lobe activity. However, the motor commands from the frontal lobe are blocked in the spinal cord so that actual movement doesn't occur.

Learning during sleep

Experiments in rats that were trained to navigate mazes showed that activity sequences in hippocampal place cells, which code for maze location, "replay" the maze navigation sequence during the rat's sleep. REM sleep deprivation in these rats disrupted this playback and the ability of the rats to retain the maze learning.

REM sleep has been shown to be important for consolidating learning. During REM sleep, what has been learned during the day and held in short-term memory is transferred to long-term memory. Short-term memory is associated with changes in synaptic strengths in the hippocampus (refer to "Regulating the Autonomic Nervous System: The Hypothalamus" earlier in this chapter). During REM sleep, these strengthened hippocampal synapses feed back and activate the areas of cortex that activated them, producing a mutually excitatory circuit in the cortex for representing the learned features.

NREM sleep

After REM sleep we transition to deep sleep through the NREM phases, labeled N1, N2, N3, and sometimes N4.

Often the sleeper then descends through the phases in order, N1 to N4, and then oscillates irregularly between phases after that. Late in the sleep period the phase sequences tend to be shallower, sometimes not reaching N3 or N4, with some brief transitions from REM to momentary wakefulness. Little is known about any difference in the function of the four NREM phases.

Brain oscillations and function

EEG rhythms are categorized in frequency bands:

- **Delta:** Up to 4 Hertz (Hz), or cycles per second
- **Theta:** 4 to 8 Hz
- **Alpha:** 8 to 13 Hz
- **Beta:** 13 to 30 Hz
- **Gamma:** 30 to 100 Hz
- **Mu:** 8 to 13 Hz (motor cortex specific)

Sleep phases are characterized by distinct changes in EEG patterns, examples of which you can see in Figure 7-8. Wakefulness is associated with beta rhythms in the EEG. Relaxation and meditation shift the EEG rhythms from beta to alpha. In the earliest stage of sleep, characteristic slow eye movements occur, technically called slow rolling eye movements (SREMs). About this time, alpha waves nearly disappear from the EEG, and theta waves begin to predominate. Stage N2 of sleep is also dominated by theta waves, but these change to delta waves in N3 and N4. N4 is the deepest stage of sleep, from which it is the most difficult to awaken.

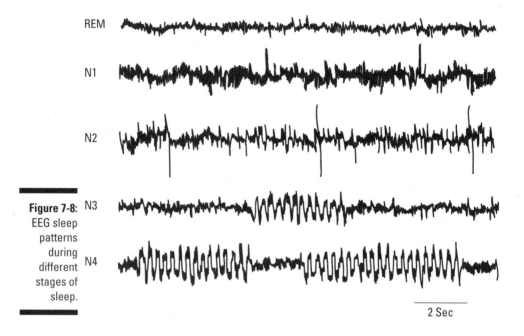

Figure 7-8: EEG sleep patterns during different stages of sleep.

2 Sec

Hypothalamic body function regulation

The hypothalamus controls many behaviors and rhythms. It receives inputs from several areas:

- Bloodstream
- Brainstem reticular formation
- Nucleus of the solitary tract
- Locus coeruleus
- Ventrolateral medulla
- Limbic system
- Septum
- Olfactory bulbs
- Cortex

The hypothalamus interacts with the autonomic nervous system by secreting neurohormones (called *hypothalamic-releasing hormones*). These hormones act on the pituitary gland, stimulating or inhibiting the secretion of pituitary hormones.

Homeostasis: Temperature, blood pressure, breathing, and heart rate

One function of the hypothalamus is to respond to substances it receives from the bloodstream from areas like the heart and digestive system. Nuclei within the hypothalamus also respond to *blood osmolarity* (total solute concentration) and plasma glucose concentration. The hypothalamus is the body's thermostat: It stimulates heat production to raise the temperature, or sweating and *vasodilation* (widening of the blood vessels) to cool it. It also creates fevers.

Neural input to the hypothalamus from the brainstem includes visceral and cardiovascular signals carried by the vagus nerve.

Autonomic hormones and behavior

Many hormones affect the hypothalamus, including insulin, angiotensin, and pituitary hormones. The hypothalamus responds to monoamine neurotransmitters, including noradrenaline, dopamine, and serotonin. The hypothalamus also controls oxytocin secretion in the mother in response to, for example, suckling.

The olfactory input — meaning smells that come in through the nose — to the hypothalamus can mediate aspects of sexual behavior. Consider the case of *pheromones,* which are odorants animals produce that have unconscious behavioral (often sexual) effects in others. (We generally aren't even conscious of detecting these pheromones.) For example, in the well-known "Bruce effect," if a pregnant mouse is exposed to the urine of a different male shortly after coitus, the pregnancy is likely to be terminated. Synchronized menstruation in women living in close proximity (such as in college dorms) has been shown to depend on odor signals (pheromones).

The insula (insular cortex)

The *insula* (insular cortex) is a portion of the cortex (actually, the mesocortex) located in the deep fissure that separates the temporal from the parietal and frontal lobes. Above the insula (bilaterally, of course) is a structure called the *operculum,* which means "lid." It's highly interconnected with the limbic system and appears to be important in assigning emotional significance to sensory input. It receives inputs from sensory areas of the thalamus and projects to limbic system structures such as the amygdala, orbitofrontal cortex, and the ventral striatum of the basal ganglia. It also projects directly to areas of the motor cortex.

Perceiving pain

The executive control of the insula includes coordinating the regulation of some aspects of homeostasis, the conscious perception and awareness of pain, and some aspects of motor control. Awareness of the amount of pain, and even imagining pain, activates the insula, particularly on the right side. It's also involved in the high-level control of the autonomic nervous system and the immune system.

Other roles

In motor control, the insula operates as an executive control center that regulates heart rate and blood pressure to levels appropriate for the level of the body's exertion and emotional state. It also appears to have a role in speech articulation and some poorly understood aspects of body awareness, emotions, and social awareness via its connections to the limbic system.

Reading Up on the Reticular Formation

The *reticular formation* is an ancient brainstem "area" that courses throughout much of the subcortex. The word *reticular* is derived from the Latin word for *net*.

The reticular formation comprises over 100 neural circuits that control essential body functions. It extends from spinal projections to the medulla, through the midbrain and pons, to reticular "zones" above the midbrain in reticular areas of the thalamus. (See "The Brainstem: Medulla, Pons, Midbrain," earlier in this chapter, for more about these parts of the brain.) The reticular formation interacts with numerous brain areas to control all life processes, such as heart rate, respiration, temperature, and even wakefulness.

Damage to the reticular formation typically results in coma or even death.

Starting with the spine

Some motor neurons in the primary motor cortex send their axons to the reticular formation nuclei in the medulla, instead of down the spine directly to alpha motor neurons. The nuclei in the medulla that receive these motor inputs then project down the spine in what are called *reticulospinal tracts* of the spinal cord. These tracts are important for maintaining balance during body movements. There are also inputs to the reticular formation from the eyes and ears through the cerebellum that integrate them for motor coordination.

The reticular formation is organized in a manner similar to the intermediate gray matter of the spinal cord, which it's continuous with at the bottom of the medulla.

Moving through the brainstem

The reticular formation in the medulla can be divided into several nuclei that extend into three major columns that run through the brainstem:

- ✔ **The median column (also known as the Raphe nuclei):** Sends axons diffusely through the neocortex that release serotonin.

- ✔ **The medial or magnocellular column (consisting of large-cell somas):** Sends projections to the medulla and midbrain, and may be involved in sleep/wakefulness control.

- ✔ **The lateral or parvocellular column:** Projects to the medulla and midbrain. It is not clear what functionally differentiates this group of nuclei from the medial group.

These nuclei send projections through the medulla and into the midbrain.

Controlling functions

The reticular formation controls the heart via its cardiac and *vasomotor relation* (dilating blood vessels) centers of the medulla. It's also involved in pain modulation, because pain signals from pain receptors in the lower body relay in the medulla nuclei that project to the cortex. Descending axons from the cortex can help to inhibit feelings of pain in the spinal cord by blocking the transmission of some pain signals to the brain.

Ascending projections from the reticular formation to the thalamus and cortex control or gate the sensory signals reaching these structures. The reticular formation is a gateway for essential functions of states of consciousness and awareness versus sleep. Other motor nuclei in the reticular formation control the ability of the eyes to track objects and central pattern generators (somewhat similar to those in the spinal cord for locomotion — refer to Chapter 6) that coordinate muscles for breathing and swallowing.

Reticular activating system

Reticular formation nuclei that modulate activity of the cerebral cortex are part of the *reticular activating system* (RAS). The RAS is a neural circuit by which the brainstem interacts with the cortex through relays in several thalamic nuclei in so-called intralaminar regions (see the following section).

The RAS also includes the tegmentum and dorsal hypothalamus. The RAS midbrain reticular formation controls transitions from relaxed wakefulness to focused attention.

The main neurotransmitters used by the RAS are acetylcholine and noradrenaline; they operate in an antagonistic manner to regulate states of awareness and consciousness by controlling thalamo-cortical activity. *Cholinergic projections* (those that use acetylcholine) from the RAS to the thalamus, basal forebrain, substantia nigra, and cerebellum are increased during wakefulness and REM sleep.

Most of the noradrenaline output of the RAS is from the locus coeruleus in the pons. These neurons project to many of the same areas to which the cholinergic RAS system projects, but with opposite effects: They're active during waking and slow-wave sleep, but not during REM sleep. The locus coeruleus also projects to the cerebral cortex and the spinal cord.

Continuing through the thalamus and cortex

Although the classic reticular formation is located in the brainstem, extensions of it exist at higher levels. For example, the thalamic reticular nucleus in the ventral thalamus almost encloses the reticular formation on its lateral extent. Also, an area called the peri-geniculate nucleus exists around the lateral geniculate nucleus, the main relay from the retina to occipital cortex. Reticular cells are mostly *GABAergic* (their axons release the inhibitory neurotransmitter, GABA) and have inhibitory effects on the cells around them.

Thalamic reticular nuclei receive input from dorsal thalamic nuclei and the cerebral cortex, in addition to inputs from brainstem reticular nuclei. Reticular areas of the thalamus project to dorsal thalamic nuclei, but not to the cerebral cortex like most thalamic nuclei.

The function of the thalamic reticular areas appears to be to modulate the information projected from other nuclei in the thalamus to the cortex. This can be limited to one sense, or between different senses. For example, although you may be concentrating on reading a sign in front of you, rapid movement toward you in your peripheral vision will almost always pull your attention toward the movement. This would also be true if you heard a loud noise behind you as well. The reticular formation controls not only whether you're awake or asleep, but also important aspects of what you pay attention to while awake.

Chapter 8

Generating Behavior: Basal Ganglia, Thalamus, Motor Cortex, and Frontal Cortex

. . . .

In This Chapter

▶ Behaving different ways with the basal ganglia

▶ Moving your muscles through the primary motor cortex

▶ Getting muscles to work like a team

▶ Moving through the thalamus to the neocortex

▶ Being a boss like the prefrontal cortex

▶ Seeing what really controls your thoughts and actions

. . . .

*Y*our mother said it, and she was right: You've got to have goals. Well the fact is that you do, because animals, including humans, do things according to goals. You may decide you want a better view of some squirrels outside. You decide to walk to the window. You decide to move your right foot first. (I didn't say they all needed to be big goals.) Actions start with a hierarchy of goals and sub-goals, translated into general and particular motor procedures. Where in your brain does all this happen?

You may think there is some place in the center of the brain that embodies the real you, that makes these decisions. Descartes thought the soul was in the pineal gland, because it's one of the few brain structures that there is only one of (instead of two bilaterally symmetrical ones). Most neurobiologists don't believe the soul is in the pineal gland, or anywhere else in the brain to which one can point. Rather, goals and decisions are distributed across many brain circuits and "bubble up" from activity across them. But some circuits have been shown to be more important than others in this process. The important brain areas for decisions about doing things include the basal ganglia, thalamus, and frontal lobes, all of which I discuss in this chapter.

The Basal Ganglia and Its Nuclei

The basal ganglia are phylogenetically old, probably as old as being four-legged (or *tetrapod*). Below the basal ganglia are the brainstem and spinal cord. These structures are adequate to control basic locomotion and regulate body processes for homeostasis. But somewhere decisions have to be made about what gait is to be used, in what direction. The basal ganglia are the original decision locus for overall behaviors. The evolution of the neocortex gave the basal ganglia many more behavioral options from which to choose.

The basal ganglia nuclei include the caudate nucleus, putamen, and globus pallidus. Always discussed with these three nuclei are the subthalamic nucleus, part of the subthalamus, and the substantia nigra, which are actually in the midbrain. Figure 8-1 shows these nuclei. The globus pallidus is divided into internal and external segments. Inputs to the basal ganglia reach the basal ganglia through relays in the caudate and putamen, which together is called the *striatum*. The output of the basal ganglia is chiefly from the internal segment of the globus pallidus and the substantia nigra pars reticulata.

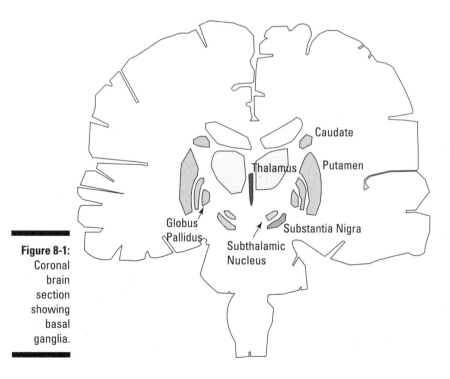

Figure 8-1: Coronal brain section showing basal ganglia.

The basal ganglia are involved in initiating and controlling movement through connections to the frontal lobe, as well as through the extra-pyramidal motor system — a distinct system from the primary motor cortex pathway in mammals that involves, for example, projections from brainstem nuclei to the the spinal cord. Both the basal ganglia and motor cortex interact with the cerebellum (refer to Chapter 6 for more about the cerebellum), an ancient motor sequence coordination center. The following section looks at the organization of the basal ganglia nuclei.

Striatum inputs and output to the thalamus

The basal ganglia interact with the thalamus and cortex in a brain circuit, part of which you can see in Figure 8-2. Excitatory (glutamate) connections are black, inhibitory (GABA) connections are gray. Most of neocortex sends excitatory connections to the caudate and putamen, or striatum. The striatum inhibits the globus pallidus external segment (GPe), globus pallidus internal segment (GPi), and substantia nigra reticulata (SNr). GPe inhibits the subthalamic nucleus (STN). STN excites GPe and GPi/SNr. The output of the basal ganglia, GPi/SNr inhibits the thalamus, which itself excites the frontal cortex. The net effect of all this is that the inputs to the thalamus that are *not* inhibited by the basal ganglia are the ones that activate the cortex.

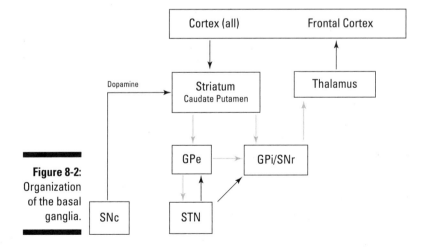

Figure 8-2: Organization of the basal ganglia.

Although the operation of the basal ganglia and related nuclei are not well understood, it is clear that the basal ganglia are involved in the selection of behaviors. Given the current inputs and brain state, the neocortex is simultaneously activating "programs" for multiple behaviors. The job of the basal ganglia is to choose one behavior over all the others.

The basal ganglia neural circuit

Several similarities exist between the organization of the basal ganglia and the cerebellum (see Chapter 6). Like the cerebellum, the basal ganglia receive inputs in the outer nuclei (caudate and putamen), which project to inner nuclei (globus pallidus). The output of the basal ganglia is chiefly from these inner nuclei to the thalamus, and it is primarily inhibitory.

Projections from the striatum give rise to two main pathways within the basal ganglia, called direct and indirect pathways:

- **The direct pathway** is the inhibitory projection from striatum to the GPi/SNr complex, which itself inhibits the thalamus. Because inhibiting an inhibition results in disinhibition, the net effect of the direct pathway is excitatory to the thalamus. This enables the cortical excitatory projections to the corticospinal tract and brainstem (refer to Chapter 7).

- **The indirect pathway** consists of neurons in the striatum projecting to the external segment of the globus pallidus (GPe), which inhibits the subthalamic nucleus (STN). This is a disinhibition of the STN. The STN excites the GPi/SNr complex, which inhibits the thalamus. This opposes the direct pathway and reduces activation of the cortex.

Both the direct and indirect pathways are modulated by the SNc, which uses the neurotransmitter dopamine. Dopamine release by the SNc amplifies activity in the direct pathway, increasing cortical activation of movement. Dopamine released by the SNc also reduces the effect of indirect pathway inhibition. The reduction of dopamine release in the case of Parkinson's disease causes people to lose their ability to initiate movement, because of both lowered activity of the direct pathway and reduced inhibition of the inhibitory indirect pathway.

Controlling Muscles: The Primary Motor Cortex

Many neurons in the motor cortex send their axons down the spinal cord and synapse on *alpha motor neurons* (the motor neurons that innervate muscle fibers; refer to Chapter 5) in a direct control pathway. This direct pathway allows fine, conscious control of muscles, particularly in the hands and fingers.

However, many other motor cortex neurons synapse on spinal interneurons and mediate their effects through spinal circuits. The primary motor cortex (Brodmann area 4; see Chapter 8) has neurons that control muscles directly through synapses on alpha motor neurons in the spinal cord. The primary motor cortex is the most posterior region of the frontal lobe, located just anterior to the central sulcus.

Among the characteristic histological features of primary motor cortex are:

✔ The primary motor cortex contains giant *pyramidal cells* (a common type of cortical neuron with a pyramid-shaped cell body) called *Betz cells* in layer V, which are less common elsewhere in the frontal lobe. Betz cells send their axons to alpha motor neurons in the ventral horn of the spinal cord in the corticospinal tract, accounting for about 10 percent of the descending projection.

✔ The primary motor cortex does not have *granule cells* that are typical in the input layer to most neocortex (layer IV). Because of this this part of neocortex is sometimes called *agranular*.

The homunculus

The primary motor cortex contains a distorted map of the body's muscles called a *homunculus*. This map is similar to the somatosensory map in the parietal cortex just posterior to (or behind) the central sulcus. The way this map functions suggests that it corresponds not to muscles as they're distributed, but to the movements mediated by those muscles. Single neurons in primarily the motor cortex can activate several muscles related to one joint and coordinate muscle activity associated with movement of the limb.

The distortion in the homunculus occurs because the size of the cortical representation of an area is proportional to the fineness of the neural control, not the area of the body. For example, the lips and face occupy a greater area of cortex than the thighs. (More than one discrete area may be associated with the fingers as well — one associated with the supplementary motor area [SMA], and the other with the premotor cortex [PMC] circuits, which are described later in this chapter.)

Population coding

Neurons in the primary motor cortex that control the arms are most active when the arms are reaching in a specific direction, but they respond for other directions near the "preferred" direction. The average of thousands of these units produces a much tighter directionality than could be specified by a single neuron via what's called a *population code*. Individual neurons can be regarded as vectors with a direction where their firing is at a maximum, and they fire proportionately less for movements in other directions. The average firing of all neurons then controls muscles to move a limb in the direction we want to move.

Coordinating Muscle Groups: Central Control

Almost every movement you make involves a sequence of at least dozens of different muscles. Try extending your arm out to the side. This movement is simple to do, but it still requires many muscles: Your trunk counterbalances the movement, and your legs muscles stabilize your body. Not so simple, is it?

Although the spinal cord is pretty good at coordinating ordinary movement, evolution has not yet programmed your body to dance the foxtrot, play hopscotch, or swim. Voluntary movements, especially new ones, require learning organized sequences of muscle commands. The next couple sections discuss the SMA internal motor control circuit that your brain uses to perform familiar tasks, and the PMC external control circuit that your brain uses to do new things.

The supplementary motor area and learned sequences

One way to look at the frontal lobe is that is has an axis of abstraction. The most abstract representations of your goals exist in prefrontal cortex, the most anterior part of the frontal lobe. The axons that drive muscles are in the primary motor cortex, the most posterior part of the frontal lobe, just anterior to somatosensory cortex, which has a matching homunculus.

The SMA is just anterior and medial to the primary motor cortex. Anterior to that (excluding the frontal eye fields) is the prefrontal cortex. Figure 8-3 shows a diagram of the cortex on the right, with the motor cortex stippled. Anterior and lateral to the primary motor cortex is the PMC.

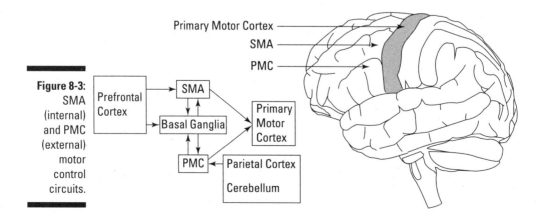

Figure 8-3: SMA (internal) and PMC (external) motor control circuits.

You can imagine that prefrontal cortex has the most abstract representation of some goal, like getting someone's attention across the room. You know that you could do this in many ways. You could call out, wave, walk over to the person, or send someone else over to her. Whatever option you choose (possibly involving input from the basal ganglia) must be translated into an appropriate sequence of commands for the specific muscles.

The prefrontal cortex is where the abstract plan originates. If you're going to do something you know how to do, you activate the SMA posterior to the prefrontal cortex, but just anterior to the primary motor cortex. Both prefrontal cortex and SMA communicate with the basal ganglia to choose what you're going to do. The SMA, which sits medially, opposite the motor areas for the limbs, then projects to the motor cortex to control exactly what muscles you're going to use.

The SMA is activated even if you just *imagine* doing something like moving your arms and legs, without actually doing it.

Externally monitored performance and the premotor cortex

When you're learning to do something new, you need sensory feedback from the parietal lobe somatosensory, visual, and even auditory areas. You also need feedback from the cerebellum, which monitors errors and learns timing sequences. When doing unfamiliar tasks, the input to the primary motor cortex comes more from the premotor cortex (PMC), which receives projections from parietal sensory areas and the cerebellum. The PMC lies more laterally on both sides of the brain to the SMA, where it is anterior to the primary motor cortex.

Besides projecting to primary motor cortex, the PMC also projects directly to the spinal cord and has reciprocal connections with the SMA. The PMC has a distinctive histological appearance — it has a granular layer IV that is distinct from the agranular primary motor cortex.

The frontal eye fields and superior colliculus

Anterior to the SMA is a cortical area called the *frontal eye fields* (FEF), which are involved in visual attention, initiating eye movements (voluntary *saccades*), which are the rapid movements your eyes make when going from one point to another, such as when you're reading. The FEF receive visual inputs in a pathway that starts with the retinal projection to the superior colliculus, which projects to the medial dorsal nucleus of the thalamus, then to the FEF cortex. The FEF contains a map that represents eye movement saccade targets. When neurons in the FEF are electrically stimulated, the eyes move to and look at areas of visual space that correspond to the stimulation point.

The superior colliculus is a midbrain nucleus that receives projections from nearly all retinal ganglion cells. In non-mammalian vertebrates, this structure is the main visual processing center, but in mammals it appears to mostly code for eye movements. Electrical stimulation of the superior colliculus, like the FEF, produces saccadic eye movements according to a well-defined map across its surface.

The Thalamus: Gateway to the Neocortex

The *thalamus,* the major part of the diencephalon, is the sensory gateway to the neocortex. The upcoming sections look at the ways in which different types of sensory input relay through the thalamus.

Reaching all the senses

All sensory input to the cortex — except some smells — relay through the thalamus. The output from the motor cortex on the way to the spinal cord or cranial nerves is also modulated by the thalamus by its inputs from the cerebellum and basal ganglia. Refer to Figure 8-1 to see where the thalamus is located (bilaterally, of course).

Seeing visual inputs

The visual input to the thalamus is the retinal projection to a region of the thalamus called the lateral geniculate nucleus (LGN; see Chapter 10 for more detail on the visual system). Although the way the LGN is organized varies considerably among mammals, most of them, including humans, have a LGN with several layers. The layers are dominated by inputs from two major types of retinal ganglion cell, which in primates are called

- ✔ **Parvocellular:** A small, continuously responding, and often color-coding cell
- ✔ **Magnocellular:** A larger, transient-responding and movement-sensitive cell

Visual neurobiologists sometimes call the LGN a "relay nucleus" because the LGN cells respond in a very similar manner to the retinal ganglion cells that innervate them. Also, the number of recipient cells in the LGN is about the same as the number of entering ganglion cell axons, giving a 1:1 input-to-output ratio.

Although the LGN relay cells don't greatly change the character of the responses passed on to the cortex, they do perform an important gating function. Inputs to the dLGN come from the brainstem reticular formation, and projections come back from the cortex to the dLGN. In fact, more synapses come back from the visual cortex to the dLGN than retinal input synapses.

These other inputs can weaken or strengthen some inputs within the visual domain, or modulate them against other senses. For example, suppose you're looking in the bushes for your yellow tennis ball. Everything yellow will jump to your visual attention. The fact that you're looking for something yellow is held in the working memory in your frontal lobes. The consciousness of your search for a round yellow ball highlights, like a spotlight, round yellow things in your field of view.

The relay neurons in the LGN project via an axon tract called the *optic radiation* to visual cortex area 17 (also called V1), at the back of the head, the pole of the occipital lobe. Most of the thalamic inputs to area 17 terminate in layer 4 of the six-layered visual cortex, as do thalamic inputs to cortex for other senses. The density of cells in the visual system is so high that cell stains in area 17 show a distinctive stripe in layer 4 and some other sub-layers. Because of this appearance, area 17 is called *striate* (for striped) *cortex*.

Listening for auditory inputs

The way auditory information reaches the thalamus is more complex than vision. The auditory nerve leaving the cochlea contains about 30,000 fibers that project to the cochlear nucleus in the brainstem at the junction between the pons and the medulla (parts of the brainstem; refer to Chapter 7). From there are the following projections:

1. **Neurons in the cochlear nucleus project to the superior olive.**

2. **The superior olive projects to the inferior colliculus in the midbrain.**

3. **The inferior colliculus projects to the medial geniculate nucleus of the thalamus.**

4. **This thalamic nucleus projects to the mid-superior temporal lobe (auditory area A1), in a region called Heschl's gyrus.**

The majority of auditory information from the left ear goes to the right cortex, and vice versa. However, unlike the visual system, some fibers that project this way in the auditory system are below the thalamus. These lower areas that receive both *ipsilateral* (from the same side) and *contralateral* (from the opposite side) ear input help to locate sound. To locate a sound, neural circuits compare the difference in loudness between the two ears, and the difference in when the sound arrives between the two ears. (See Chapter 10 for more on the auditory system and sound localization.)

Sampling taste inputs

Taste information from the tongue proceeds to the thalamus via two pathways: Information from the front and sides of the tongue projects via the chorda tympani nerve, while taste receptors at the back of the tongue project via the glossopharyngeal nerve. There are also some taste receptors in the mouth and larynx that project centrally through the vagus nerve. These three nerves project to the nucleus of the solitary tract in the brainstem (medulla), which projects to the ventral posteromedial nucleus of the thalamus (VPM). The VPM projects to cortical taste processing recipient zones in the insula and frontal operculum cortex.

Some taste information is also projected to the orbitofrontal cortex where, combined with smell information, it gives rise to the finer senses of food flavor. Tell that to your foodie friends at their next dinner party!

Feeling out touch inputs

The sense of touch involves multiple types of tactile perception, including vibration, motion across the skin, deep skin indentation, and skin sense modalities that are not really touch but other senses, such as temperature and pain. Touch information is tranduced by skin sensors that are the axons of dorsal root ganglion cells outside the spinal cord. Information from these sensors is relayed to the thalamus (ventral posterior nucleus) via two pathways:

- ✔ **The dorsal column–medial lemniscal pathway:** This pathway has large fibers that mediate fine-touch senses.
- ✔ **The spinothalamic pathway:** This is the pathway that transmits information about pain, temperature, and coarse touch.

Sniffing out olfactory inputs

Compared to the other types of sensory input, olfaction (the sense of smell) is the odd one out. Odor information from the olfactory bulb projects directly not only to several non-thalamic areas, but also to the cortex. Areas of the brain that receive direct inputs from the olfactory bulb include the amygdala, the orbitofrontal cortex, the piriform cortex, and the entorhinal cortex. The amygdala, orbitofrontal cortex, and piriform cortex project to a thalamic nucleus called the mediodorsal nucleus, which projects back to the orbitofrontal cortex (see Chapter 11 for more detail on the olfactory system).

Paying attention to the pulvinar

The *pulvinar* is a set of nuclei in the most posterior region of each thalamus. The subdivisions are medial, lateral, anterior, and inferior, each of which consists of several nuclei.

The superior colliculus projects to medial, lateral, and inferior pulvinar subdivisions and appears to be involved in mediating the focus of attention in the visual system, and controlling eye movements to prominent locations. These areas have extensive reciprocal connections with early visual cortical areas. For example, the dorso-lateral pulvinar interacts with posterior parietal cortex (the "where" or "how to" dorsal visual pathway). Medial pulvinar nuclei have extensive connections with premotor and prefrontal cortical areas, cingulate cortex, as well as posterior parietal cortex.

The pulvinar is larger and more extensively connected in humans compared to other mammals. It constitutes about 40 percent of the thalamus in humans, but is almost nonexistent in rodents and many other mammals. Pulvinar lesions in humans cause visual attention deficits.

Moving through motor pathways

The ventral lateral and ventral anterior nuclei of the thalamus make up its motor portion. The ventral lateral nucleus receives motor information from the globus pallidus internal segment of the basal ganglia, the substantia nigra pars reticulata, and the cerebellum. The ventral lateral nucleus projects to the motor cortex and the premotor cortex.

The motor portion of the thalamus projects information to the motor cortex for coordination, as well as planning and learning movements.

Reticular zones of the thalamus

The reticular formation that begins in the brainstem extends to the thalamus. The brain has a thalamic reticular nucleus, but reticular areas typically surround nuclei or extend into intralaminar zones. Neurons in the reticular areas are mostly *GABAergic* (use the inhibitory neurotransmitter GABA), and they work to modulate or gate functions on the nearby areas. They're almost exclusively interneurons that don't project out of the thalamus.

The thalamic reticular areas receive *afferent* (inward) input from the brainstem reticular formation and cortex, and project to various thalamic nuclei within the thalamus to regulate the flow of information through these to the cortex. The cortical input tends to select ascending inputs according to what is most salient or prominent within a sense, whereas the brainstem reticular input tends to switch attention between senses according to threats and immediate contingencies.

Focusing on Goals with the Prefrontal Cortex

The frontal lobes are the center of goal pursuit. Neurons in the primary motor cortex at the most posterior part of the frontal lobes send axons down the corticospinal tract to synapse on alpha motor neurons, which in turn drive muscle fibers. Anterior to the primary motor cortex are the SMA and PMC areas (refer to "Coordinating Muscle Groups: Central Control," earlier in this chapter) that organize and sequence groups of muscles to accomplish movement goals, such as running while bringing your tennis racquet back in readiness to stop and hit a forehand.

Anterior to SMA and PMC, which constitute Brodmann area 6 (BA6), is the region called the frontal eye fields, involved in visual attention. Everything anterior to these areas is called the *prefrontal cortex*. The frontal lobes constitute about 40 percent of the neocortex, and most of the frontal lobes consist of prefrontal cortex. The following sections explore what goes on in the prefrontal cortex.

Making plans with the lateral prefrontal cortex

The lateral prefrontal cortex is the maker of plans. Let's say it's the first day of fall and you decide you need a warmer coat. You need to make plans that include checking your budget, going to a store, going to the right part of the store when you get there. You could accomplish all these things in many ways, and you'll find many distractions around every action you take. Your prefrontal cortex processes sensory experience in light of your goals and sub-goals to direct your behavior. In order to do this it has to maintain a representation of your goals and interpret what's going on around you in light of those goals.

Neurons in the lateral prefrontal cortex receive projections from nearly the entire rest of the brain. These neurons feed back to the neurons that activate them. In the case of the coat you need, you may have decided it should be light colored and less than $200. Your prefrontal cortex maintains a resonant circuit in which the neural representations of these attributes in other parts of the brain remain mutually active. When you get to the store, you inhibit yourself from looking at dark coats, or coats costing more than $200.

Your behavior, including all your movements, is controlled by the set of goals represented in your prefrontal cortex. When this brain area is damaged, behavior becomes stimulus driven, not dependent on internal goals.

Processing emotions with the orbitofrontal cortex

Many of our plans and beliefs are rational and calculated. We may purchase a coat that we can afford and that will keep us warm. Any of a number of coats may satisfy this need equally. But we have other beliefs and behaviors that elicit strong emotions: Our love for our spouse or children moves us to take life-threatening risks for them. We're revolted when we witness animal cruelty. We're nervous when driving in rush-hour traffic.

The *orbitofrontal cortex* is the most ventral and anterior part of the prefrontal cortex. It's extensively connected to the amygdala, which is involved in memory for emotionally important events.

Damage to the orbitofrontal-amygdala system can result in sociopathic behavior in which the person is unable to feel empathy. It can also result in reckless behavior, such as excessive gambling, because the affected person doesn't have the normal fear associated with placing large, financially dangerous wagers.

Anterior and posterior cingulate cortex

The cingulate cortex is a sheet of mesocortex lying just above the corpus callosum and below the neocortex. The division between the anterior and posterior cingulate is about at the location of the central sulcus. Here's what each does:

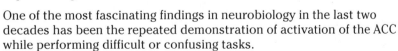

✔ **Anterior cingulate cortex (ACC):** The most dorsal portion (toward the front of the brain) of the ACC has reciprocal connections to prefrontal, motor, and parietal cortices. It is believed to be an executive controller that allocates processing priority among the connected brain areas. The ventral ACC has connections with the amygdala, insular cortex, hypothalamus, and nucleus accumbens. The ventral ACC is involved in processing emotional stimuli.

One of the most fascinating findings in neurobiology in the last two decades has been the repeated demonstration of activation of the ACC while performing difficult or confusing tasks.

✔ **The posterior cingulate cortex (PCC):** The area implicated in pain awareness and episodic memory. It's connected to the prefrontal cortex, the orbitofrontal cortex, and the parahippocampal gyrus (which feeds the hippocampus). The PCC is thought to be a crucial area in the "default mode" network of the brain. This network is active when a person is not concentrating on a specific task.

You find out much more about the frontal lobes and the rest of the neocortex in Chapter 9.

Knowing, or Not Knowing, Who's In Control

This chapter explains that motor activity can be driven by extrapyramidal inputs from the reticular formation of the medulla and pons that modulate motor activity without directly innervating motor neurons. Neurons in the reticular formation are, in turn, modulated by the basal ganglia, cerebellum, and sensory areas of the cerebral cortex, particularly the parietal lobe. This pathway is involved in reflexes, locomotion, and balance.

The chapter also talks about how neurons in the primary motor cortex, which directly activate alpha motor neurons, can themselves be activated by either the SMA or PMC cortical areas, both of which receive inputs from the prefrontal cortex and the basal ganglia.

So, who's in charge? It depends on the circumstances. If you trip while walking, the extrapyramidal system may control your arms, legs, and trunk. If you're trying to hit a high backhand tennis shot that you rarely practice, you may depend on your PMC. Turing the knob and opening the door to your house — which you do every day — probably mostly activates your SMA.

But you may feel that you perform some movements entirely voluntarily, decided by the real "you" somewhere in the brain, like deciding to get up and get some ice cream from the freezer. Certainly you're aware of this thought stirring you to action. But maybe the thought existed before you were aware of it? Perhaps you were slightly hungry, but you hadn't clued in yet. Perhaps a sound you heard or something you saw had an association with eating ice cream that you had forgotten. Your blood sugar may be low, or some unconscious brain activity may have re-created the fact that you bought a new ice cream flavor yesterday but hadn't remembered until now.

Cold-blooded vertebrates that have basal ganglia but little or no neocortex have a limited repertoire of complex behaviors that generally don't depend much on learning. Mammals in general, primates in particular, and humans specifically have a large number of complex behaviors, and they learn new ones throughout their lifetimes. Nevertheless, the selection among these behaviors remains embedded in old neural circuits, including the basal ganglia, but now within complex memories and hierarchical goal systems.

The control system is hierarchical and distributed, but only one motor program can control the muscles at a time. You can't hit a forehand and a backhand at the same time — you have to choose. You're aware of the choice, certainly, but not everything that may have gone into it.

Chapter 9

Topping It Off: The Neocortex

. . . .

. . . .

*I*f you picture the hierarchy of brain processing, the neocortex is at the summit. It's the neural circuit area that is most enlarged in mammals, and it allows us to set goals, change our minds and plans when we need to, and store memories that inform future decisions. Thanks to the development of the neocortex, humans evolved into the intelligent (well, mostly) and adaptable creatures we are today. In this chapter, I tell you all about this important part of the brain.

You're probably aware that your brain has two sides, or *hemispheres* — one left and one right. The left side of the brain generally receives inputs from and controls the right side of the body, while the right side of the brain interacts with the left side. In this chapter, you meet your two hemispheres and I tell you more about what they do. I also discuss the differences that exist between the male and female brain.

Looking Inside the Skull: The Neocortex and Its Lobes

When we look at a human brain from above or from the side, we see virtually all neocortex, with the cerebellum sticking out from the back of the brainstem below the occipital lobe. Neurobiologists divide the neocortex into four lobes (see Figure 9-1):

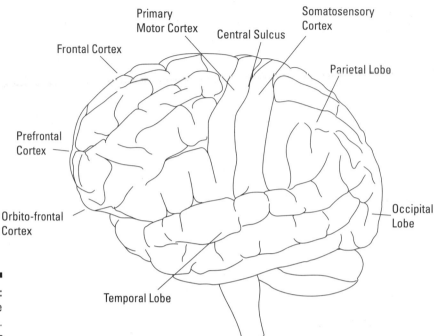

Primary
Motor Cortex

Somatosensory
Cortex

Central Sulcus

Frontal Cortex

Parietal Lobe

Prefrontal
Cortex

Orbito-frontal
Cortex

Occipital
Lobe

Figure 9-1:
Lobes of the
neocortex.

Temporal Lobe

✔ **Frontal:** The frontal lobe is the output of the brain because its most posterior part is the primary motor cortex, which controls voluntary movement. It extends from the most anterior part of the brain behind the forehead to a groove near the middle of the brain called the *central sulcus.* Anterior areas of the frontal lobe (prefrontal cortex) are concerned with plans and contingencies. These areas project to premotor areas such as the supplementary motor area and premotor cortex, which then project to the primary motor cortex. Neurons in the primary motor cortex project directly to motor neurons throughout the head and body.

✔ **Parietal:** The parietal lobe begins at the central sulcus and extends posteriorly to the occipital lobe at the back of the head, and to its ventral border with the temporal lobe. The parietal lobe does sensory processing of visual, auditory, and *somatosensory* (relating to bodily sensations) inputs. One of the main functions of the parietal lobe is processing sensory inputs to enable sensory feedback for movement. It's also essential for our awareness of personal space and the space around us.

✔ **Temporal:** The temporal lobe has (at least) three main divisions:

  • The superior portion of this lobe processes auditory information that then projects to higher-order levels in the parietal lobe.

  • The inferior temporal lobe processes visual information for object identification in what's called the "what" pathway, which allows us to identify objects.

- The medial wall of the temporal lobe has a high-level visual area at the anterior pole called the *fusiform face area* that processes faces and other complex visual stimuli. The medial temporal lobe also has projections to the hippocampus for memory and limbic lobe structures such as the insula.

✔ **Occipital:** The occipital lobe is almost totally visual. It contains the primary visual cortex V1, and several higher-order visual areas such as V2 and V3. Although neurons in the occipital lobe are driven by visual input from the retina-dLGN pathway (refer to Chapter 8), V1 can still be activated in blind people when they're tasked with identifying somato-sensory patterns, such as when reading Braille.

Although the central sulcus forms an obvious division between the frontal and parietal lobes in most human brains, the parietal and occipital and temporal lobes have no such obvious border between them.

Most functional brain areas extend down into the *sulci* (grooves), which comprise a large percentage of the total neocortical area (about 2,400 square centimeters, or about 2.5 square feet). Functional areas may extend over different *gyri* (ridges or folds) and sulci. In general, we can't say that one function is restricted to one particular gyrus or sulcus.

Illustrations of the brain typically show sections (cuts) that can be in one of three right-angled planes, as shown in Figure 9-2:

✔ **Horizontal section:** A horizontal section is, as its name implies, parallel to the ground.

✔ **Sagittal section:** A sagittal section is a cut from front to back. The most common sagittal section is along the midline of the brain, dividing it into roughly mirror-symmetrical left and right halves.

✔ **Coronal section:** A coronal section cuts the brain in a plane roughly parallel to the forehead (in the plane of the corona that is often around the head in medieval religious paintings).

Each of these section planes has advantages for showing areas of the neocortex and various subcortical structures. One thing that they all show is that the neocortex consists of a thin 2- to 4-millimeter gray area on the surface, with a much larger white area below. The gray matter is where the neuronal cell bodies are located in the neocortex, whereas the white matter is almost pure axon tracts.

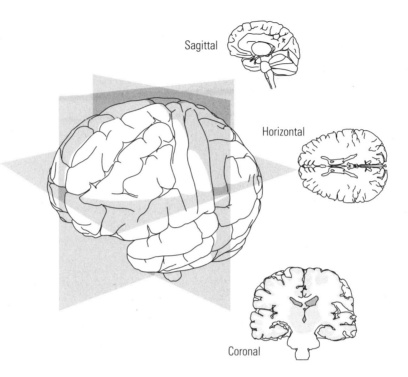

Sagittal

Horizontal

Figure 9-2:
Three ways
to section
brain.

Coronal

Noticing uniform structure and circuits

One of the most important organizational principles of the neocortex is that it has a standard, six-layered structure almost everywhere. Figure 9-3 shows a small region of the neocortex consisting of a sulcus between two gyri (left). The gray matter is a thin 2- to 4-millimeter-deep sheet of neurons sitting on top of the white matter axons.

Big brains

The larger the brain, the more white matter it has. Why? Suppose that in the brain, every neuron were directly connected to every other neuron. If the number of neurons were to grow, the number of axons would have to increase as the square of the number of neurons. Connecting every one of the 100 billion neurons in the human brain to every other neuron would require a white matter volume the size of a house!

The brain solves this problem by having any given neuron connected to a few thousand other neurons (on average), with the densest connections to nearby neurons, so that most axonal lengths are short. A finite number of major axon tracts project information long distances in the brain. Information is highly compressed in these projections. For example, about one million visual axons from the thalamus drive about 200 million cortical neurons in V1.

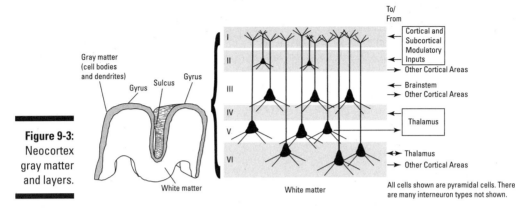

Figure 9-3: Neocortex gray matter and layers.

Axons in the white matter are of three major types:

- ✔ Axons from subcortical parts of the brain projecting to the neocortex
- ✔ Axons from the neocortex projecting to subcortical structures
- ✔ Cortical–cortical connections

The right side of Figure 9-3 is an illustration of the gray matter. The fundamental neuronal type in the neocortex is the pyramidal cell, which is the only cell type illustrated in the figure. The axons of the pyramidal cells comprise virtually all the long-distance excitatory *glutamatergic* (using glutamate) connections in the neocortex. Numerous other cells (not shown in Figure 9-3) make up the local interneuron population. Most of these, other than the excitatory stellate cells, are inhibitory, and use GABA as a neurotransmitter (see Chapter 3 for a discussion of neurotransmitters).

The types of cells in the six layers and in the inputs into and out of these layers are pretty much the same across the neocortex. This is remarkable given that the neocortex processes inputs from very different senses and produces movements all using the same neuronal circuit.

Communicating with the diencephalon and the rest of the nervous system

Cortical–cortical connections typically terminate in layers I and II. These cortical–cortical axons arise from these two layers as well as layers III and VI. In sensory areas, inputs to cortex usually come from the thalamus into layer IV. Layer VI also projects back to the thalamus.

Figure 9-4 shows a few of the connections between thalamus and cortex, and within cortex, in what is sometimes called a *canonical neocortical circuit.* Thalamic relay cells send excitatory connections to cortical layer IV stellate cells, which excite neurons in layers above and below layer IV. Other cortical interneurons (not shown in Figure 9-4) carry both feed-forward and feedback inhibition within the cortex. Intracortical circuits also exhibit mutual excitation that must be balanced by inhibitory pathways.

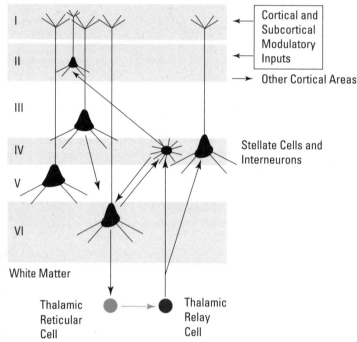

Figure 9-4:
Thalamic–
cortical
connections.

Cortex layer VI (typically) feeds back to the thalamic reticular area cells that may inhibit thalamic relay cells. Connections to other cortical layers usually arise and terminate in upper layers.

Neurobiologists generally assume that, given a common circuit, the neocortex produces a common neuronal computation on its input. A given area of cortex seems to be able to process a set number of inputs. This implies that when more sensory cells are in an area of skin, or retina, or anywhere else for higher *resolution,* the brain uses more cortical area to process the larger number of inputs.

More complex computations require more cortical areas. Each area processes the input from the lower area, extracts some information, and sends its output to the next area, building up a hierarchy of selectivity. In the visual system, for example, as one moves from V1 (primary visual cortex) to V4 and higher levels in the ventral object identification "what" stream for identifying objects and faces, receptive fields get larger and can include most of the visual field. However, selectivity gets higher for particular features, such as responding only to faces.

Using a single circuit for all sensory and motor neural computation is one of the most remarkable traits of mammals. Many neurobiologists believe that it's the key to mammals' success and the ultimate generator of human intelligence and consciousness. How the neocortex arose in relation to the rest of the brain is the subject of the next section.

Getting to the Brain You Have Today: The Neocortex versus Your Reptilian Brain

The idea of an evolutionarily layered *triune brain* (the model developed by American neuroscientist Paul D. MacLean) is a historically popular account of how the brain functions. The triune brain consists of three sequentially evolved systems:

✔ **The reptilian complex (basal ganglia):** Thought to have arisen first, and believed to control typical instinctual behaviors, such as territorial aggression and dominance

✔ **The paleomammalian complex (limbic system):** Thought to control emotion and motivation for feeding and reproductive behavior

✔ **The neomammalian complex (neocortex):** Arising in mammals, this system is thought to permit abstract planning and, ultimately in humans, language

Although many details of the triune brain idea are not quite correct, it does explain brain function based on evolution and hierarchical control. Previous chapters of this book deal with the function of the *basal ganglia* (reptilian brain — refer to Chapter 8) and *limbic system* (paleomammalian brain — refer to Chapter 7). Here, we look at the *neocortex* (neomammalian complex).

The two major ideas about how the neocortex relates to the rest of the brain may appear to be contradictory, but may not actually be:

✔ The first idea, taken from the triune brain and similar models, is that the neocortex sits at the apex of a controller hierarchy. It sets the big-picture goals and procedures, and allows lower levels to take care of the details.

✔ The second idea views the neocortex much like a set of subroutines in a computer program. The "main" procedure in subcortical areas is actually the sequence controller, but the neocortex "calls" subroutines (particular computational areas of neocortex) for doing detailed calculations at high resolution.

Which of these views is right? I argue that both are correct, and that the neocortex and some subcortical areas may interact to control behavior.

Imagine you're deciding to take a trip. The decision involves information that you have in your neocortex about various ways to travel, such as by car or by plane. The decision also involves goals about what you expect to gain from the trip, and your current state of affairs (money in your bank account, vacation time). Dealing with all this conflict almost certainly involves the anterior cingulate cortex (which is mesocortex, not neocortex) and the thalamus. In a sense, these various motor programs "bid" on carrying out the task, with subcortical brain structures using memory and information from the neocortex to decide exactly what to do. An illustration of this is shown in Figure 9-5.

Deciding How to Go from Point A to Point B

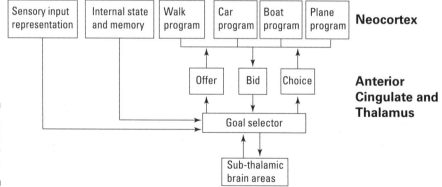

Figure 9-5:
Neocortex:
controller or
subroutine?

This is a hierarchical system because the details of how to carry out tasks in various ways reside in the neocortex. If you were monitoring brain activity while a person was taking a plane from point A to point B, you would say that areas of the frontal lobe of the neocortex were controlling the procedure. But also true is that the method of transport you use (a plane) and the alternatives you take within that method (which flight to take, choosing the window or aisle seat) are decided by lower-level brain systems with input from the neocortex. In that sense the relationship between subcortical and cortical levels is more like the former calling subroutines in the latter.

Looking at how cortical areas developed

The neocortex develops by precursor stems cells migrating along the radial glia from the neural plate in an embryo's outermost layer of cells — the *ectoderm*. This generation region is called the *ventricular zone,* because it's next to the ventricles. Neural stem cells located in the ventricular zone are called *progenitor cells.* Progenitor cells divide asymmetrically, with one daughter cell remaining a progenitor, while the other cell migrates and differentiates into glia and neurons.

The first progenitor cells to specialize are glia whose fibers are radial and span out from the ventricular zone to the outer, pial surface. These radial processes provide scaffolding for later progenitor cell divisions to migrate outward from the ventricular zone to their destination layer. The last progenitor cell division produces daughter cells that differentiate into glial or *ependymal cells* (special glial cells that line the ventricles).

The developmental sequence is "inside out," with layers closest to the neural plate (starting with layer VI) developing first. Later, stem cells' daughters migrate through the developed layers to differentiate in more superficial layers.

The radial glia are thought to determine how cortical minicolumns are organized. A *cortical minicolumn* is a vertical column through the cortical thickness, comprising about 100 neurons. Its diameter is about 30 to 40 micrometers. The human brain has about 200 million minicolumns.

Evidence suggests that minicolumns may be narrower and denser in autistic children than they are in children who are developing normally.

Enlarging the frontal lobes for complex behavior

Mammals increased their brains' abilities to do complex computations by developing and expanding the neocortex. One aspect of the success of the neocortex is its uniform organization. The same neural circuit is used to increase resolution in everything from processing visual detail to sequencing muscle movements.

Neocortical resolution is enhanced in two ways:

- ✔ **The area devoted to a task increases the resolution at which a limited number of computations are done *within in a particular area.*** For example, in the visual system, animals with larger numbers of retinal ganglion cells have a primary visual cortex with more area — so much so that the area of visual cortex per ganglion cells is about the same. Within the primary visual cortex, attributes such as orientation, *binocular stereopsis* (where each eye gets a slightly different image due to its position), and color are among the characteristics that are extracted everywhere within one area.

- ✔ **Resolution is increased in the *kinds of discriminations* that can be performed by *increasing the number of distinct cortical areas involved.*** Each area does a limited set of feature extractions. These features are fed into the next area, which starts with those features as a basis and extracts even more complex features.

In evolution, this ability of cortical tissue to expand its area for discriminating higher resolutions, and expand in multiple areas for more complex kinds of discriminations, allowed mammals to dominate among land animals. Mammals that depended on their sense of smell increased olfactory areas, while visual animals increased visual ones.

Setting and accomplishing goals

Primates (monkeys, apes, humans) increased the neocortex — specifically, the frontal and prefrontal cortex. Figure 9-6 shows the relative sizes of the neocortex in the cat, rhesus monkey, chimpanzee, and human. The prefrontal cortex in each is in a darker shade. Prefrontal cortex increases as a percent of total cortex, as well as in absolute area, from non-primates to primates, and from monkeys to apes to humans.

As I discuss in Chapter 8, the prefrontal cortex is the seat of abstract planning, goals, and reasoning. It's also the home of working memory, allowing us to keep complex ideas in mind. For example, if you're setting the table for dinner, your brain needs to access the sequence of tasks that will take you from start to finish, as you're doing each task. Prefrontal cortex moves us from having actions that are largely reactive and dependent on stimulus to having plans that are more flexible and driven by our goals.

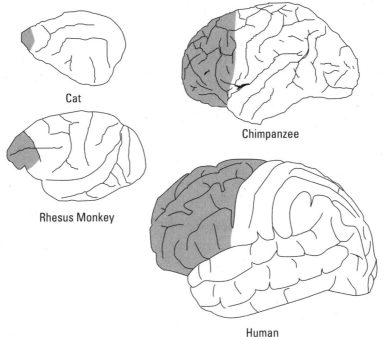

Cat

Chimpanzee

Rhesus Monkey

Figure 9-6:
The evolution of the prefrontal cortex.

Human

The prefrontal cortex is the entire frontal lobe anterior to the following areas:

- **Primary motor cortex:** Neurons in this area send their axons down the spinal cord and synapse on alpha motor neurons that activate muscle fibers.

- **Supplementary motor and premotor cortices:** These areas organize groups of muscles to accomplish specific tasks.

- **The frontal eye fields:** This area controls eye movements and is involved in visual attention.

The frontal lobe overall constitutes about 40 percent of the neocortex, and most of that is prefrontal. The prefrontal cortex is divided into dorso-lateral prefrontal cortex and ventro-medial (orbitofrontal) cortex. These two frontal-lobe areas are the topic of the next sections.

Making Decisions: The Lateral Prefrontal Cortex

Humans don't always live in the present. We think about the future — such as considering where to go for lunch tomorrow — and we think about the past — such as when cringing at an embarrassing moment that happened the night before. This ability allows people to make plans with a complex hierarchy of goals and subgoals, and modify these plans as we carry them out if things don't go as expected.

The *dorso-lateral prefrontal cortex* enables the brain to represent information that is not in your current environment, right in front of you. It's generally associated with what's called *working memory* (what you purposely keep in your mind to complete a task). Working memory is necessary not only to remember what you're doing, but, equally importantly, to prevent you from being distracted by irrelevant stimuli and thoughts. This ability to use a representation of your goal to stay focused underlies all higher executive functions.

Keeping it all in mind

The function of the prefrontal cortex is executive because it controls the flow of information in other brain structures. For example, suppose a friend asks you for directions to a local restaurant. Neurons in the prefrontal cortex must maintain an auditory image of the spoken request, translate this auditory image into an image of the restaurant, and then, while maintaining that image, begin constructing images of the streets and turns between here and there. All the time you're giving directions, you must maintain an image of the goal of the directions, and where you are in the sequence of steps.

Changing your plans

People with damage to their frontal lobes have particular trouble changing strategies according to circumstances. A common neurological test for frontal lobe damage is the Wisconsin Card Sorting Test.

For this test, cards in a deck have varying numbers of objects that are of particular colors and shapes. Subjects are told to draw cards one a time and guess how to sort them. The examiner keeps a secret rule in mind, such as "sort by color," and only tells the person whether his or her choice is right or wrong. Virtually all people, including frontal-lobe patients, quickly figure out what the rule is and begin to sort properly after a few tries. However, after the patient gets a certain number right, the examiner changes the secret rule (for example, sort by number of objects on the card). After a few tries, most people figure out that the rule has changed, but frontal-lobe patients persevere and have great difficulty on the rule switches.

The ability to follow complex abstract goals involves making a series of decisions about what actions are currently appropriate for that goal, and which are not. For example, if you're driving in slow traffic to an appointment and running late, one response is to drive faster. Full frontal-lobe development causes you to weigh the usually minor problem of being late against the possibility of a speeding ticket or, worse, car accident.

If you've ever griped about teenage drivers, you won't be shocked to know that axons in the frontal lobes are the last parts of the brain to be fully myelinated (wrapped with a glial process, such as from an oligodendrocyte), usually not until the end of the teenage years. So, a teenage driver is someone controlling a car without a fully developed frontal lobe.

Dialing that number: Working memory

The concept of a working memory is derived from an older concept of short-term memory. The classic example of short-term memory is holding a phone number in mind just long enough to dial it.

The reason phone numbers have seven digits is because of research by George Miller, a cognitive psychologist at Princeton University, on short-term memory. His research showed that seven digits was about the maximum amount most people could remember for a short period of time.

The Atkinson–Shriffin idea of the memory proposed in 1968 is one of the classic models of memory. It follows a sequence of three steps:

1. **Sensory (iconic) memory:** The dorso-lateral prefrontal cortex establishes a visual image or sequence of sounds in a buffer, called a *sensory* or *iconic memory*. The memory is specific to the sense you experienced it with (visual or auditory).

2. **Short-term memory:** You hold the iconic memory in your mind just long enough to use it. As this iconic memory is fading, the process of attention and rehearsal can retain about seven items in a short-term memory store.

3. **Long-term memory:** With sufficient rehearsal, or through encountering the image or sound sequence again, the memory begins to move into long-term memory.

Late 20th-century memory research revealed several problems with the Atkinson-Shriffin model. One is that information can get into long-term memory without consciously being rehearsed in short-term memory. But a more fundamental problem is with how things get into the focus of attention associated with short-term memory. The classic model supposes that this comes only from the most immediately recent sensory experience.

However, suppose I asked you to tell me about your first car. You would summon information about the car from your long-term memory, a neural buffer that allows you to answer factual and hypothetical questions about the car. Most neurobiologists believe this is the same buffer used in classical short-term memory. They also believe that this buffer is located in the frontal lobes — specifically, the lateral prefrontal cortex.

Neurons have been recorded in the lateral prefrontal cortex that appear to have the properties necessary for representing working memory. The following test has been done with monkeys, who are non-human primates. The monkey was presented with an image for less than a second. He was trained to wait until a "go" signal, and then he could do something based on the stimulus to get a reward. Neurons recorded in the lateral prefrontal cortex didn't fire during the stimulus; they only began firing when the stimulus was removed, and continued firing the entire time until the go signal (this was a variable interval). These neurons then stopped firing at the go signal when the monkey reached for the reward.

Another property of neurons in the lateral prefrontal cortex is that they're connected with virtually the entire rest of the brain. Although we don't know the connectivity of the neurons described in the monkey test, we can imagine the following scenario: If the stimulus is a green square in the upper-left corner of a card, active neurons in visual cortex that code these properties would be set up in a reverberant circuit by the lateral prefrontal neurons. In this way, the prefrontal neurons controlled the existence of the monkey's mental image of the green square in the upper left, which he used to press the right key to get the reward.

Recalling that number: Long-term memory and executive control

One of the most famous projects in the history of neuroscience is Lashley's search for the *memory engram,* the location in the brain of memories. Lashley, an American psychologist working in the early 20th century, found that when any particular part of a rat's brain was marked by lesions, its memory of how to run a maze remained intact. So, he concluded (mostly erroneously) that memories were not stored in any one part of the brain, but distributed throughout the brain.

Lashley's conclusions were wrong mostly because he didn't understand rat biology. Rats have multiple sensory representations of a maze that they can use to re-navigate it. They can remember it visually, recall the smell of various portions, remember moving in straight lines versus turns, and perhaps even recall certain sounds associated with the maze. Small brain lesions are likely to take out only one sensory modality. Even large brain lesions are unlikely to take out all of them. The rats' navigation system is multiplexed and, therefore, redundant, but it's not distributed throughout the brain.

However, within one sensory modality, the situation is more complicated. Data about the function of the hippocampus show that it's very important to forming long-term memories. But long-term memories aren't stored in the hippocampus; instead, they're stored in the cortical areas that were originally active in processing the stimulus that a person is remembering. (Refer to Chapter 7 for more about memory and the hippocampus.)

It's unclear how the cortical system that represents a stimulus changes so we can store it as memory, all the while preserving our ability to factually represent new stimuli. The process of creating long-term storage involves reciprocal activation from the hippocampus and seems to occur particularly during REM sleep. Presumably, the areas of the sensory system that were originally activated by the sensory input are the ones altered, but we do not, in fact, know in any detail. (Refer to Chapter 7 for more about the different stages of sleep and their effects on our brains.)

Doing the Right Thing

Have you ever caught yourself remembering something funny, and then realized that you were actually chuckling out loud? You probably have — we all do — but wouldn't it be awkward if that happened during a business meeting or in the middle of a church service? We all experience various urges. Most of these urges are okay in some circumstances, but highly inappropriate in other circumstances. The next sections look at how we know which behaviors are appropriate, and how we suppress those that aren't.

Responding with the orbitofrontal cortex and learned emotional reactions

Virtually all mammals are born fearing certain things, such as snakes, very large birds, spiders, and heights. Many of these fears are probably present in non-mammalian vertebrates as well, and may be built into portions of the limbic system.

Other fears, however, are not innate and we need to learn them, such as fear of exposed electric wires or a certain expression on your boss's face. Knowing to avoid the dangers of complex human society requires

✔ The ability to accurately represent the circumstances that present a threat

✔ The ability to remember the salient aspects of threat circumstances so that the memory will guide future behavior

Earlier in this chapter I discuss the lateral prefrontal cortex in the context of working memory (refer to "Dialing that phone number: Working memory," earlier in this chapter). Working memory maintains current and past sensory input and goals, which allows us to carry out our plans.

The orbitofrontal cortex also holds a kind of working memory. However, the orbitofrontal cortex is particularly concerned with behavior that has a learned or social dimension with negative costs (embarrassment or shame, for example). It also interacts with consciousness indirectly by giving you an intuitive, gut feeling that something is about to go wrong.

Damage to the lateral prefrontal cortex results in the inability to alter plans or strategies according to circumstances. Damage to the orbitofrontal cortex results in the inability to inhibit inappropriate behavior. For example, patients with orbitofrontal damage typically engage in risky behavior such as gambling or unsound investments. Some tend to use excessive and inappropriate profanity and otherwise act in a way that makes them social outcasts. Patients with severe orbitofrontal damage may be unable to experience empathy for the pain of others, and in extreme cases, can be sociopaths.

Another orbitofrontal damage syndrome is called *utilization behavior.* If some of these patients are left alone in a room with a bucket of paint and a paint-brush, they may begin painting the walls. Orbitofrontal damage takes away a person's ability to have a "gut feeling," which we all get when experiencing the urge to do something we know is inappropriate given the circumstances. The orbitofrontal cortex seems to be particularly involved in representing the memory of situations that may have negative outcomes, particularly social situations. The representation function of the orbitofrontal cortex depends on its interaction with its specific memory device, the amygdala.

Getting that bad feeling: The amygdala, emotional learning, and cortical connections

The lateral prefrontal cortex holds the context of a given situation in working memory, so the hippocampus can generate a context-sensitive memory of the most important parts of an experience. Just anterior to the hippocampus is another structure in the limbic system called the *amygdala.* The amygdala works with the orbitofrontal cortex to learn and recall situations that warn us of negative consequences.

Patients with amygdala damage have difficulties with things like

- Learning that certain situations predict bad consequences
- Identifying fearful facial expressions
- Reacting normally and automatically to gruesome or threatening scenes — such as the scene of a car accident or a gun being pointed at them

The difference between orbitofrontal and amygdala damage is the learning aspect. Patients with damaged amygdalae can have normal fear responses to intrinsically threatening scenarios such as snakes or heights. But they don't learn or experience fear of things normal people learn to fear, such as risky gambling bets and socially inappropriate behavior. Patients with orbitofrontal damage may even lack fear responses to things they rationally know are dangerous.

Going with your gut

One aspect of behavior that sums the frontal lobe is *approach-withdrawal behavior.* You can think of many situations as things to either avoid or seek out, because things to avoid have negative consequences, while things to seek out have rewards.

A left-right brain asymmetry seems to exist with approach-withdrawal behavior. The left prefrontal cortex appears to be approach oriented, so damage to this area tends to cause depression and withdrawal. The right prefrontal cortex appears to be withdrawal oriented, so damage to it can cause, at least in some cases, manic behavior.

The contrast seems to be stronger for the orbitofrontal than the prefrontal cortex. The orbitofrontal cortex communicates its "computation" of approach-withdrawal judgments unconsciously, through gut feelings. This shows that emotions don't just stem from some evolutionarily old part of the brain that is inferior to the rational portion. In fact, emotions can be the result of complexly represented, very real, learned experiences. Even if an emotion isn't communicated by a rational, verbal thought representation, gut feelings themselves can be quite rational.

Gut feelings can tell you when your behavior in a social group is unacceptable, even when no one tells you. Although you aren't aware of it, your brain is constantly processing the facial expressions, tones of voice, and body language of those around you. Similarly, when learning to play a new game, you may get the feeling that your strategy won't work out, even if you can't rationally explain the feeling. The orbitofrontal-amygdala system provides an intelligence that cannot be put into words for situations involving rewards and risks. This intelligence is highly complex and certainly not a throwback to a more primitive brain.

Seeing Both Sides: The Left and Right Hemispheres

When you look at a human brain you can see an obvious mirror-symmetry between the left and right halves. As I mention throughout this book, the left half of the brain tends to deal with the right side of the body, and vice versa.

Nothing is perfect. If you look carefully at any particular brain, it will almost never be totally symmetrical in the pattern of its gyri and sulci.

Figure 9-7 shows a view from the side of the left half of the brain (top), and a mid-sagittal section of the interior of the right half of the brain (bottom). The numbers are the designations according to the German anatomist Korbinian Brodmann in the early 1900s.

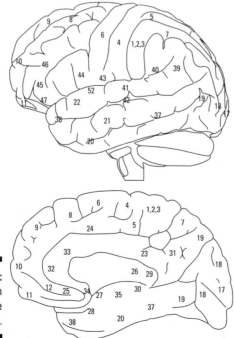

Figure 9-7:
Brodmann areas of the neocortex.

Although the two brain hemispheres are nearly mirror-symmetrical in how they look, asymmetries do exist between the left and right hemispheres. Virtually all right-handed people (greater than 95 percent) and the majority of left-handed people (about 60 percent) have most of their language function on the left side of the brain. The right hemisphere is much more competent at handling spatial skills. Since the French physician Pierre Paul Broca found language localized to the left hemisphere in the 1800s, neurobiologists have wondered about the origin and meaning of left–right functional brain asymmetries.

Specializing for language

Two areas of the brain known to be left-specialized for language are Broca's area (around areas 44 and 45 in Figure 9-7) and Wernicke's area (near the area marked 39 in Figure 9-7). Broca's area is in the frontal lobe, near the premotor cortex area that controls the speech apparatus. As its location implies, it's particularly important for producing speech.

Broca's area

Two reasons exist for why Broca's area is on one side only:

- ✓ Speech involves control of muscles like the tongue and vocal cords on the center line of the body, whose operation in speech uses symmetrical motor control on both the left and right sides.

- ✓ Interhemispheric communication is slow, making it particularly difficult to produce rapid speech. And given the brains' symmetrical control aspects, one side of the brain came to dominate speech production.

Wernicke's area

Wernicke's area is at the junction of the temporal and parietal lobes, near the angular gyrus. This area is a high-order audio-processing region and receives input that starts in the primary auditory cortex (Heschl's gyrus in mid-superior temporal lobe) and passes through high-order auditory association cortex around the primary cortex. Damage to Wernicke's area does not interfere with rapid speech production, but the speech produced doesn't make sense. Damage to this area also compromises speech comprehension.

Interestingly, the homologous area of the right hemisphere to Wernicke's in the left appears to be involved in processing meaningful intonations in speech. Patients with damage to this area can understand speech, but they lack the ability to "get" ironic and other tones of voice.

Taking in the big picture: Spatial processing

The right side of the brain appears to be superior to the left in processing visual imagery and visual attention. Damage to the right parietal lobe prevents people from paying attention to things in the left visual field. After a stroke in that location, a patient may forget to shave the left side of his face, or hit the left side of the garage with her car.

An area in the right medial temporal lobe called the *fusiform face area* is crucial for recognizing faces. However, damage to the homologous area on the left side doesn't affect facial recognition.

Managing with two brains in one head

Several years ago, pop psychology was full of ideas to help us "get in touch" with the creative right sides of our brains that had been supposedly repressed by formal education's emphasis on left-brain activities. Fortunately, much of this talk has died down. It's preposterous, for example, to think that writing poetry or fiction, a left-brain language skill, does not involve high creativity.

The reality about brain lateralization is that the beginnings of such specialization are phylogenetically very old, appearing even in birds. Song production in songbirds relies more on structures in the left sides of their brains that the right, for example. Lateral specialization is more extreme in humans, mostly because of language. But each side of the brain gives us unique capabilities, and we use both sides. This is an advantage, as I discuss in the next section.

Appreciating the style of each hemisphere

Instead of thinking of the right hemisphere as good and the left as bad, or the right as creative and the left as not, consider what scientific evidence says about the difference between the two sides. Some of the original findings about hemispheric asymmetry suggested that the right hemisphere is more holistic, and the left is more analytical.

Holistic processing

Holistic processing deals with the "big picture" and categorizes by the whole. For example, you can recognize your friend's face even if he shaves off his moustache or puts on sunglasses. In fact, in a casual encounter with someone you know, you may not even notice these changes. The right hemisphere appears to operate in a case-based style of reasoning, identifying people by matching the current stimulus to the set of people you know.

Analytical processing

Analytical processing is rule based. It looks at particular features individually. For example, if you were asked to describe a stranger at a crime scene, you would likely be asked to go through a set of attributes: height, weight, skin color, gender, age, and so forth. The police would search for their suspect based on this set of criteria.

Processing by rules

The relevance of this to brain operation is that language is a rule-based system. It's a sequence of discrete words with definable meanings that get strung together according to rules of grammar. The word definitions and grammar types must be put together to extract the meaning. This is a left-brain type of skill. Some have argued that it's similar to using the dominant right hand (controlled by the left hemisphere) to perform a sequence of specific steps to make a tool or throw a fastball.

Remembering the layout of a scene, however, requires a more literal memory of spatial relationships — describing a scene isn't easy to do using rules because you have to account for metrics such as distances and sizes. The holistic right brain seems to be able to discriminate differences between faces, or between poodles and terriers, even though the parts of the objects being compared are more or less the same, and more or less in the same locations, as one would describe using language. For example, a rule-based description of a face would go something like this: Fred has two eyes above a nose in the middle, above a mouth, also in the middle. This description doesn't help you to distinguish Frank from Fred.

Epilepsy and split brain surgery

The so-called "split brain" operations that were done in the late 1950s to limit epileptic seizures revealed a lot about differences between brain hemispheres in humans. The operations typically involved completely sectioning the *corpus callosum* (the 200-million-axon fiber tract that connects the neocortex on the left with the right). At first, after the operations, the patients showed almost no difference in behavior, except that they had far fewer seizures. I remember reading a magazine article at the time quoting a neurosurgeon who said (I hope jokingly!) that perhaps the function of the corpus callosum was to conduct epileptic seizures from one side of the brain to the other.

More careful experiments showed that information about stimuli transiently presented to the left visual field, which goes to the right half of the brain, cannot reach the left hemisphere. The split-brain subject cannot verbally say anything about the stimulus. However, he can point to a matching picture with his left hand, controlled by the informed right brain. These patients were also much better at solving spatial puzzles with their left hands, controlled by the right hemisphere, than by their right hands.

Gender and the Brain

Economist Larry Summers famously got himself in very hot water when, as president of Harvard University in 2005, he suggested that given the differences between male and female brains, it may be no accident that most professors in departments like physics were male. So, what are the differences between male and female brains, and what do these differences mean?

Sizing up the male and female brain

The first difference that we cannot dispute is average brain size. Males have an average brain volume of about 1,260 cm^3; women, around 1,130 cm^3. Although the brain does scale with physical size, the brains of men average about 100 g more than those of women of the same size. However, given the large variation in brain size and measures of intelligence, a 100 g difference is "in the noise" and wouldn't mean any significant difference in intelligence.

Zeroing in on certain areas

Gender differences are more obvious in particular brain regions. Males average greater volumes in the neocortex, cerebellum, and amygdala, while women have a relatively larger hippocampus. Men may have a higher ratio of gray to white matter compared to women. None of these differences would statistically predict significant differences in intelligence, however.

Lateralization

Another relatively well-documented difference between male and female brains is the extent of lateralization, or lateral specialization. Many imaging studies, for example, show that females display more bilateral activation while doing various tasks. Females also generally recover better than males from brain damage during development and strokes in adulthood that damage the brain unilaterally.

This laterality data is probably what got Summers in so much trouble. If male brains are more lateralized, they are — in a sense — more specialized. The downside is that males are more susceptible to brain injury, but the upside may be some advantage in right-brain specialized skills. Test data consistently show females do better than males in language skills, and males do better than females in spatial skills. At present, we don't know how much of this result is cultural and how much is due to brain laterlization differences.

Thinking in different styles

Another way some researchers parse gender brain differences with respect to lateralization is to postulate that humans may tend to have either a left- or right-brain "style" of thinking.

The classic example of right-brain style versus left-brain style is giving directions. The left-brain style is to give the sequence of lights, intersections, and turns to get from one place to another. The right-brain style is to describe a general map of the area with accurate distances, but not so accurate intersection counts. The left-/right-brain style argument posits that males and females can have left- or right-brain styles, but a much larger percentage of males are right brained.

A somewhat derivative argument from the specialization idea associated with laterality is the bell-curve argument Suppose the average IQ of all women and men is exactly the same. But when lateral specialization works well it causes some males to excel, and diminishes capacity in others when it doesn't. Thus, both tails of the male curve extend farther above and below the mean IQ. If the lower IQ tail tends to produce people who go to prison because they can't cope with society, and the upper tail produces geniuses, then almost all the people in prison and almost all the professors in spatial skill areas will be male based on the wider bell curve for men versus women, as the argument goes.

Of course, these arguments are based on ideas that IQ is a solid predictor of a person's success — which it isn't. Moreover, besides having verbal and spatial IQ, many other types of intelligence exist that do not fit so neatly into either of those categories, such as artistic abilities and social skills.

Knowing the role of hormones

Male and female brains show their differences because of gender-specific hormones, such as testosterone, estrogen, and oxyctocin that affect brain development and function.

In mammals, female is the default developmental phenotype in sexual differentiation (as opposed to birds, where male is the default). This means that without either testosterone or estrogen, the mammal's body plan will develop as female. Development of a male body plan requires what is called *defeminization*, as well as *masculinization*. Hormones affect these processes in the following ways:

- ✔ **Testosterone:** In females, elevated levels of testosterone can cause brain masculinization during development, such as larger size and greater white matter. Circulating testosterone after development affects spatial ability, attention, and memory functions. Reduced testosterone levels that happen in males is a risk factor for Alzheimer's disease.

- ✔ **Estrogen:** Low estrogen levels during development aren't associated with unusual brain effects in females. In adult women, however, low estrogen levels are sometimes associated with depression, particularly at postpartum, perimenopause, and postmenopause periods. Normal males have some estrogen, and abnormally low estrogen levels in males have been associated with obsessive-compulsive disorder.

- ✔ **Oxytocin:** Oxytocin is a hormone involved in sexual reproduction, particularly around childbirth. It's important in maternal behaviors, social behavior, and female orgasm. Oxytocin promotes what is sometimes colloquially called "mother bear" behavior in females — highly protective behavior toward offspring and relatives, and high aggression toward outsiders.

Autism and the extreme male brain

Autism occurs more often in males than in females, by more than a 4:1 ratio. Children with autism are socially withdrawn and may fixate on unusual stimuli like the sound of a fan whirring. Some autistic children demonstrate savant skills. The *extreme male brain theory* suggests that autism is an extreme case of a male brain that is much better at *systemizing* (focusing on and detecting patterns) than empathizing with other people. This theory is related to the idea that autistic children lack an adequate "theory of mind," which allows people to understand that other people have feelings and intentions.

Autism is a spectrum disorder, which means it has multiple causes and is expressed in many ways. The extreme male brain theory may be more useful in describing some cases of autism than others.

Part III
Perceiving the World, Thinking, Learning, and Remembering

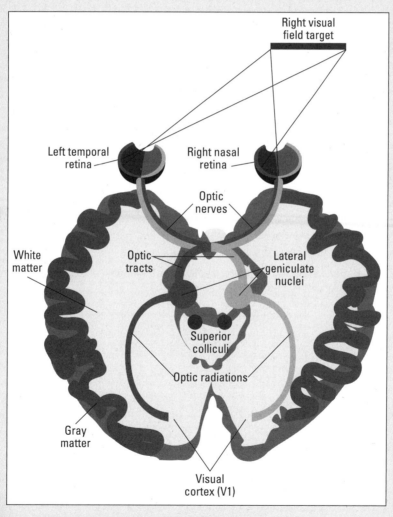

Right visual field target

Left temporal retina

Right nasal retina

Optic nerves

White matter

Optic tracts

Lateral geniculate nuclei

Superior colliculi

Optic radiations

Gray matter

Visual cortex (V1)

In this part . . .

- ✔ Uncover how we see and hear the world by studying vision and audition.

- ✔ Consider the other main senses — feeling, smelling, and tasting.

- ✔ Think about how the environment changes the brain through learning and memory.

- ✔ See how the brain is a hierarchical control system by looking at the frontal lobes and executive brain.

- ✔ Recognize that language, emotions, lateralization, and thought deal with high-order brain processes.

Chapter 10

Looking at Vision and Hearing

*Y*ou see with your eyes and you hear with your ears, right? Well, yes, but without the brain, you'd never be able to look at a beautiful sunset or listen to a favorite song.

Vision is a process. It starts with retinal photoreceptors capturing photons that go through complex analysis in the cortex and other brain areas. The brain produces neural images that represent different aspects of the visual world, such as the color, movement, and location of the edges. *Audition* (hearing) is a similar process, beginning with sound waves creating auditory action potentials in the inner ear. This chapter covers the neural responses involved in sight and sound.

Imaging and Capturing Light: Vision

The eye has evolved tissues that act like the optical elements of a camera. The lens of the eye acts like a camera's lens, and the *pupil* of the eye, which is the opening through which the light enters, acts like a camera's aperture.

The *cornea* is the outermost clear layer at the front of the eye, which controls light coming into the eye. The cornea is mostly responsible for focusing your vision with light, and does about 70 percent of the job. Light hits the cornea, which *refracts* (bends) that light onto the eye's lens, which is slightly denser than the surrounding tissue (and, therefore, has a higher index of refraction). Figure 10-1 illustrates how this all works. The lens is responsible for the other 30 percent of the eye's focusing. It can change shape to adjust the focus for near and far objects, a process called *accommodation.*

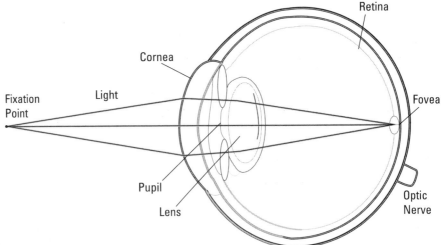

Figure 10-1:
Focusing
light by the
eye.

The image formed by the cornea, lens, and pupil is projected onto the *retina,* the neural lining inside the eye. This is where the real action in vision begins. The following sections outline what happens in the retina to convert the optical image to several neural images.

Making movies on the retina: Optics and eye movements

An important difference between the eye and a camera is that the eyes are moving continually. The eyes make large movements, called *saccades,* about three to four times a second. Even during so-called *fixation,* in between saccades, the eye still makes various small movements, called *microsaccades, drift,* and *tremor.*

All this movement is actually necessary for us to see. The result of experiments with stabilized images, where scientists use an apparatus that keeps the image from moving on the retina, is that after a few seconds all vision disappears. The retina adapts to constant light, and only responds to changes.

All this eye movement presents a problem: How do we perceive the world as stationary when the retinal image is always jumping around? The answer is that the brain takes into account the eye movements it commands with the associated image movements. If the eyes move, the image should move in a stationary world. If the eyes track a bird flying across the sky, the bird image stays relatively fixed on the retina, but we know the bird is moving.

This constant movement of our eyes, bodies, and the world around us presents another problem with respect to balance. The brain's knowledge of eye and body movements is combined with the output of the *vestibular system* (the semicircular canals in the ear, which I tell you more about at the end of this chapter) to tell us our orientation and movement.

If you spin around for a while or go into microgravity space, the semicircular canals in your ears can send the wrong message about your orientation. The disagreement between your visual and vestibular system can make you nauseous.

Converting photons to chemical reactions: Photoreception

Light is focused by the eye's optics on the retina, a sheet of neurons lining virtually the entire inside of the eye. The retina consists of several layers of cells that are highly conserved across vertebrate evolution. Figure 10-3 shows a diagram of these layers.

Photons are the quantum units of light that are absorbed by photoreceptors. *Photoreceptors* are specialized neural cells in the retina that convert light into electric current, which in turn modulates the release of the neurotransmitter glutamate. This process is called *phototransduction*.

Photoreceptors have four main structural parts:

- ✔ The **outer segment** contains the photopigment in disk-like structures, and a high concentration of cyclic nucleotide-gated sodium channels.
- ✔ The **inner segment** contains mitochondria and machinery for transporting *rhodopsin* (a red-colored, light-sensitive pigment) made in the cell body.
- ✔ The **cell body** contains the nucleus and the sites where protein is manufactured.
- ✔ The **synaptic terminal** is where glutamate is released onto second-order cells (bipolar and horizontal cells).

Two main types of photoreceptors exist:

✔ **Rods:** These photoreceptors work in very dim light for night vision. At night, only enough photons are present for rods to respond. Because all rods have the same absorption function, you cannot have color vision because the signal from the rods contains no information about the color (technically, wavelength) of the photons absorbed. The human retina has about 120 million rods.

✔ **Cones:** These photoreceptors function only in brighter light, such as daylight. You have three different types of cones: red, green, and blue. Although, like rods, cones do not individually signal the wavelength of the photons absorbed, the brain can deduce wavelength from the ratio of activity of different cones. If something is red, for example, the red cones are relatively more activated than the green or blue cones. The human retina has about 6 million cones.

When a photoreceptor absorbs a photon of light, a cascade of events occurs to send a message to other neurons in the retina:

1. When the molecule rhodopsin (in rods, similar molecules exist in cones) absorbs a photon, it transitions (or changes stereoisomer form, meaning it has the same chemical composition but a different structure) from a kinked form called 11-cis retinal to a straight form called all-trans retinal.

2. The all-trans retinal uncouples from the protein opsin to which it was bound. The unbound opsin activates a protein in the outer segment called *transducin,* which causes transducin to dissociate from *GDP,* and bind guanosine triphosphate (GTP). The GTP complex activates phosphodiesterase that breaks down an internal second messenger called *cyclic guanosine monophosphate* (cGMP) into 5'-GMP.

3. cGMP is a second messenger that promotes the opening of cyclic nucleotide-gated sodium channels open in the outer segment of the photoreceptor. The reduction in the intracellular concentration of cGMP reduces the number of open sodium channels.

4. Closure of the sodium channels causes hyperpolarization of the photoreceptor due to the ongoing potassium current in the inner segment that pulls the membrane potential down toward EK more effectively.

5. The hyperpolarization of the photoreceptor causes a structure at its base, called the *pedicle,* to release less *glutamate,* the photoreceptor neurotransmitter. The photoreceptor pedicle is very similar to a conventional axon terminal except that, instead of individual action potentials releasing puffs of neurotransmitter, light absorption continuously modulates the release of glutamate.

6. The modulation of glutamate release drives other cells in the retina. Specifically, the outputs of photoreceptors drive two main types of cells called *bipolar* and *horizontal cells.* These cells are discussed in the next section, and illustrated in Figure 10-3.

Dark currents and synaptic release

In the dark, cGMP concentrations in photoreceptors are high, which means the percentage of open sodium channels in the outer segment is very high. In the inner segment, a large number of potassium channels are continuously open. The dark current is the simultaneous entry of sodium in the outer segment and exit of potassium in the inner segment. When the outer-segment sodium channels are closed by the light, the excess potassium current in the inner segment hyperpolarizes the cell and reduces the release of glutamate from the photoreceptor terminal (the sodium-potassium transporter pump works to counteract the effect of this current to maintain the normal cell low sodium–high potassium concentration imbalance). Glutamate release is thus high in the dark, when the photoreceptor is depolarized, and lower in the light, when it is less depolarized.

In *vertebrates* (animals with backbones, like humans), photoreceptors hyperpolarize to light in the same way I describe in the previous paragraph. However, some invertebrates, like squids, have photoreceptors that depolarize to light using different photochemistry.

Photoreceptor adaptation

One form of light adaptation is the switch from rods in dim light to cones in bright light. However, both rods and cones themselves adapt to environmental light. Cones can function in light levels from deep shadow to snow reflection. Rods adapt over a range of 2 log units of background intensity. These adaptational processes allow the photoreceptors to generate relatively large signals for changes in light level, instead of communicating the absolute light level to detect salient objects in the visual world by contrast transitions that are independent of overall light level.

Photoreceptor distribution in the retina

When considering photoreceptors, the eye is not like a camera in the following respect: In a camera, the resolution of the image sensor (film or chip) is the same everywhere. But the photoreceptor distribution in the retina is highly nonuniform, especially for cones. Figure 10-2 shows this distribution.

The cones are much smaller and more densely packed in the central retina, particularly in the fovea (central 1 degree of highest visual acuity), compared to the periphery of the retina. The rods are more evenly distributed, but still higher in the central retina than the periphery, except for the fovea, where they're completely absent.

Photoreceptors do not send an image of the world directly to the brain. Instead, they communicate with other retinal neurons that extract specific information about the image to send to higher brain centers. The following sections explore that communication.

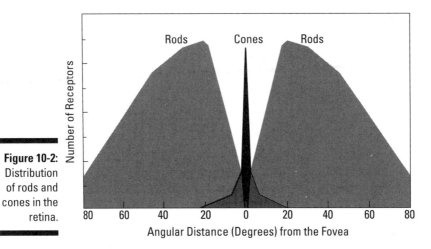

Figure 10-2:
Distribution
of rods and
cones in the
retina.

Joining the Nervous System: Photoreceptor Output

The photoreceptors release glutamate from their synaptic terminals at a synapse that is common in the retina but rare elsewhere, called the *ribbon synapse*. The cells that receive this glutamate are bipolar and horizontal cells (see Figure 10-3). These synapses are located in a layer called the outer plexiform layer (*plexiform* is a technical word for synaptic).

The output of photoreceptors is to two different types of cells, bipolar and horizontal cells. Bipolar cells carry the signals to ganglion cells, the output cells of the retina. Horizontal cells modulate the signal from photoreceptor to bipolar cells.

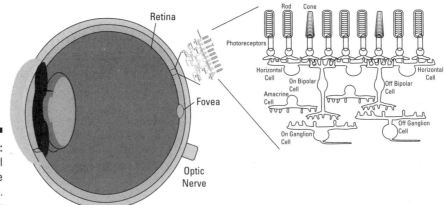

Figure 10-3:
The neural
circuit in the
retina.

Horizontal cells mediate a kind of lateral inhibition, making the photoreceptor output to the bipolar cell reflect not the actual light level, but the difference between the light level at the photoreceptor and that of the surrounding photoreceptors. This is called *local contrast,* and it's a much more useful signal by which to detect objects than the absolute light level.

Horizontal cells also mediate a kind of adaptation. Although photoreceptors themselves adapt to the overall light level, an additional neural circuit adaptation happens at the outer plexiform layer. Bipolar cells, which generate a large signal but over a small dynamic range, are kept in their responsive range by horizontal cells.

Converting light to contrast: Bipolar and horizontal cells

The signal from the photoreceptors is a modulation of their glutamate output. Horizontal cells compute an average of the light intensity in every region of the image, and, through their inhibition, cause the signal from the photoreceptors to the bipolar cells to be the difference between the amount of light hitting the photoreceptor, and the amount of light in the surrounding region. The result is that more glutamate released for parts of the image darker than the average across the image, and less glutamate is released for parts of the image brighter than the average across the image.

Two types of bipolar cell respond in opposite ways to the glutamate released by photoreceptors. These two bipolar cell types are called *depolarizing* (or "On") bipolar cells and *hyperpolarizing* (or "Off") bipolar cells. I explain why there are these two types with opposite responses next.

Making symmetry with On and Off bipolar cells

Figure 10-3 refers to two types of bipolar cell, "On" and "Off." Those terms refer to how photoreceptors release more glutamate in the dark, and less in the light.

On bipolar cells have a metabotropic receptor for glutamate that is inhibitory (called MgluR6) because it opens non-selective *cation* (positively charged) channels. The reduction of glutamate release because of the light disinhibits these bipolar cells, so they're excited by light.

In all but the darkest environments, the light input to the retina is a small modulation both above and below the ambient light level. Detecting objects means detecting this modulation, not the ambient light level. Right from the beginning two parallel pathways are established in the retina. One is excited by stimuli lighter than the background (On bipolars); the other is excited by stimuli darker than the background (Off bipolars). These parallel channels are maintained through the thalamus.

Integrating patterns in space and time

Bipolar cells adapt so they communicate the difference between the activity of photoreceptors to which they are directly connected and the surrounding photoreceptors through a process called *lateral inhibition*. Horizontal cells mediate lateral inhibition.

Lateral inhibition helps to reduce instances of the retina sending redundant signals. Suppose you're staring at a green car. You don't need all the cells responding to different parts of the car to report with high precision that the car is exactly the same shade of green all over. The retina uses horizontal cells to allow photoreceptors to communicate to bipolar cells the difference between the light they receive and the surrounding light.

Coloring it in: Photons and color vision

Color vision requires having receptors with different *spectral sensitivities* (the probability of absorbing light as a function of the wavelength of that light). This is because the same molecular cascade that modulates glutamate release happens no matter what the wavelength of the photon that is absorbed. (Refer to the section "Converting photons to chemical reactions: Photoreceptors," earlier in this chapter.) So, if you have only one photoreceptor type, you can't tell from its output if it received a small number of photons with a wavelength that is well absorbed, or a larger number of photons absorbed with a lower wavelength percentage — you'd have the same total absorption regardless of wavelength.

Color vision takes advantage of the fact that different visual pigments have different spectral sensitivity curves. So, the probability of absorbing a photon is a function of its wavelength. Figure 10-4 shows the cone spectral sensitivity curves and the probability of absorbing a photon as a function of wavelength (the rod curve is also in the diagram in light gray). At wavelength A, 530 nanometers (nm) the activity of the green cone is about 10 percent greater than the red cone, with the blue cone near zero. At wavelength B (560nm) the red cone activity is about 10 percent greater than green. Every wavelength results in a unique ratio of activity of the three cones.

The other thing color vision needs is for the signals from different cone types to be kept separate until the retina can compare the ratio of activity between cones. This is exactly what happens in color-opponent ganglion cells in the retina. The activity of one cone type — say, red — is opposed to the activity of another type — say, green — so that the ganglion cell is excited only by red light and inhibited by green. Color opponency is a second parallel visual pathway, after On versus Off in the bipolar cells. (Refer to the earlier section, "Making symmetry with On and Off bipolar cells.")

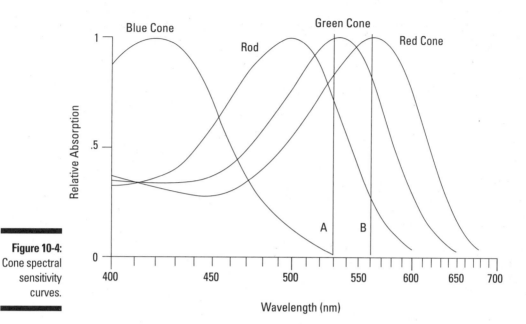

Figure 10-4:
Cone spectral
sensitivity
curves.

Mismatching your socks: Color blindness and anomalies

Animals like humans and other primates that have three cones are called *trichromats* (three colors). So, what's special about having three cones — why not two or four? Most mammals and many partially colorblind humans have only two cones, and are called *dichromats* (two colors). A dichromat will only have really good color discrimination in the area where the spectral sensitivities of the two cones overlap considerably, so that the ratio of the outputs of the two cones changes a lot with any change in wavelength. With three cones good wavelength discrimination occurs in more of the spectrum. Humans and other primates appear to have developed trichromacy by splitting the ancestral long-wavelength cone into green and red cones, giving good color discrimination for ripe red fruit against a green leafy background, among other things. Some vertebrates have four cone types, and some invertebrates have even more. Fooling those eyes would require matching the entire spectral distribution almost exactly.

Humans who are missing a cone type are colorblind, although the term is a misnomer because these people are color deficient in only part of the spectrum. The most common colorblindness means missing a red cone (*protanope*) or green cone (*deuteranope*). This occurs in about one in 20 men, but only one in 400 women. The gene for the red and green cones is on the X chromosome. Because women have two copies, they need two defective genes to have this colorblindness. But because men have only one X chromosome, one mutation gives the defect to a man.

If you're missing the blue cone, you're a *tritanope*. This is much less common than red-green colorblindness. Tritanopes do not see well at all in the blue end of the spectrum because they lack the blue cone that is sensitive there.

Because of certain congenital conditions and retinal degenerations, some people have no *rods* (the photoreceptors that respond in dim light) and are night blind.

Making nerve pulses in the retina

Earlier I discussed how the message from light gets into bipolar cells, of which we have two classes — On and Off — plus bipolar cells that are specific to different cone types. (We also have rod bipolar cells, which are only the On type.)

Bipolar cells carry their contrast and color signals forward to the next layer of retinal processing before the brain. Their outputs are in a second synaptic layer in the retina where they connect to the dendrites of two kinds of post-synaptic cells: amacrine and ganglion cells.

Sculpting the message with amacrine cells

Amacrine cells are laterally interacting neurons that work in the inner plexiform layer something like horizontal cells work in the outer plexiform layer (which I discuss at the start of this section). The amacrine cells conduct inhibitory signals from the surrounding bipolar cells so that the ganglion cell responds to the difference between the light in its area and the surrounding area. This action reduces the amount of redundant information that ganglion cells must transmit. However, amacrine cells do much more than lateral inhibition.

Most mammalian retinas have about ten distinct types of bipolar cells. These include On and Off bipolar for each of the two or three cone types, a rod bipolar, and a few other types that gather input either widely or narrowly.

But from this limited number of bipolar cells — all with very similar responses — emerges 20 or more ganglion cell classes. These ganglion cell classes respond to different colors, or movement, or the presence of long edges, or corners. Over 30 classes of amacrine cells create all these ganglion cell classes. Most classes of amacrine cells use GABA as a neurotransmitter, but some use glycine, acetylcholine, dopamine, and almost every neuromodulator transmitter known, such as somatostatin, VIP, and substance P. Only about half of the 30 classes have been functionally identified in any detail.

Seeing in different colors

Abnormal color vision occurs when a person has cones with a different spectral sensitivity than a "normal" person. This produces poorer color vision in most cases, but in some cases, it produces better color vision. Specifically, because a woman has two X chromosomes, she can be effectively a tetrachromat (four colors) if she has two different genes for the same cone but with different spectral sensitivities.

Projecting a neural image with ganglion cells

On (depolarizing) bipolar cells, which are excited by light, and Off (hyperpolarizing) bipolar cells, which are inhibited by light, are connected to matching ganglion cells called On-center and Off-center ganglion cells, respectively. Just as several photoreceptors are connected to one bipolar cell (outside the fovea, at least), several bipolar cells are input to one ganglion cell.

Color and fine detail

In most mammalian retinas are two classes of ganglion cells (On and Off) whose response is very much like that of their bipolar cell input. These ganglion cells have brisk-sustained responses, meaning that they have high firing rates that are well modulated by small changes in light intensity. In primate retina, the major class of brisk-sustained ganglion cells is called *parvocellular* (which means small cells). These ganglion cells tend to code for color and fine detail, and are by far the most numerous ganglion cells in the human retina. The fovea has only a specialized set of parvocellular ganglion cells, called *midget ganglion cells.* In this system, a single photoreceptor is connected almost entirely to one bipolar cell, which is connected to one ganglion cell, although lateral interactions with horizontal cells still happen. This is what produces very high acuity in the human fovea.

Movement and low contrast

However, amacrine input sculpts the responses of most other ganglion cell classes. The second most important ganglion cell class (besides On and Off parvocellular) are called On and Off *magnocellular* (large cells), which are selective for motion and low contrast. Parvo- and magnocellular ganglion cells (known by other names in other species) constitute the major projection to the lateral geniculate nucleus of the thalamus in virtually all mammals.

Specific features

Amacrine cells also produce ganglion cell classes that respond only to specific features from the visual input, and which project to particular areas of the brain. For example, some ganglion cells respond only to motion in a certain direction and help you track moving objects or keep your balance. Other ganglion cells sense only certain colors; still others indicate the presence of edges in the scene. These other ganglion cells project to brain areas such as the superior colliculus, accessory optic and pretectal nuclei, and the suprachiasmatic nucleus.

Covering distance with action potentials

Within the retina, the processes of photoreceptors, horizontal, bipolar, and most amacrine cells extend less than 1 millimeter. These distances can conduct neural signals without action potentials (refer to Chapter 4), but the messages ganglion cells send from your eye to your brain have to travel many centimeters. Action potentials are the means by which ganglion cells convert their analog bipolar cell input into a digital pulse code to transmit to at least 15 retinal recipient zones in the brain.

Sending the Message to the Brain

Earlier in this chapter, I discuss how parallel visual pathways that extract different information start in the outer retina with photoreceptors. These photoreceptors have different absorption curves, and On and Off pathways. The population of about 20 ganglion cell classes establishes 20 parallel pathways leaving the retina. Information about each point in visual space is extracted by all these classes, everywhere except the fovea. In the fovea, only a specialized set of parvocellular ganglion cells, called *midget ganglion cells,* exists, that projects to the dLGN.

The retina is part of the central, not peripheral, nervous system. It just happens to be outside the skull, because optical imaging through the skull bones would not work very well.

The human retina projects primarily to the dorsal lateral geniculate nucleus of the thalamus (dLGN, which I discuss in the next section), which projects to occipital lobe of the cortex. Many subcortical brain areas also process unconscious aspects of visual behavior, such as controlling eye movements.

Relaying at the thalamus

The main output of the retina is through the parvocellular and magnocellular ganglion cell classes to the dLGN of the thalamus. Figure 10-5 shows how the retinal ganglion cell axons leave each eye as the optic nerve, but then combine a few centimeters later at a structure called the *optic chiasm,* which means "optic crossing." Here, some of the ganglion cell axons from each eye cross at the chiasm and go to the other side of the brain, and some don't.

As you can see in Figure 10-5, the part of the right retina closest to the nose (called the *nasal retina*) receives images from the right visual field, while the part of the right retina farthest from the nose (called the *temporal retina*) receives input from the left visual field. At the optic chiasm, the axons sort themselves so that the information received from the nasal retina (right visual field) projects to the left thalamus, while the temporal retinal axons that receive light from the left visual field project to the right thalamus. The same rearrangement occurs for the left eye, of course, so that the right thalamus has ganglion cells from both eyes that see the left visual field, and the left thalamus has axons that see the right visual field. The nerves leaving the optic chiasm are called the *optic tracts.* The major destination of the optic tracts is the dLGN.

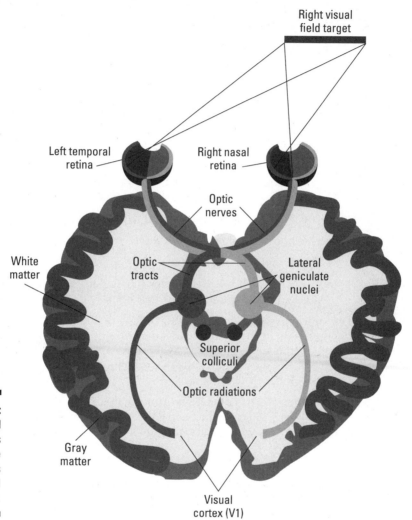

Figure 10-5:
Retinal
projections
to the
thalamus
and visual
cortex.

In the dLGN, each thalamic relay cell receives inputs from one or a few similar ganglion cells; for this reason, these ganglion cells are often called *relay cells.* The dLGN is layered, and some layers receive inputs only from parvocellular ganglion cells, while others receive inputs only from magnocellular cells. Although the relay cells in the thalamus respond very much like their parvocellular or magnocellular ganglion cell inputs, other inputs to the dLGN from other parts of the brain (including visual cortex) allow gating functions that are associated with attention. These inputs modulate the strength of a neuron's responses to any particular stimulus based on the context — the importance of that stimulus.

Parallel processing in diverse visual centers

The most important visual destinations of retinal ganglion cell axons are as follows:

- **The dLGN:** This is the most important destination.

- **The superior colliculus:** This is the second most important visual target. It controls eye movements.

- **The accessory optic system:** This destination consists of several areas that are involved in attention, eye movements, and the coordination of vestibular with visual input for balance. The optic system consists of

  - The medial terminal nucleus (MTN)

  - The lateral terminal nucleus (LTN)

  - The dorsal terminal nucleus (DTN)

  - The pretectum, whcih includes the nucleus of the optic tract (NOT), pretectal nucleus (PO) and posterior pretectal nucleus (PP)

- **The suprachiasmatic nucleus (SCN):** This retinal target receives inputs from ganglion cells that have their own photopigment, respond directly to light, and need to be driven by photoreceptors. This nucleus, because of inputs from these photosensitive ganglion cells, controls our circadian rhythms. (Refer to Chapter 6.)

- **The Edinger-Westphal nucleus:** This area receives inputs from photo-receptive ganglion cells that signal the current overall light level. This nucleus controls your pupil's dilation.

Fanning Out in the Occipital Lobe

The thalamic relay cells send their axons to the visual area of the neocortex at the back of the head — the occipital lobe. This fiber tract of axons leaving the dLGN is called the *optic radiation* because the axons look like they're "fanning out" from a bundle. This pathway mediates almost all the vision of which you are conscious (versus vision functions, such as pupil contraction and dilation, which you're neither conscious of nor able to voluntarily control).

Layering and concurrent processing in V1

The area of the occipital lobe that receives the input from the thalamic relay cells is called "visual area 1" (V1). It's also referred to as "area 17" (refer to Chapter 9), and "striate cortex," because of a dense stripe in this area that appears in histological stains. After the signal reaches neocortex, visual processing pathways diverge in numerous ways, because this area has about 1.2 million ganglion cell and dLGN relay axons. These cells drive about 200 million cortical cells in V1 and start to become specialized, such as only responding to edges that have a certain orientation (horizontal, vertical, or other), or very specific colors. In other words, a few ganglion cells in the retina ultimately drive hundreds of V1 neurons.

Selecting for orientation and movement

The hundreds of V1 neurons extract local features that exist across a small region of the retina. David Hubel and Torsten Weisel of Harvard University first showed that V1 cells are almost all sensitive to the orientation of the stimulus that excites them. This means that these cells don't fire action potentials unless the image contains a line or an edge. Several ganglion cells — in a line and of a particular direction — are activated to represent the image.

All stimulus orientations (vertical, horizontal, and everything in between) are represented in V1. And so, a small group of ganglion cells in a restricted area of the retina must give rise to a much larger number of V1 cortical cells. These cells respond only to a particular orientation of an edge in that area.

Other V1 neurons only respond to certain directions of motion, as though a particular sequence of ganglion cells had to be stimulated in a certain order. As with orientation, all directions are encoded, each by a particular cell or small set of cells. Other V1 cells are sensitive to the differences between the image that the right eye sees compared to what the left eye sees. This *binocular disparity* is because the eyes are located in slightly different places on the head.

Area V1 represents all these different extracted features in *columns.* One column has neurons sensitive to a particular orientation and eye dominance. As one moves across the cortex, the orientation preference changes from vertical to horizontal, then back to vertical. The set of neighboring columns spanning all orientations and (approximately perpendicularly) going from left to right eye dominance is sometimes called a *hypercolumn.*

Streaming the Message to the Temporal and Parietal Lobes

Neurons in area V1 project to other areas of the cortex, and these areas go on to project to many other areas. Virtually all of the occipital lobe and most of the parietal lobe and inferior temporal lobe are comprised of visual neurons that respond to specific patterns of visual inputs. Area V1 is at the posterior pole of the occipital lobe. Just anterior to V1 is area V2, and anterior to V2 is V3. Neurons in these areas tend to respond in similar ways.

After V2 and V3 comes the V1-3 complex. It gives rise to two major pathways: the dorsal stream and the ventral stream. The way the neurons in these pathways respond to stimulus, and the vision problems that arise if these pathways are damaged, show that they have important functional differences.

Seeing complex shapes and colors in the ventral stream

The *ventral stream* is the projection of V1-3 into the inferior aspect of the temporal lobe (called *infero-temporal cortex*). The ventral pathway is typically called the "what" pathway. Parvocellular ganglion and dLGN neurons are the main drivers of this pathway.

Cortical areas in this stream have neurons that prefer particular patterns or colors (almost all neurons in ventral stream area V4, for example, are color selective). As you move in an anterior direction along the inferior temporal lobe, you find neurons that respond only to increasingly complex patterns — such as the shape of a hand. Near the pole of the temporal lobe is an area called the *fusiform face area* that contains neurons that respond only to faces.

People with damage to the fusiform face area typically cannot recognize any faces, including their own.

Seeing where and how-to in the dorsal stream

The *dorsal stream* is the projection of V1-3 into the parietal lobe. Magnocellular ganglion and dLGN neurons are the primary drivers of this pathway. Cortical areas in the dorsal stream include areas called middle temporal (MT) and medial superior temporal (MST). These areas are dominated by neurons that respond only to movement in a particular direction, or a particular pattern of movement. In MST, for example, some neurons that respond to image movement are created by self-movement, such as tilting the head, resulting in the rotation of the entire visual field, and by optic flow, which is the expanding motion pattern generated by forward movement, such as typically shown in movies for spacecraft traveling through star fields. The dorsal pathway also encodes the pattern of *motion parallax,* in which close objects appear to shift more than distant objects when you move your head from side to side.

The dorsal pathway is necessary for doing things that rely heavily on vision, such as catching a ball, running through the woods without bumping into trees, and even putting a letter in a mail slot. (Damage to this area results in *apraxis* — the inability to skillfully do those kinds of tasks.) The parietal lobe dorsal pathway is concerned with movement *patterns,* rather than with identifying features and things. A famous patient with rare bilateral damage to MT could not cross the street or pour a cup of tea because she couldn't understand motion trajectories. Her life was like living in a strobe-lit disco.

Communicating between dorsal and ventral streams

Despite the difference in the functions of the dorsal and ventral streams, they do communicate — or crosstalk — with each other. Here are two examples:

- ✔ **Deciphering structure from movement:** In "structure from motion" experiments, researchers illuminate only a few reflector spots on various body parts of actors. By watching motion patterns, observers can tell that the dots are on the bodies of people, what the people are doing, and even the people's gender. Observers are able to know all this because motion-detecting neurons from the dorsal pathway must send information to object-analyzing neurons in the ventral pathway.

- ✔ **Perceiving depth:** Depth perception is another example of dorsal-ventral pathway crosstalk. The visual system estimates distance to objects in the environment using a variety of cues. Some of these cues are based on patterns (such as depth cues like overlap), and other cues involve movement, such as motion parallax. Ventral pathway pattern-based cues must be combined with dorsal pathway motion-based cues to create the whole picture and judge depth.

Seeing without meaning: Agnosias

Agnosias (a term coined by Sigmund Freud) are losses of specific visual abilities, usually because of damage in high-order areas of the visual cortex. Examples of these visual losses include the following:

- ✔ **Blindness:** Damage to the retina, dLGN, or V1 typically results in a total loss of vision.

- ✔ **Pattern vision:** Damage to ventral stream areas causes one to lose pattern vision, such as facial agnosia where a person cannot recognize faces.

- ✔ **Sense of color:** Another well-studied ventral stream agnosia is a loss of color sense, called *achromatopsia,* due to damage to area V4 in the ventral stream. Unlike more common colorblindness, which comes from the retina, people with achromatopsia report that they can see differences between areas of different colors, but not the colors themselves. They say everything looks like "different dirty shades of gray."

⮞ **Motion detection:** Damage to area MT in the dorsal pathway causes a motion detection defect called *akinetopsia*.

⮞ **Left-sided vision:** Damage to the parietal lobe, particularly on the right side of the brain, results in *hemineglect,* in which people do not see or pay attention to anything in their left visual field.

Listening In: Capturing Sound Waves

Hearing, like vision, captures energy from the environment. Our ears detect vibrations in the air that are created by objects vibrating in the world around us (unless you're underwater — in which case they're vibrations in water). When objects vibrate, they create a series of high- and low-pressure pulses in the air that travel through the air in waves. Sound is the perception we generate by receiving and processing this energy.

Our auditory system is unbelievably sensitive. The threshold for the auditory system to detect pressure waves in the air is very close to the threshold of the air motion itself. You can't do much better than that. Our sense of hearing allows us not only to detect that sound exists, but also what made it, what it means, and from where it came.

Good vibrations: Gathering and transmitting sound to the brain

Before involving the brain, the auditory system has three major structures: the outer ear, the middle ear, and the inner ear. Figure 10-6 shows its anatomy. The outer and middle ears involve mechanical transformations of sound waves to help detect and discriminate sounds. The inner ear is where neurons respond to sound and produce a neural image that gets sent to the brain through the auditory nerve.

Tuning and directing in the outer ear

As I explain at the beginning of this chapter, the eye has camera-like mechanical elements that focus the light on the retina and control its intensity via the pupil. In the same way, the auditory system has mechanical elements that capture, direct, and amplify sound.

The first mechanical transformations happen in the outer ear. The outer ear has three parts: the pinna, the auditory canal, and the eardrum (which transitions to the inner ear).

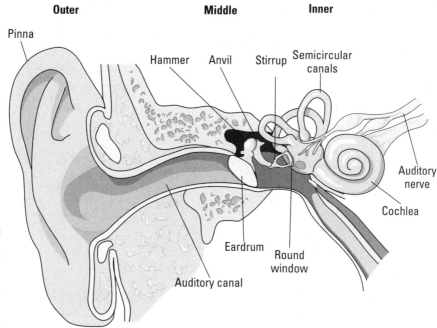

Figure 10-6:
The anatomy
of the
auditory
system.

The first part of the outer ear that sound waves encounter is the pinna. *The pinna* is the technical name for what is commonly called the ear. The pinna "captures" and filters the sound waves and directs them via the auditory canal to the eardrum. Specifically, the pinna does two things to sound:

- ✔ It concentrates sound by reflecting it from the larger pinna area to the smaller auditory canal opening.

- ✔ It changes the frequency content of the incoming sound based on the direction it came from. The pinna's complex shape helps us to know the direction.

Each person's pinna is slightly different. As we grow and develop, we "learn" our own pinna's directional frequency transform function to better localize sound.

The pinna reflects the sound waves into the auditory canal. The auditory canal has a resonance (at which it transmits better) at midrange frequencies that are important for hearing human voices. When sound reaches the end of the auditory canal causes the eardrum to vibrate. The eardrum is attached to the three bones of the middle ear.

Amplifying in the middle ear

On the other side of the eardrum from the auditory canal are three tiny bones called the *hammer* (Latin name: *malleus*), *anvil* (Latin name: *incus*), and *stirrup* (Latin name: *stapes*), which constitute the middle ear. The vibrations of the eardrum drive the hammer, which drives the anvil, which drives the stirrup, which is attached to the *oval window* (part of the inner ear) at the entrance to the cochlea. (I discuss the cochlea in the next section.)

The hammer, anvil, and stirrup are the smallest bones in the body.

These three bones comprise a lever system. The ball-like head of the hammer — where it connects to the anvil — is the fulcrum in this system. An eardrum movement that has larger vibrations but weaker force causes a smaller but stronger movement of the stirrup. This leverage system exists because fluid in the cochlea, which is going to be vibrated, is stiffer than air at the eardrum.

Another mechanical advantage in the eardrum to oval window system is that the area of the eardrum is larger than the area of the oval window. That means the force per area is amplified by this ratio, as well. The total leverage ratio of the middle ear bones and difference in eardrum versus oval window area produces a leverage ratio roughly around 20 to 1.

Toning up: Frequency transduction in the Organ of Corti

Sound pressure waves travel from the middle ear to the oval window of the cochlea, which is filled with fluid. The cochlea is where auditory receptors (hair cells) are located. When the oval window vibrates, it creates pressure waves in the cochlea that bend the *cilia* (auditory hair cells inside the cochlea). This generates action potentials in the auditory nerve.

The cilia that extend into the cochlea fluid are derived — evolutionarily — from motor-type cilia, such as those that some single-celled organisms use to move. (The outer segments of photoreceptors are also derived from cilia-type cell extensions.) Auditory hair cells are so sensitive to small vibrations that they respond to deflections of their cilia by widths the size of an atom.

Within the auditory hair cell are specialized ion channels that are activated when the cilia bend. These ion channels depolarize the hair cell and cause the axon terminals of the auditory nerve fibers at the other end of the hair cell to fire action potentials. These action potentials travel on the 30,000 auditory nerve axons to the cochlear nucleus.

The *Organ of Corti* is the apparatus inside the cochlea that contains the hair cells that respond to sound. The Organ of Corti contains two types of hair cells: inner and outer. There are fewer inner hair cells than outer ones, but the inner hair cells make more connections to the auditory nerve, so they generate most of the sound transduction. The outer hair cells have an important function, which is to control the stiffness of the membrane near the hair cell cilia. This boosts the hair cell response to low amplitude sounds, particularly at high frequencies, but weakens the response for very loud sounds to prevent hair cell damage.

Auditory neurons resemble — in structure — mechanoreceptors in the dorsal root ganglia of the spinal cord (refer to Chapter 6) whose axon terminals transduce stimuli into spikes that travel back toward the cell body. In the auditory system, the cell body of the auditory neuron whose axons make up the auditory nerve is in the cochlear nucleus in the brainstem. The cochlear neurons have an axon that projects to the superior olive, carrying the auditory message higher in the brain.

The cochlea has a spiral structure that causes high-frequency vibrations to be concentrated near the oval window, while low-frequency vibrations travel to the end of the spiral. This means that the auditory nerve is frequency coded, and different fibers respond best to particular frequencies. The auditory nerve codes frequency in two ways:

✔ Fibers are active according to their location on the cochlea (more important for high than low frequencies).

✔ For low frequencies — fewer than 500 Hertz (Hz) — the nerves can fire at the frequency of the sound. This can't occur for higher frequencies in the human hearing range (20 to 20,000 Hz) because neurons can't fire action potentials faster than about 500 Hz. The hair cells fire at a particular phase of the sound, such as the peak amplitude, in a process called *phase locking* that is important for later neural circuits to determine location by interaural time difference.

Auditory fibers also code for the amplitude of the sound by the number of action potentials per sound wave. They also code for amplitude by having hair cells with different thresholds, so that some only fire to very loud sounds.

The auditory nerve has no explicit code for locating sound — unlike the retina, for example, where position on the retina corresponds precisely to visual field angle. Instead, in the auditory system, the auditory cortex computes the location of the sound in space by combining information from the two ears. This is something like how the visual system computes depth — not explicitly represented on the two dimensional retina, but via binocular difference detectors in visual cortex.

Channeling Sounds to the Brain

Auditory nerve fibers don't project directly to the thalamus like retinal ganglion cell axons do. Instead, they relay twice before reaching the auditory thalamic area, called the *medial geniculate nucleus.* The auditory nerve action potentials that reach the cochlear nucleus cause an action potential in the cochlear nucleus bodies, which in turn causes an action potential in a second axon that crosses the body midline and projects to the superior olive in the pons.

Comparing and relaying in the superior olive, inferior colliculus, and thalamus

Most axons from the right cochlear nucleus cross over to the superior olive nucleus on the left; action potentials from the left project to the superior olive on the right. However, a few axons stay ipsilateral, so that some areas in the superior olive and around it have binaural input. This binaural input is part of the mechanism for localizing sound.

Relay cells in the superior olive project to the inferior colliculus, located just below the superior colliculus in the midbrain. The inferior colliculus neurons project to the medial geniculate nucleus of the thalamus. Virtually all the projections after the contralateral projection to the superior olive are ipsilateral. So, the medial geniculate on the right side of the body receives input mostly from the left ear, and the medial geniculate on the left side of the body receives input mostly from the right ear.

Localizing by intensity and delay comparisons

Neural comparisons between the outputs from each ear make up the neural coding for localizing sound. In the auditory system, neural mechanisms sensitive to the differences in sound volume and arrival time between the two ears mediate how horizontal sound is localized. These computations require precise timing, so they must occur very early in the auditory processing stream, as close to the two cochlear nuclei as possible. Locating sound elevation is done primarily by the change in frequency content by different reflections from the pinna, as I mention earlier in this chapter.

Relaying at the medial geniculate nucleus of the thalamus

Medial geniculate neurons respond similarly to the responses in the auditory nerve. In this sense, the thalamic relay for the auditory system is similar to that for vision. (Refer to "Relaying at the thalamus" earlier in this chapter.) Typical functions that gate for attention in the thalamus occur in the medial geniculate, as in other thalamic areas. For example, if you hear a suspicious noise, your attention will be drawn to that noise and other similar sounds.

Analyzing sounds in the superior temporal lobe

The medial geniculate nucleus projects to the superior temporal lobe at an area slightly posterior to the middle of the superior sulcus — known as Heschl's gyrus. This area is called the primary auditory cortex, or A1. A1 has a *tonotopic map,* in which position on the cortical surface corresponds to the frequency to which neurons respond.

In visual cortex, patterns composed of image segments at different locations are put together to define visual objects in the world. In the auditory cortex, patterns of frequencies are assembled to indicate meaning, such as the word *hello* or the sound of car keys jangling.

Sound localization also is processed by neurons in A1 using subcortical timing and intensity comparisons. Lesions in A1 may prevent a person from locating the direction of a sound.

Perceiving tones in music and voices

Around auditory area A1 are several higher-order areas, referred to as *auditory association areas*. Neurons in these areas respond best to complex or environmentally relevant sounds such as chirps or rattles, rather than pure tones.

The selectivity for higher-order patterns in auditory areas is a common theme in cortical processing. At lower sensory levels, most neurons respond to most stimuli — the neural image is carried by a relatively small number of axon transmission lines. But in the cortex, neurons become pickier. They prefer more complex patterns, and only a minority of cortical neurons responds to any particular sound. But many more neurons are available to parcel out this sparser representation in which similar sounds drive completely different cells. We achieve these specific neural responses by learning and experience. Learning gives neurons the ability to differentiate complex stimuli based on few characteristics, such as vocal utterances corresponding to words.

Music is a complex stimulus for audio processing. A clinical syndrome called *amusia* is associated with bilateral damage in higher-order auditory areas. People with this condition can't recognize melodies, although they can understand speech and other complex sounds around them.

Understanding language

Wernicke's area is located at the border between the superior, posterior part of the temporal lobe and the parietal lobe (around Brodmann area 22). This area is crucial for processing speech. People with damage to Wernicke's area have problems understanding language, and the language they produce is often gibberish.

Wernicke's area, in the sensory cortex, has many connections with another language area in the frontal lobe, Broca's area. Broca's area is located just anterior to the primary motor areas that control the tongue, vocal cords, and other parts we need for speaking. Damage to Broca's area makes producing speech and understanding complex sentences (such as passive-voice constructions) difficult.

Both Wernicke's area and Broca's area are on the left side of the brain in about 95 percent of right-handed people and about 60 percent of left-handed people. Damage to the brain area on the right that is mirror symmetric to Wernicke's area causes problems with processing meaningful tones in spoken language — the changes in tone and rhythm. People with this damage have trouble distinguishing sarcasm from a question.

Losing Hearing

Hearing loss can range from complete deafness to the loss of only some frequencies, or some hearing loss at all frequencies.

Deafness or hearing loss can be congenital (a person is born that way) or the result of disease or damage. An impact (such as putting a cotton swab too far in the ear) or even a loud noise can damage the eardrum. Loud noise can also kill auditory hair cells.

Conductive versus neural hearing loss

Conductive hearing loss occurs when sound vibrations are not mechanically transmitted from the eardrum to the cochlea. *Neural* hearing loss is mostly due to damage to the auditory hair cells, typically from loud noises. However, tumors or strokes that affect any part of the auditory pathway can cause neural hearing loss as well.

Inner ear infections can cause conductive deafness by destroying the three middle ear bones (refer to "Amplifying in the middle ear," earlier). One cause of conductive hearing loss is *otosclerosis,* the growth of spongy masses on the middle ear bones. This is a hereditary conductive hearing loss that can happen between the ages of 15 and 40. A pregnant woman with rubella (also called German measles) can transmit the virus to her baby, causing the child to be born deaf.

Items entering the auditory canal can physically damage eardrums, as can high pressure, such as diving into deep water.

Eh? Aging, environment, and hearing loss

As we age, our high-frequency sensitivity (*presbycusis,* which occurs in almost everyone, particularly males) declines. Young people can hear in the range of 20 to 20,000 Hertz, but the elderly hear little above 15,000 Hz.

Some age-related hearing loss is probably inevitable, but the most frequent cause of hearing loss in older people is due to damage to the auditory hair cells. The louder the noise, the more quickly it damages a person's hearing.

Being exposed only once to very loud sounds — such as standing by the speakers at a rock concert — can cause significant hearing loss no matter your age. On the other hand, consistently working in a loud environment such as a construction site can cause hearing damage that accumulates over decades.

Auditory hair cell damage is permanent.

Aiding hearing: Amplifying and replacing

Hearing aids can treat conductive hearing loss and some neural loss. Hearing aids are devices that amplify sound, usually matching in a complementary way the hearing loss profile. This is why good hearing aids are custom programmed.

If a person has severe neural loss, amplifying sound is useless because nothing is left to transduce it. Wihin the last few decades, over 100,000 auditory prostheses have been installed in people with profound deafness. These are linear sets of about 30 electrodes threaded into the cochlea to electrically stimulate the cochlear fibers and restore some hearing. This works well because of the cochlea's inherent different frequency sensitivity along its length.

Cochlear inserts cannot treat deafness that is caused by damage higher in the nervous system. Electrode arrays are being developed with the intent to implant them into brain structures in the auditory pathway. But so far, they're experimental and not generally available.

Ringing and tinnitus

The perception of ringing in the years is called *tinnitus*. Chronic tinnitus is psychologically debilitating and has led some patients to suicide. It has multiple causes that include ear infections, allergies, reactions to certain drugs, and exposure to loud noise (tinnitus is common among rock musicians).

Muscle spasms in the ears cause *objective tinnitus*. The condition is diagnosed with special ear-specific instruments that detect the actual noise. *Subjective tinnitus* cannot be diagnosed objectively. It can have numerous causes and is typically associated with hearing loss. Tinnitus can appear suddenly and then disappear within a few months.

One treatment for tinnitus has people wear noise-producing earphones that mask the ringing sound with electronically generated white noise. In extreme cases, people need to have the auditory nerve surgically destroyed to get some relief, but this compromises normal hearing.

Balancing via the Vestibular System: "Hearing" the Fluid Sloshing in Your Head

The vestibular system gives us our sense of balance. It starts with the three semicircular canals and otoliths in the inner ear, which are organs sensitive to gravity and acceleration. These canals are oriented in three right-angled planes. Hair cells in these canals work like nearby cochlear hair cells. However, instead of responding to sound vibrations, they respond to the movement of fluid in the cochlea that happens when you move or turn your head. The moving fluid acts on a structure called the *cupula,* which contains the hair cells that convert the physical movement to vestibular nerve action potentials.

The semicircular canal system transduces rotational movements while the otoliths sense linear accelerations such as occur during the beginning of forward movement. The vestibular system projects to neural structures that control eye movements, which generates the *vestibulo-ocular reflex* — a compensatory eye movement that allows us to see stable images.

The three semicircular canals are called the horizontal (lateral), anterior (superior), and posterior (inferior) semicircular canals. The vestibular nuclei project to the cerebellum, spinal cord, thalamus, reticular formation, and to the nuclei of cranial nerves III, IV, and VI. These nerves allow the muscles to compensate for things such as uneven terrain, so that we keep our balance. Some nuclei combine vestibular with visual signals from directionally selective ganglion cells that also inform the brain about rotations and translations.

The vestibulo-ocular reflex (VOR) stabilizes images on the retina when you move your head by producing an opposite, compensatory eye movement. The VOR reflex does not require visual input; it happens even when the eyes are closed. A related reflex, called the *optokinetic reflex* (OKN), is mediated by inputs from directionally selective ganglion cells in the retina. The test for this reflex typically involves having the subject view horizontally translating stripes, the normal response to which is that the eyes smoothly track the stripes for a few hundred milliseconds, and then snap back to a more central position, in a repeated cycle.

Meniere's disease is a condition of the cochlea and semicircular canals that affects hearing and balance. It likely has multiple causes, but at this point the disease is poorly understood.

Chapter 11

Feeling, Smelling, and Tasting

The skin is your protective barrier between you and the rest of the world. It is the largest organ in the body in terms of area, and acts as an insulator that helps keep your body temperature constant. You get a lot of information through receptors for touch, temperature, and pain that are nearly everywhere in the skin.

Smell and taste are senses also tell you a lot about the world. Is that food safe to eat? Are you near a toxic substance? These senses also work together, and are strongly associated with memory.

In this chapter, I explain how these three senses work, and how touch sensations, odors, and tastes from the outside world enter the body and project to the brain so you can recognize them.

Getting in Touch with the Skin

You feel all sorts of different touch sensations — tickle, pressure, movement — with your skin. You can also perceive other kinds of sensations with your skin, such as temperature and pain. For different touch, temperature, and pain perceptions, you have different kinds of skin receptors.

Feeling your way with mechanoreceptors

The skin senses are called *somatosensation.* The *somatosensory receptors* in the skin allow us to have two senses of touch:

- **Passive touch:** When something contacts your skin. Passive touch receptors allow you to identify this contact, such as a mosquito landing on your arm, or the feel of the back of the chair in which you're sitting. (Perhaps at this very moment?)

- **Active touch:** Most active touch happens with your hands and fingertips. This sense is precise enough that you can hold an egg in your hand without damaging or dropping it. Different kinds of receptors in the skin mediate the many skin perceptions and active touch senses you feel.

The sense of touch, or *somatosensory perception,* for most of the body (below the head) is relayed through the spinal cord, to the thalamus, and then to a strip in the parietal lobe where a "touch" (somatosensory) map of the body exists.

The skin's structure

The skin has two major layers with different properties:

- **Epidermis:** The outermost layer of the skin that you can see is the *epidermis* (*dermis* means "skin" and *epi* means "on or above"). The epidermis consists of several layers of dead cell "ghosts" that provide your body with mechanical protection from the outside world. Cells at the bottom of the epidermis, where it meets the dermis, are constantly dividing, migrating outward, and dying to replace the dead layers as they wear off.

By dragging your fingernail lightly along your skin, you can easily remove a layer or two of epidermis. It doesn't hurt because these cells are dead and have no pain receptors.

- **Dermis:** Below the epidermis is the *dermis,* the living layer of the skin that contains almost all somatosensory receptors, including the mechanoreceptors I tell you about next.

Quick touch versus pressure

Mechanoreceptors are skin receptors that respond to various kinds of pressure. They are sensitive to different characteristics of force that make contact on the skin, such as a force's rate of change and intensity. Mechanoreceptors are located in the dermis layer of the skin. Figure 11-1 shows how mechanoreceptors work in the skin. Small receptive fields are usually associated with shallow mechanoreceptors (those that are near or even intrude into the epidermis), whereas receptors located deeper in the dermis typically have larger receptive fields.

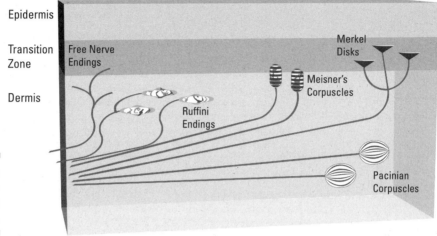

Figure 11-1:
Mechano-
receptors
in the skin.

Almost all somatosensory receptors are within the dermis, with only an occasional receptor found in the epidermis.

Skin receptors are very different from the visual and auditory receptors (refer to Chapter 10), which have cilia-derived specializations for transducing light and sound energy. Skin receptors are axonal endings (refer to Chapter 3) of neurons whose cell bodies are located in dorsal root ganglion of the spinal cord (for skin below the head). These axonal endings produce action potentials when they are mechanically deformed. The action potentials travel what would be in most neurons the retrograde direction toward the soma. At the T-junction in the dorsal root ganglia, the action potentials then proceed in an orthograde direction where they make synapses in the spinal cord gray area for both local reflex circuits and projection up the spinal cord to the thalamus.

Localizing touch

Four distinctive anatomical types of touch receptors are called mechanoreceptors (refer to Figure 11-1):

- ✔ **Merkel disks:** These disk-shaped receptors for pressure are located typically near the border between the dermis and the epidermis. They respond to relatively constant pressure over small areas of the skin.

- ✔ **Meissner's corpuscles:** These receptors also respond to pressure over small areas, but they can respond to more rapid changes in pressure than Merkel disks. The sensation evoked when the Meissner corpuscles are stimulated is called *flutter*.

- ✔ **Ruffini endings:** These receptors respond to skin stretched over large receptive fields. They're important because they detect forces likely to tear the skin.

Lose it and use it

Active touch requires feedback from the skin, as well as position and force receptors in the joints and muscles. Losing feeling in a limb is so disabling that people without feeling from a limb refuse to use it, even if the motor neuron control circuitry is actually intact. A treatment called "constraint induced therapy" (CIT) forces a patient to use their "paralyzed" arm while the other "good" arm is temporarily restrained in a sling. With practice patients often achieve the necessary dexterity for common two-armed life tasks such as tying shoes.

✔ **Pacinian corpuscles:** These are the fastest responding of all the touch mechanoreceptors. They tend to be located deep within the dermis. They have a connective tissue wrapping derived from Schwann cells — similar to the glial wrapping around axons — that causes the receptor to respond to rapid changes in pressure. Pacinian corpuscles mediate the perception of tactile texture. If you drag your fingertips across a coarse surface like sandpaper, these receptors mediate how you assess the coarseness of that surface.

Figure 11-1 also shows free nerve endings, which I discuss next.

Avoiding pain: Axonal endings for temperature and skin damage

In addition to touch sensations, the skin also senses temperature and pain. Receptors for temperature and pain are axon terminals called *free nerve endings*. Unlike other mechanoreceptors, free nerve endings aren't surrounded by any structure (refer to Figure 11-1).

Some free nerve endings are like mechanoreceptors that generate action potentials in response to force, except for extreme force that is potentially damaging and perceived as pain. A receptor type that has transient receptor potential (TRP) channels responds to a variety of potentially damaging stimuli, including temperature and high force.

Temperature receptors

Free nerve endings for temperature have ion channels that open in response to particular temperatures. Different types of temperature receptors respond best to particular temperatures, like different cones in the retina respond to different wavelength ranges (refer to Chapter 10). Warmth receptors

Feeling no pain

Attitude and mood can strongly alter the feeling of pain. Distraction or necessity can cause us to ignore or not even feel pain, while anxiety can intensify the perception of pain associated with stimuli that cause it. Being able to influence pain sensation with the mind is well documented in cases such as soldiers ignoring significant wounds, yogis tolerating extreme cold, and women feeling reduced pain in childbirth from hypnosis.

respond best to temperature ranges above body temperature (98.6 degrees Fahrenheit), while cold receptors respond best to temperature ranges below it. You can judge temperature quite precisely by sensing the unique ratio of activity of different receptors types that are activated at any particular temperature. Extreme heat, cold, or skin pressure, however, activate receptors that are interpreted as pain.

Complex aspects of pain

What different types of pain receptors have in common is that they're activated by stimuli indicating that the skin is about to be damaged. Some pain receptor types also respond to chemical damage from acids or bases, and mechanical damage (such as damage caused by a cut).

 Although pain is usually associated with something dangerous happening to a particular part of your body, pain can arise from other causes, many of which are unknown. Chronic pain that is not associated with any identifiable physical source can cause long-lasting depression. The brain has no known map for pain, like the maps in the brain for other skin senses. Instead, central nervous system pathways for pain are spread out and have many effects.

Running high on endorphins

Many drugs can reduce pain without causing a person to lose consciousness and without numbing the area that hurts. This is possible because the pain system in the brain uses a unique set of neurotransmitters. *Endogenous opioids* are neurotransmitters that are morphine-like substances called *endorphins* ("endogenous morphines").

Opioids — like morphine and heroin — reduce pain by mimicking the action of the neurotransmitters that the body produces naturally to control pain. The body produces endorphins during childbirth and distance running. Opioid drugs like heroin bind these same receptors and, at normal physiological doses, produce similar effects.

When ingested in large doses, opioid drugs produce a "high" and are highly addictive. The drug naloxone antagonizes the effects of these opioids and is often given to addicts to reverse the effects of heroin they've injected.

Endorphins are also responsible for many cases of the placebo effect. The *placebo effect* is when a patient is given an inert substance that has no pain-blocking potential but, because the patient believes it's a real pain reduction drug, he perceives that the drug is reducing his pain. Naloxone reduces the placebo effect. This means that the placebo effect isn't just psychological; it has a physiological component that involves cognitive stimulation — from belief — of the body's internal endorphin production.

Easing pain with distraction

Cognitive distraction — focusing your mind on something else — can often reduce pain. The Melzack and Wall gate theory is a hypothesis about this idea. According to the gate theory, ordinary mechanoreceptors in the skin messages activate some of the same relay neurons in the spinal cord that receive inputs from pain receptors (in the *substantia gelatinosa,* a cell body area in the spinal cord near the dorsal root where somatosensory input axons synapse). When only pain receptors are activated, their signals pass through the gate and reach the brain. However, if mechanoreceptors are sufficiently activated, they can block the neural gate and suppress the pain signal to the brain. These gate neurons also receive descending inputs from cognitive activity (that is, by distracting yourself) that can close the pain gate.

Losing the pain sense

We can all agree that feeling pain is a major, well, pain. So, would we be better off without it? Definitely not. We know pain is necessary because of what happens to people who have lost this sense. For example, in *peripheral neuropathy,* pain receptors in the peripheral nervous system die or become inactive, often as a result of vascular problems associated with diabetes. Loss of pain sense can also result from strokes and other brain damage.

People with peripheral neuropathy tend to injure themselves without knowing. They burn themselves severely while cooking, and break bones during routine physical activity. People who can't feel pain can also ignore skin lesions until they become serious infections. The sense of pain is essential for preventing harm to the body.

Locating your limbs with skin, muscle, and joint receptors

How does your brain know where your limbs are and what they're doing? *Proprioception* is the term for knowledge of limb position, while the sense of *kinesthesis* concerns information about limb movement. Some information about your limb positions comes from mechanoreceptors in the skin around your joints, which gets stretched when your limbs move. Other joint information comes from Golgi tendon organs and muscle spindles.

Golgi tendon organs are located at the junction between the muscle and the tendon that attaches it to a bone. Golgi tendon organs give feedback about the force of muscle contraction. Joint receptors for position have many similarities to skin mechanoreceptors, except that they're located in the joints and the tissues around joints. These send information to the spinal cord about joint position and movement. Free nerve endings report extreme and painful joint positions (refer to the heading "Avoiding pain: Axonal endings for temperature and skin damage," earlier in this chapter).

Spinal processing and cranial nerves

For most of the body, sensory input is transduced by the axons of dorsal root ganglion cells that synapse in the spinal gray area. The output of these receptors participates in monosynaptic and polysynaptic reflexes (refer to Chapters 5 and 6), and is also relayed to the thalamus (see the next section). Sensory receptors in the skin of the head project to the brain via numerous cranial nerves such as the trigeminal nerve for the face, along with some upper cervical nerves for the back of the head (refer to Chapter 7).

Sending the message to the thalamus

Two major pathways project skin information to the brain from the body below the head:

✔ The *spinothalamic pathway* is a phylogenetically old, small fiber tract that mediates several reflexes, such as withdrawal. The spinothalamic pathway relays sensory information from the skin to the brain about temperature and pain (lateral section of the tract) and coarse touch (anterior-ventral section of the tract). Axons in this tract *decussate* (cross) within the spinal cord, rather than in the brainstem, and relay with secondary neurons in the substantia gelatinosa or the nucleus proprius. These nuclei project to the rostral ventromedial medulla, which projects to several somatosensory thalamic nuclei. These thalamic nuclei for the spinothalamic pathway project to somatosensory cortex, cingulate cortex, and insula.

✔ The *lemniscal pathway,* whose axons are larger in diameter than the spinothalamic tract, carries fine-touch sensory information and proprioceptive information for active touch. The axons of this pathway are large diameter and myelinated. After ascending the spinal cord, axons of this tract synapse with neurons in the cuneate and gracile nuclei of the medulla. These nuclei relay to the ventral posterolateral nucleus of the thalamus (ventral posteromedial nucleus for sensation from the head via cranial nerves).

Relay neurons in the thalamus may have antagonistic center surround receptive fields (a central region where stimulation increases neural firing, surrounded by a region that reduces it) — something like those found in the visual system — but otherwise their responses are similar to their inputs from the spinal cord and cranial nerves. The thalamic neurons project to primary sensory cortex, located just posterior to the central sulcus in the most anterior part of the parietal lobe, as well as to the insula and cingulate cortex.

Recognizing What We Touch at Somatosensory Cortex

The somatosensory part of the thalamus (the ventral posterior nucleus) projects to a narrow strip of cortex just posterior to the central sulcus, making it the most anterior part of the parietal lobe (see the left side of Figure 11-2). The parts of the body closest to the ground when we're standing (the feet and legs) are represented most medially, while the fingers and face representations are more lateral.

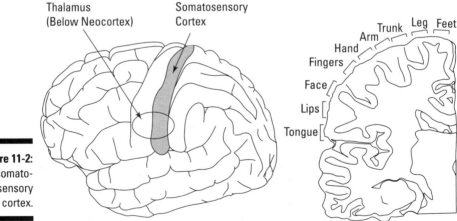

Figure 11-2:
The somato-sensory cortex.

Mapping senses with the homunculus

The topographic map of the skin on the cortex is called the *homunculus*. The term means "little man," and the map is actually shaped somewhat like the human body. The right side of Figure 11-2 shows where major body areas are represented on a coronal section of the somatosensory cortex.

This map isn't perfect. For example, the area of the homunculus that responds to stimulation of the fingers is near that for the face. Also, the homunculus representation on somatosensory cortex is clearly distorted. The fingers take up much larger areas of somatosensory cortex than, say, the skin on the abdomen, which is a much larger skin area.

Two principles explain the distortion in the homunculus:

- ✔ **Different areas of the skin have very different receptor densities.** The skin in the fingertip, for example, has many more receptors per area than the same areas in the skin on the stomach or back. This allows you to have high two-point discrimination in your fingertips so you can manipulate objects precisely.

- ✔ **In the way the neocortex is organized, a given area of cortex processes inputs from about the same absolute number of receptors.**

Skin areas with high receptor density, such as the fingertips, get proportionally more cortical area than the skin areas with low receptor densities. The neocortex is a constellation of millions of interconnected minicolumns, all with nearly the same neural circuitry. Each of these minicolumns can handle about the same number of inputs. Where the external receptor density is high, there will be more cortical area compared to other areas where density is lower.

Specialized somatosensory areas

The assessment of what is the primary projection area in the neocortex for somatosensation is complicated in somatosensory cortex because this sense includes multiple, different types of skin sense — different types of mechanoreception, temperature, and pain senses.

Primary somatosensory cortex is essentially Brodmann area 3, which receives the largest direct thalamocortical projection, although direct projections may go to Brodmann areas 1 and 2 as well. Area 3 has been subdivided into areas 3a and 3b, with 3b being the best candidate for the major primary somatosensory cortex because it receives significant direct inputs from the thalamus. Neurons in 3b are selectively responsive to typical tactile skin stimuli, whereas neurons in 3a appear to receive proprioceptive inputs about joint position and muscle forces.

Brodmann areas 1 and 2 are generally now considered high-order somatosensory areas that receive most of their input from area 3b rather than directly from thalamus. Neurons in Brodmann area 1 respond to stimulation of Pacinian corpuscles (refer to the "Localizing touch" section, earlier in this chapter) that encode some aspects of texture information. Area 2 has neurons that are involved in active touch for determining the shape of objects.

Inputs to somatosensory cortex, like other neocortex, project into layer IV. Neurons in this layer generate excitation and inhibition in other layers. Somatosensory cortex, like other sensory cortex, shows a columnar organization, with neurons that have similar response properties grouped together.

Perceiving pain

The primary cortical areas that receive pain receptor projections have been difficult to locate. The spinothalamic tract ends in the VPM, VPL, intralaminar, and medial dorsal nuclei of the thalamus. The ventral and medial dorsal thalamic nuclei that receive input from pain fibers project directly to secondary cortical areas. For example, the perception of pain tends to be associated with activity in the insula and anterior cingulate cortex. Pain axon projections also go to the lateral nucleus of the amygdala and the hippocampus. Activating the amygdala is associated with immediate emotional responses.

The somatosensory cortical areas for the hands and fingers are located close to areas for the face (refer to Figure 11-2). The phenomena of "phantom limb" feelings (including pain) that some people experience after having a limb amputated may occur because neural projections from the face invade the neighboring part of the cortex that was once devoted to the limb. Face sensation that activates these inappropriate inputs may be interpreted as pain in the limb, even though the limb is no longer there.

Pain is also complex because it can be strongly influenced by psychological factors. Men tend to be less tolerant of chronic pain than women are, though men are more tolerant of acute pain. Athletic training and strong motivation to obtain some goal can significantly reduce the disabling effects of pain. Pain tolerance generally increases with age. Different cultures also tend to have different levels of pain tolerance — cultures that encourage emotional expression typically report lower pain tolerance.

Sniffing Out the World around You

Whereas senses like vision and hearing require the detection of energy (light photons and sound waves), *olfaction* (smell) involves detecting actual substances from the world. You smell using your nose, which also filters, warms, and humidifies the air you breathe and analyzes that air for odors. The nose has olfactory receptors in its "roof." The olfactory receptor neurons have cilia that stick down into the mucus that lines the roof of the nose that respond to different odors. Figure 11-3 shows the location of the olfactory receptors in the nose, and the olfactory bulb that I discuss a bit later.

Most mammals use a larger percentage of their brain for olfactory processing compared to humans. A dog might have a billion olfactory receptors, comparable to the neuron count in the rest of its brain. Humans have 10 million olfactory receptors (compared to 125 million photoreceptors) in a 100 billion neuron brain.

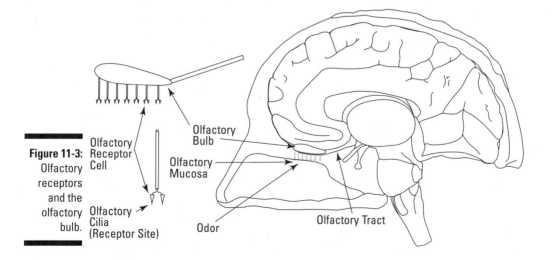

Figure 11-3: Olfactory receptors and the olfactory bulb.

Olfactory Receptor Cell

Olfactory Bulb

Olfactory Mucosa

Olfactory Cilia (Receptor Site)

Odor

Olfactory Tract

Nosing around: Olfactory receptors

Olfactory receptors function much like metabotropic receptors (refer to Chapter 4), except that a molecule from the world binds to the receptor. This binding causes a second messenger cascade inside the cell that results in the release of intracellular messengers that bind on the inside of other receptors and open other channels.

To recognize the myriad substances that we smell every day, we elaborate approximately 1,000 different olfactory receptor types. Every odor binds to a different subset of these receptors so that each odor has a unique receptor activity signature. The brain identifies the odor by comparing the activity of different receptors.

Exploring the olfactory bulb

Humans have about 10 million olfactory receptors. However, unlike cones in the retina that come in three varieties (refer to Chapter 10), olfactory receptors come in about 1,000 different types. This is because of the myriad chemical differences that exist in the odorants we can detect based on their molecular shapes and charge distributions. The immune system faces a similar issue in responding to foreign invaders by their binding to many possible receptor sites. Most olfactory receptors respond to many odorants, so that odors are encoded by the pattern of activity of multiple receptor types.

Olfactory receptors project to the olfactory bulb just above the back of the nose (refer to Figure 11-3) where about 1,000 to 2,000 different recipient zones, *olfactory glomeruli,* are located. Most glomeruli receive inputs predominantly from a single receptor type. The pattern of activity across the glomeruli constitutes the signature for that odor.

Most odors that we encounter actually contain a complex mix of odors. Coffee aroma, for example, contains at least 100 different kinds of odor molecules. This means that the odor of coffee generates more than 100 different signatures simultaneously in the olfactory glomeruli. Your brain still needs to do a bit of processing before you can recognize what you're drinking.

The problem of multiple odorants is mitigated somewhat by the fact that different odorants have different transit times across the olfactory mucosa. Each sniff produces a synchronized input to the nose, so that the odorant responses are spread out over time. This is sometimes referred to as the *chromatographic theory of odor perception.* Proteins in the mucosa called *olfactory binding proteins* help some non-soluble odorants enter and transit the mucosa to reach the receptor cilia.

Olfactory receptors die, and new ones are continuously regenerated, even in the adult nervous system. This differs from other sensory systems where the death of receptors is usually permanent.

The regenerative ability of olfactory receptors has led some neurobiologists to attempt to transplant olfactory mucosa neurons (mostly the olfactory ensheathing cells, a kind of epithelial stem cell in the olfactory system) into damaged areas of the brain or spinal cord. The hope is that the transplanted olfactory cells will regenerate and convert into spine or brain neuronal types to integrate functionally into damaged neural circuits. Recently more research emphasis has been placed on using stem cells, particularly converted cells from the same individual, for transplants.

Reaching the cortex before the thalamus

The projections of the olfactory bulb are unique among the sensory systems because they go directly to several areas of the cortex without first relaying through the thalamus. The result of direct projections to structures such as the amygdala is that you often have an immediate emotional response to some odors before you're consciously aware of their identity. Some olfactory information does reach the thalamus directly, and indirectly, however. Figure 11-4 shows the overall olfactory projection scheme.

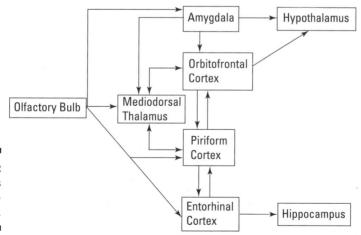

Figure 11-4: Projections of the olfactory bulb.

The olfactory bulb projects to these areas of the brain:

- ✔ **The amygdala:** The amygdala mediates emotional responses to odors and projects to the hypothalamus to mediate hormonal responses to odors.

- ✔ **The entorhinal cortex:** Projections to the entorhinal cortex, amygdala, and hippocampus allow you to remember odors, particularly if they were part of an important experience.

- ✔ **The piriform cortex:** The projection to the piriform (pear-shaped) cortex is an ancient pathway, which makes unconscious and reactive odor discrimination possible. The piriform cortex is allocortex lying just ventral to the amygdala and contiguous with the entorhinal cortex.

- ✔ **The orbitofrontal cortex:** The orbitofrontal projection (through the medio-dorsal thalamus) mediates conscious odor discrimination. Some odor information also merges with taste here to give the perception of flavor.

- ✔ **Mediodorsal thalamus:** This is the olfactory area of the thalamus, which is reached indirectly by a relay projection from the olfactory cortex, rather than from the olfactory bulb directly.

In the other sensory systems, peripheral receptors project to the thalamus, that then projects to a succession of cortical areas. The lower and higher cortical areas then project to memory structures such as the entorhinal cortex and hippocampus after cortical processing to identify what we're sensing. Smell is different from the other senses in that smell often intrinsically generates an emotional response. Many smells are either immediately disgusting or displeasing (such as feces or spoiled food) or pleasing (such as flowers or chocolate cake).

The olfactory system has an evolutionarily older pattern with a direct projection to cortical and memory structures (from the bulb). This pathway mediates quick responses to elemental smells, such as something rotting. The amygdala is located anterior to the hippocampus and has a similar memory function to it, except that it processes emotionally salient memories. In the case of olfaction, it stores memories for which a smell was the trigger for emotional salience, such as the odor of a particular food before you get sick.

The amygdala projects to the olfactory thalamus and frontal lobe. The direct projections from the olfactory bulb to the amygdala appear to be part of a neural circuit that mediates learning associated with approach/withdrawal behavior for smells. A single negative incident can trigger lifelong aversion to spoiled food — even if the food is not spoiled.

A "high road" pathway through the mediodorsal thalamus mediates responses that depend on more nuanced identification of odors that requires higher-order cortical processing to identity before being stored in our memory. This is the smell processing that doesn't generate an immediate limbic-like behavioral response, but which mediates conscious aspects of odor detection, as occurs in all other senses.

The difference between the overall anatomical structure of the olfactory system and other sensory systems may be due to its early evolution in mammals. Most mammals are more olfactory than primates, and olfactory-induced behavior is generated directly (the proposed function for the limbic system). Olfactory processing that was not directly linked to behavior happened when a phylogenetically newer thalamic pathway was created. The pathway was created by projecting from olfactory cortex to thalamus, which then projected back to cortex, in a manner similar to the other senses.

Smelling badly versus smelling bad

The inability to perceive odors is called *anosmia*. It is most often a result of damage to the olfactory mucosa and olfactory receptors. Temporary anosmia typically is caused by mucosa inflammation from infections such as cold viruses or minor head trauma. Olfactory neurons are among the few central nervous system cells that regenerate constantly, so receptors are always being repopulated. Continuous exposure to noxious substances that damage the tissue can reduce or destroy the sense of smell. A less than total loss of smell is called *hyposmia,* which can occur for specific odors. We all adapt to odors, particularly our own (so we may be unaware of our offense when not showering often enough).

Congenital anosmia is a lack of the sense of smell from birth. This is usually genetic. Some people have a greater than normal sense of smell, referred to as *hyperosmia*. Women typically have a better sense of smell than men do.

Permanent loss of smell may occur from death of olfactory receptor precursor neurons. Like other senses, it also can occur from damage to the olfactory nerve or damage to olfactory brain areas. Schizophrenia, Parkinson's, and Alzheimer's diseases are sometimes associated with hyposmia or anosmia.

Communicating with pheromones

Smell contributes to sexual behavior both consciously and unconsciously. For example, the menstrual cycles of women who live together or near each other tend to synchronize unconsciously through smell. Odors induce an attraction toward the opposite sex, as the multi-billion-dollar perfume industry proves.

The nose contains a specific organ of smell near the vomer bone called the *vomeronasal organ*. This organ appears to have receptors for human sexual odors that are unconsciously processed by non-thalamic odor pathways. The biological term for a communication odor that influences species-specific behavior is a *pheromone*. Some (though diminishing) controversy exists about the appropriateness of this term for human odor communication.

Nevertheless, humans produce similar odors via glands similar to those in other mammals; these odors act on similarly located receptors, have similar central projections, and result in similar unconscious behavioral effects.

Tasting Basics: Sweet, Sour, Salt, and Bitter Receptors

Humans, like all animals, must be able to discriminate between non-toxic and toxic plants, ripe and unripe fruit, and fresh and spoiled meat during eating. Because what you taste is already in your mouth about to be ingested, you need to make these discriminations rapidly and accurately.

Receptors for taste reside mostly on the tongue in structures called *papillae* (see Figure 11-5) that appear as little bumps on the tongue. The tongue has four types of papillae: fungiform, foliate, circumvallate, and filiform. The central portion of the tongue has almost exclusively filiform papillae; taste does not occur there (the filiform papillae don't have taste receptors but have a mechanical function in some species that use rough tongues to *rasp,* or grate, ingested food). Fungiform, foliate, and circumvallate papillae contain taste receptor cells. These papillae are located at the tip, sides, and back of the tongue, respectively.

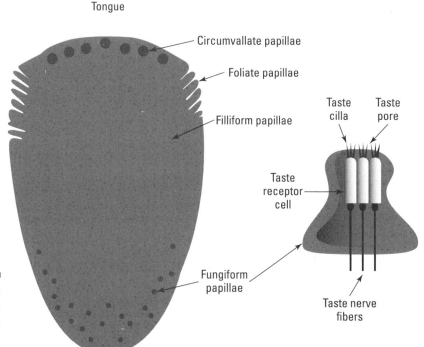

Figure 11-5: Taste receptors on the tongue.

Traditionally, when we think of the sense of taste, we think of four basic tastes:

- **Sweet:** The sweet taste comes from receptors that respond to sugars (such as glucose and fructose), the source of energy for metabolism. Many human taste receptors respond almost exclusively to sugar.

- **Salt:** Salt (NaCl) constitutes the major solute in the fluid throughout our bodies. A large number of taste receptors also respond almost exclusively to NaCl salt. However, other salts, such as potassium chloride (KCl) also activate the same receptors.

- **Sour:** The sour taste is the detection of acidity, so that sour receptors react to H+ ions. Sourness is a characteristic of foods that many people enjoy, such as lemons, but it can also indicate spoilage. So, the reaction to the sour taste is complex and depends on learning.

- **Bitter:** Bitterness, like sourness, is sometimes a sign of food being unripe or toxic. The prototypical bitter substance is quinine. We learn that the occurrence of bitter taste in some foods means they should be avoided, while other foods may contain bitter spices but are okay to eat.

In addition to the four traditional tastes, many neurobiologists now include a fifth basic taste, *umami,* a meaty, MSG-like taste that comes from the Japanese term meaning "savory and pleasant taste." This receptor responds to the amino acid L-glutamate. Also, some evidence shows CO_2 receptors activated by carbonated liquids.

Most taste receptors respond to different tastes, and most taste buds have several different types of receptors. The taste buds contain about 10,000 taste cells. Receptors for all the basic tastes are located in all papillae types (fungiform, foliate, and circumvallate) throughout the tongue. However, the tongue has regional differences in the percentage of receptors, such as relatively enhanced taste for sweet at the front of the tongue and bitter at the back.

Coding for taste: Labels versus patterns

Taste information in the tongue is projected to the brain via the chorda tympani and glossopharyngeal nerves, which I discuss later in this section. Some of these nerve fibers will receive inputs almost exclusively from similar receptors, such as salt fibers, while others receive a mix of inputs from different receptor cell types.

An important historical debate in neurobiology is about whether the "code" used by the taste system was "labeled line" or "distributed." The labeled line proponents suggested that most taste axons were selective for specific tastes, whereas the distributed theory argued that fibers represent tastes by the pattern of firing across fibers. This feature selection versus general filter argument is present in ideas about sensory coding throughout the nervous system.

The evidence about labeled line versus distributed coding is complex. Some receptors for saltiness and, to some extent, sweetness appear to be highly specific, so our brains can consider activation of these receptors as labeled line receptors reporting the presence of salt or sweet. On the other hand, a large percentage of taste receptors respond to some degree to salt, sweet, sour, and bitter tastes, leaving it to the higher brain centers to identify taste from the ratio of receptor activation distributed across a number of receptors. What's unique about taste is that the combination of labeled line and distributed coding strategies exists in the same nerve.

Understanding the umami problem

The taste umami is based on receptors that have been discovered for L-glutamate. These receptors also respond to guanosine monophosphate (GMP) and inosine monophosphate (IMP). The perception generated when these taste receptors are activated is described as "pleasant" or "meaty" with a sensation of coating the tongue. However, the umami taste is pleasant only within a narrow concentration range, which also depends on the salt concentration. Some older people like when agents get added to food that generate the umami taste because of their generally lowered taste and smell sensitivity.

Although the Japanese scientist Kikunae Ikeda proposed umami as a basic taste in 1908, its status was debated until the mid-1980s. The ribonucleotides GMP and IMP amplify the umami taste and are used to increase the palatability of many foods because of the synergistic effect between GMP and IMP and glutamate.

Supertasters

Some people are far more sensitive to taste than others. They're called "supertasters." About one third of women but only 10 percent to 20 percent of men are supertasters, and they're less common in Caucasians than in other ethnic groups. Besides having lower taste thresholds and better taste discrimination generally, supertasters have a heightened taste response to bitterness. This makes some supertasters picky eaters, but many picky eaters are not supertasters.

The supertaster ability is associated with several factors:

- An increased number of fungiform papillae

- The TAS2R38 gene that codes for bitter taste

- The ability to taste substances called PROP (propylthiouracil) and PTC (phenylthiocarbamide) that have no taste to non-supertasters

Tasting with the Brain

Each taste bud has five to ten taste receptor cells (Figure 11-5 shows only three), with most taste buds having at least one of each of the five basic receptor types. The first stop for taste information in the brain is the rostral part of the nucleus of the solitary tract (NST) in the medulla. Two tracts carry this information: The chorda tympani (a branch of the facial nerve) carries signals mostly from fungiform papillae in the anterior two-thirds of the tongue, while the glossopharyngeal nerve sends information from foliate and circumvallate papillae, and a few rearward fungiform papillae in the posterior third of the tongue.

Projecting taste to the thalamus

The nucleus of the solitary tract (NST) projects to the thalamus, but also to the reticular formation, hypothalamus, and parasympathetic preganglionic neurons. Neurons projecting from the NST of the medulla mediate gag and cough reflexes. Figure 11-6 shows the projections for taste.

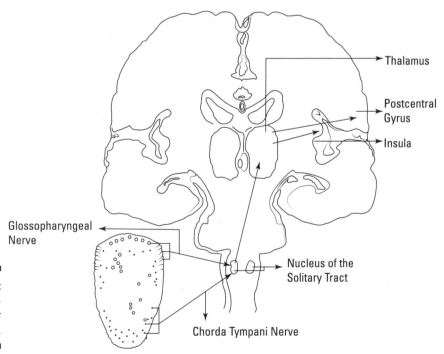

Figure 11-6: Central projections for taste.

Thalamus

Postcentral Gyrus

Insula

Glossopharyngeal Nerve

Nucleus of the Solitary Tract

Chorda Tympani Nerve

The taste portion of the thalamus to which the NST projects is the ventroposteromedial thalamus (VPM). Reciprocal connections between this thalamic area and the cortical processing areas for taste mediate conscious awareness of the taste sensation. Lesions in the VPM cause *ageusia,* the loss of the sense of taste.

Discriminating taste in the cortex

The VPM thalamus projects to the insula and frontal operculum cortex (refer to Figure 11-6), both of which are primary cortical taste areas. The insular lobe is hidden behind the temporal lobe at the junction of the parietal, frontal, and temporal lobes. The opercular cortex (operculum means "lid") is located just above the insula. The insula and operculum cortex are evolutionarily old and participate in cortical circuits that are also affected by olfaction and vision. These cortical areas are involved in satiety (which I discuss a bit later), pain, and some homeostasis functions.

The cortex can discriminate small differences in taste to allow neural activity to be modified by experience, which enhances your ability to detect and discriminate taste. You learn over your life very subtle food preferences based on taste and smell. You associate other factors with food as well. Food texture, which is communicated by mechanoreceptors while chewing, is an important component of eating.

Even people who congenitally lack both taste and smell still enjoy eating. Careful attention to food texture is part of the fare of all high-quality restaurants.

Combining taste and smell for flavor

The insula and opercular cortices project to the orbitofrontal cortex. Here, some neurons receive inputs from the olfactory system as well. Neurons receiving both taste and smell information mediate the perception of *flavor,* the complex "taste" derived from a combination of taste and smell. Much of the sense of taste is derived from odors emitted while chewing food that reach the nasal mucosa. Most people are unable to identify the tastes of chocolate or coffee with their noses blocked, for example.

The insula and opercular cortices also project to the amygdala, which mediates memory for emotionally salient experiences. The amygdala projects back to the orbitofrontal cortex. This cortical pathway allows you to associate the sight, smell, and taste of very specific foods with your experience before and after ingesting them.

Losing taste through injuries

Although some people are born without a sense of taste (ageusia), total lack of the taste sense is very rare. A very poor sense of taste *(hypogeusia)* is more common. This may actually be caused by damage to the olfactory mucosa, which is an anosmia leading to hypogeusia because of the involvement of smell with taste. Hypogeusia is rare as a congenital condition, but it may occur as a result of nerve damage, such as to the chorda tympani nerve, from disease or injury. Temporary hypogeusia often occurs during some cancer chemotherapies. Aging tends to reduce sensitivity to bitter tastes, which explains why children find some vegetables strongly bitter that are much less so to their parents.

Feeling full

Eating is partly controlled by satiety mechanisms that modulate the sense of taste. An adaption mechanism in the taste receptors themselves and a central brain mechanism mediate satiety:

- ✓ *Sensory-specific satiety* occurs in taste and olfactory receptors themselves. It tends to suppress your appetite specifically for the taste of what you're consuming, acting on a fast time scale.

- ✓ *Alliesthesia* is the name for the central satiety mechanism. As you eat and grow full, what you're eating loses its desirability because of the brain mechanism that indicates you're getting full. The mechanism for this is seen in the reduced firing of orbitofrontal taste/smell neurons to the specific odor of a food after you've eaten a lot of it.

Several gastrointestinal hormones regulate appetite via their actions on the brain. These mediate satiety not so linked to specific foods. Gut-derived hormones include ghrelin, insulin, CCK, pancreatic polypeptide (PP), and peptide YY (PYY). These hormones stimulate specific areas of the hypothalamus and brainstem. They also modify the sensations that are transmitted by the vagus nerve to the nucleus of the solitary tract (also called the *nucleus tractus solitarius* [NTS]). The hypothalamus and brainstem control appetite via interactions with higher brain centers, such as the amygdala and cortex.

Monitoring Internal Body Functions with Internal Chemoreceptors

Olfaction and taste involve *chemoreception,* the detection of substances that enter the body. The body has receptors that detect concentrations of many important substances within it, such as glucose and CO_2. Many of these receptors are in the hypothalamus where the blood–brain barrier is weak, allowing them to access neural receptors there. Other internal chemical detection sites include the subfornical organ and the organum vasculosum of the lamina terminalis. These are called circumventricular organs where neurons can sense chemicals from both blood and CSF.

Examples of substances detected by internal chemoreceptors include osmo-larity and sodium concentration for fluid balance. A host of other receptors exist for peptide hormones, such as endothelin and relaxin, angiotensin, steroids, glucocorticoids, and monoamine neurotransmitters noradrenaline, dopamine, and serotonin (5-hydroxytryptamine).

Chapter 12

Memory and Learning

· ·

In This Chapter

▶ Adapting our behaviors according to environment

▶ Being unaware of implicit memory

▶ Keeping memories for the long and short term

▶ Looking at brain structures for memory

▶ Getting all fired up about learning

▶ Losing your memory

▶ Visualizing a trick for better memory

· ·

*T*he good thing about making mistakes is the opportunity to learn from them. Learning allows us to change our behavior for the better based on past experience. We can do this thanks to short-term and long-term memory, which enable the brain to retain information and experiences.

In the nervous system, learning happens through changes in the neural circuits that process sensory information or organize motor output. A major challenge for neurobiology is to understand how neural circuits that process sensory information and organize motor output also dynamically learn.

I'm assuming you picked up this book to learn about neurobiology. And in this chapter, I talk about how learning works, by discussing what's going on in your brain that allows you to learn and store information, and retain and create memories.

Evolving with Adaptation and Instinct

Evolution is a gradual process during which organisms are shaped by their environment. Organisms that have beneficial traits pass on their genetic information to later generations more effectively than organisms without these beneficial traits. In this way, the environment naturally selects the organisms that are most fit for that particular environment. *Development* is the time during which the brains of individual organisms change in response to their environment. The changes that occur during evolution and development are different from what we call "learning," and are generally referred to as "adaptation" or "plasticity." However, plasticity and adaptation are similar to the learning process in that they all involve changes to the nervous system's functional structure.

Moving through evolution

Evolution produces an organism that has a nervous system with complex instincts for feeding, fighting, fleeing, and mating. Environmental stimuli — such as the sight of food or a rival — tend to trigger instinct-driven behavior. These instinct-driven responses are almost robot-like and are genetically built into the organism's limbic system.

Going into development

Development refines genetically built-in stimulus-response behaviors. The longer the developmental period of the organism, the more attuned and differentiated is its nervous system to the particular environment.

Humans have a much longer developmental period than most other animals. During this developmental period, we're not very good at anything except learning. The summit of this developmental climb is acquiring language, a learning that is unique to humans.

Development is typically characterized by critical periods. All humans crawl, walk, and talk about the same time. If, for whatever reason these skills are not acquired at the normal developmental time, they're often poorly mastered for the rest of the life of the organism.

Looking at learning

During development, there are large-scale changes that allow an organism to interact appropriately with their environment. Following the critical period, smaller-scale refinements to this basic neuronal scaffold occur throughout life that constitute learning. *Plasticity* is the ability to adapt to our environment during development. Learning can occur at any age. In the past, neurobiologists believed that learning occurs only by changing synaptic weights in an otherwise statically wired nervous system because it was thought that there was no adult neurogenesis. Recent evidence, however, suggests that even in adults, neurons can be produced in brain areas like the hippocampus, and this neurogenesis is important for learning.

Many different types of learning use different mechanisms and occur at different times in one animal's life. Some of these different types of learning are similar between humans and other animals, and these similarities have allowed neurobiologists to learn a lot about how learning works in our brains. Figure 12-1 shows the different classifications of learning and memory, which I explore throughout this chapter.

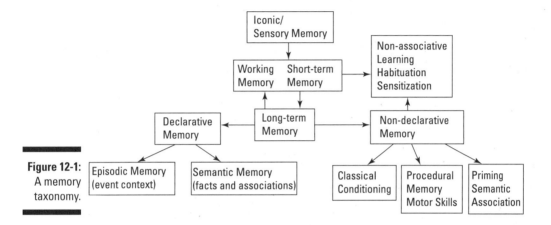

Figure 12-1: A memory taxonomy.

Implicit (Non-Declarative) Memory

Exposure to the environment can cause changes in the nervous system. The process by which this happens is typically called *learning,* and the result, *memory.* But there are different kinds of memory. We're conscious of some effects of experience, such as learning someone's name. This type of memory is called *explicit memory.* We also learn things, such as how to hit a tennis ball better, that we cannot describe verbally. This is one type of memory called *implicit memory,* or *non-declarative memory.*

The process by which a stimulus from the environment becomes a memory starts with the initial neural image registered by your sensory system that is called *iconic/sensory memory* (refer to Figure 12-1). For example, if you see a red Corvette, you can, for a few seconds, see an almost exact image of it in your mind. (Didn't you just picture a red Corvette after reading the words?)

This sensory image is closely linked to the perceptual domain in which you initially register it, such as a feeling of touch for a skin sensation, or a flavor for a taste. (Refer to Chapter 11 for more about the senses.) The iconic realistic image you hold in your mind fades very quickly. That's because of changes in the activity of the neurons that are close to the transduction of the stimulus. How these neurons change with constant or repeated stimulation is the next topic.

Getting used to habituation

All sensory receptors adapt to a constant or continually repeated stimulus. This adaptation is called *habituation*. For example, when you first sit down in a chair, you're aware of your behind hitting the chair seat, but after a few minutes, your awareness of the chair fades.

Habituation occurs in all sensory systems. Most sensory systems have mixes of slowly adapting and rapidly adapting receptors. Habituation allows you to be sensitive to change, but not distracted by a constant stimulus that's no longer important to you. How could you concentrate on reading this book, for example, if you were as acutely aware of the chair seat and back pressing against you now as when you first sat down? The initial somatosensory message helped you sit gently, but now that you're sitting, it's no longer necessary or useful for you to be aware of it.

Habituation can also occur at higher levels in the nervous system than the sensory receptors. This higher-level habituation can also be reversed, which is then called *dishabituation*. Dishabituation typically results from the effect of another novel stimulus that reverses some of the habituation to the first, habituated stimulus. For example, you might habituate to the slight feeling evoked by an insect on your arm, but if the insect were a mosquito and it bit you, you would dishabituate to similar future stimuli and probably slap at its source on your skin.

Responding to sensitization

Sometimes your brain can learn to react to a stimulus very quickly. If you're outside during mosquito season, you may not notice the first few mosquitoes that land on your legs. But after one bite, you become hypersensitive to the mosquitoes and can swat at them quickly, before they get a good bite in. This is called *sensitization*. You become sensitized when a normally neutral stimulus becomes paired, and predictive of, a painful consequence, so that you react more strongly to it. Sensitization is useful in many situations and usually occurs in the neural processing chain where the initial stimulus signal is mixed with the representation of the painful consequence. (You see or feel the mosquito on your leg and know that it means you'll be terribly itchy later, so you swat at it almost without thinking.)

Habituation and sensitization both occur unconsciously, although the behavior that sensitization provokes can be realized consciously. They are referred to as *non-associative learning:* a change in behavior due to repetition of specific stimuli. Sensitization occurs in all animals, even invertebrates, so neurobiologists know a lot about the cellular mechanisms involved.

Kandel's habituation work

The cellular bases of habituation and sensitization were studied in the gill withdrawal reflex of the sea hare *Aplysia californica* by Eric Kandel and colleagues, for which he won a Nobel Prize in Physiology or Medicine in 2000.

He showed that the gill withdrawal was a two-component reflex involving both central ganglia and peripheral neural processes, and exactly which neurons participated in the reflex and its habituation.

Preparing for priming

Priming is another form of implicit memory. If you've ever heard of subliminal advertising, you're already familiar with the concept. In subliminal advertising, the thought was that if one of every 24 movie frames flashed "buy popcorn," the audience could be induced to do so without consciously being aware of the message. Subliminal advertising was banned — but then it was shown not to be particularly effective anyway.

Subliminal stimulation is an example of priming, however priming has actually been shown to work. For example, I ask you to play a word-association game, and I give you the word *bank*. You could come up with words related to *bank* either as it refers to rivers or as it refers to money. However, if before giving you the word I showed you an image of a river, but so fast that you were unaware of it, your responses to the word *bank* would be reliably biased toward river, not money, associations.

Priming involves long-term memory not because the effect of a subliminally flashed image (the *prime*) reliably lasts for a lifetime, but because the effect of a prime activates the long-term memory system, including our world knowledge semantics. This semantic system is sometimes referred to as the *perceptual representation system*.

Conditioning classically and operantly

In contrast to non-associative learning (habituation and facilitation), *associative learning* involves behavioral change caused by animals associating temporal relationships between stimuli and responses or motor behavior. Classical conditioning and operant conditioning are types of associative learning, which I explore in the next two sections.

Classical conditioning

Classical conditioning is the type of associative learning famously studied by the Russian scientist Ivan Pavlov, and is often called *Pavlovian conditioning*. Classical conditioning starts with the phenomenon common to all animals in which either a noxious or pleasant stimulus, called the *unconditioned stimulus* (US), produces an appropriate response (avoidance or approach), called the *unconditioned response* (UR). This is typically an appropriate, species-specific reaction — for example, you touch something hot and immediately withdraw your hand from it.

In classical conditioning, a temporal pairing can be created between a neutral stimulus, such as a sound or light, that signals the US. This is usually because the neutral stimulus is presented about the same time as the US (or slightly earlier). This new, initially neutral stimulus is called the *conditioning stimulus* (CS). Because the US always produces the UR, now that the CS is paired with the US, the animal learns that the CS *predicts* the UR. Although the CS produces no response itself initially, after a number of pairing trials, called *conditioning,* the CS elicits the same response that the US always elicited. The repetition and the response create the conditioned response (CR).

Although what we call classical conditioning is typically done in psychology or neurobiology laboratories, classical conditioning actually occurs naturally throughout our lives. If you answer cellphone calls while driving and you often almost get in accidents, you learn (hopefully) to associate answering phone calls with negative consequences, and begin to avoid this behavior. If you like fast-food hamburgers, the sight of golden arches may make you salivate.

Operant (instrumental) conditioning

Operant or *instrumental conditioning* involves the pairing of rewards or punishments with some antecedent behavior. (The term *operant conditioning* was coined by B. F. Skinner, one of its most influential practitioners.) Operant conditioning is based on spontaneous behavior. This behavior can be associated with consequences that may reinforce or inhibit future recurrences of that behavior.

Pavlov's dog

In Pavlov's classic experiments, he measured a dog's salivation (the UR) when he gave it food (the US). He then paired ringing a bell (the CS) with the presentation of the food. After several pairings, the bell itself elicited salivation (the CR). The mechanism of classical conditioning depends on the fact that the CS signals or predicts the US. Classical conditioning allows animals to generate appropriate behavior to novel environmental stimuli if they're predictive of something either rewarding or painful.

For example, suppose you want to train a rat to press a lever at one end of a cage. When you first put a rat in the cage, it moves around and explores its surroundings — the spontaneous behavior. Whenever the rat moves toward the end of the cage where the lever is, a food pellet is dropped down a chute into the cage. At first, this is done just when the rat moves in the right general direction, but later, it's done only when the rat actually goes to the cage wall with the lever. This is called *shaping*. In the last phases, the rat gets the pellet only for moving very close to the lever, for touching the lever, and finally for pushing the lever.

Operant conditioning can use either rewards (reinforcement) or punishment, each of which may be linked to positive or negative consequences of some behavior. Reinforcement causes some behavior to occur more frequently, whereas punishment causes a behavior to occur less frequently.

In the terminology of reinforcement and punishment, each can be used in two different ways. Positive reinforcement is when a behavior is followed by something rewarding. Negative reinforcement (called *escape*) is when a behavior is followed by the removal of an aversive stimulus.

Punishment is distinct from reinforcement. Positive punishment is when a behavior is followed by an aversive stimulus, such as a shock. Negative punishment is when a behavior is followed by the removal of a positive stimulus, such as access to food.

Behaviors generated by operant conditioning may be lost through what is called *extinction*. Extinction results from changing the conditions so that the operant consequence associated with the previously conditioned behavior no longer happens. This causes the behavior to occur less frequently, and it may return to the spontaneous level before the conditioning started.

Like classical conditioning, operant conditioning occurs in the real world. Driving to a certain area of town that has a number of good restaurants may lead you to stop there and enjoy good meals. This may translate to going to one of the restaurants after just getting on the road that leads to that part of town, or just getting in your car. The chain of associations leading to obtaining illicit drugs appears to be a powerful component of addiction.

Learning motor sequences: Procedural memory

What used to be called *motor memory* — remembering how to ride a bicycle, for example — is now called *procedural memory,* because some forms of it don't actually involve muscle contractions. Procedural memory is typically the acquisition of skill in performing action sequences. Often conscious awareness is involved in the initial acquisition, but not in the performance afterward. When you ride a bicycle, most of the time you do so without knowing exactly where your feet are and what steering and posture adjustments you're making.

If you refer to Figure 12-1 earlier in this chapter, you can see that procedural memory is classified as a non-declarative, long-term type of memory. It's established by practice — repeating an action sequence until the sequence can be "automatically" well executed without conscious awareness.

One reason procedural memory is not called *motor memory* is that some procedure-like skills are learned by similar mechanisms that don't involve actual movement. One example is planning chess moves. Each chess piece "moves" according to certain rules. When practiced chess players learn the piece move sequences, they activate neural circuits in the cerebellum that are similar to those used for motor learning. Skillful players can imagine a sequence of moves using this learned neural circuitry without actually putting their hands on a chess piece and physically moving it.

A hallmark of procedural memory is the lack of conscious awareness of the steps that make up the overall action sequence. Moreover, attempting to bring these steps to awareness generally interferes with performing the well-learned sequences, rather than helping. One model for procedural memories is that of a causal chain, where completion of one phase of the action sequence directly causes the beginning of the next phase, without voluntary intervention of any kind. This knowledge has been referred to as "knowing how" versus conscious types of memory that involve "knowing what."

Procedural memory often involves the cerebellum, a crucial part of the brain for sequence learning (refer to Chapter 8). The cerebellum is a feed-forward controller that stores entire action sequences and chains from the current state to the next state without the necessity of slow sensory feedback. Instead, sensory feedback is used during the learning phase for setting up the action sequence so that appropriate limb movements are made in a coordinated manner in the proper sequence.

The Long and Short of It: Immediate versus Permanent Memory

Most sensory input that causes receptor activity in our bodies does not reach conscious awareness, and most of what reaches conscious awareness is not stored permanently in our brains. We have multiple memory systems that act on multiple time scales for different purposes. In terms of time scale, memory can be divided into sensory/icons, short term and long term.

Sensory/iconic memory

When a photographer takes your picture with a flash, it often generates an afterimage. The afterimage is caused by the flash "bleaching" or temporarily depleting photopigment in the retinal area that received the flash. When you look around afterward, the response of this retinal area is so different from the rest of the retina that the area stands out in a kind of neural relief that you can see.

Normal vision consists of a sequence of saccadic eye movements made at a rate of about three to four per second. Although the "neural image" produced at each fixation is nowhere nearly as dramatic as a photoflash afterimage, evidence exists for such an image at multiple levels of the nervous system. Access to this image is best if you close your eyes after looking at something, or stare at a featureless expanse.

Fleeting iconic memories

Briefly lasting neural afterimages are called *sensory* or *iconic memory.* They're literal — a picture (vision), sound sequence (hearing), or eidetic (mental) representation in other senses such as touch, taste, or olfaction.

Visual iconic memory lasts only a few seconds. Auditory iconic memory appears to last much longer, on the order of 10 to 20 seconds, perhaps because of the intrinsic nature of language communication. Twenty seconds would be long enough to store most sentences, for example. Much less is known about the length of somatosensory, taste, and olfactory iconic memories.

Seeing iconic memory in action

One of the best illustrations of iconic memory is the Helmholtz covert memory experiment. In this experiment, an array of 25 or more letters is flashed. The observer is told immediately after the flash to recall as many letters as possible in one location (say, upper right). The observer can reliably recall about five to seven letters, and no more, from any indicated location.

How is it that, despite only being able to recall at most seven letters, the observer can recall seven from any location among 25 or more letters? The answer is that the observer has some sort of rapidly fading iconic memory for the entire array. Once the observer directs his covert attention toward some portion of it, and begins verbalizing its contents, he can get through about seven items before the iconic neural image has faded.

Working/short-term memory

In the covert attention example that I explain in the previous section, the observer was able to verbalize about seven items before the iconic memory faded. The process of verbalization entails considerable processing: converting the visual image to discrete letter objects, identifying the letters, looking up the letter names, and producing verbal output (even if sub-vocal). This conversion to semantics has an enormous consequence. The semantically identified letters can now be rehearsed using a common mechanism that permits them to be retained indefinitely by repeating their names again and again. This indefinite, rehearsal-mediated retention is called *short-term memory.* Continued rehearsal in short-term memory can trigger memory processes that generate long-term memories that can last a lifetime.

The lucky seven of short-term memory

Short-term memory has the limit of seven items, and that limit is quite interesting. Although a person can remember about seven different letters, she can also remember about seven different familiar words, which obviously entails more than seven letters. Plus, if you select short, proverb-like sentences, you'll find that observers can remember about seven of these sentences (in other words, way more than seven letters).

What's going on here? The answer is *chunking.* The seven slots in short-term memory aren't slots for memory items, but slots for memory addresses, or what computer science calls *pointers.* The pointer points to any sort of memory configuration that has an identity with learned, strongly self-reinforcing internal components. Letters of the English alphabet are well learned and stored as single semantic identities, whereas this would not be true for most English speakers for Chinese characters. Well-known English words also exist in memory as single entities, recoverable if some letters are partly obscured. The same is true for some short sentences, like sayings such as, "Thou shalt not kill," which has a pointer that generates the entire string given part of it.

Working memory

The short-term memory mechanism is common to processing inputs across the senses. You can rehearse and remember about seven letters you see or hear. You can also place in short-term memory contents from your long-term memory. For example, suppose you were told that you were going to be asked questions about your seven best friends in high school. It might take some time and thinking to come up with this list, but after doing so, you could rapidly answer questions about any of the seven people. Because this and sensory-input short-term memory share many properties, the term *working memory* is most commonly used for a consciously retained list of items maintained by rehearsal.

Explicit (declarative) memory

Sufficient rehearsal in short-term memory can cause a memory to be long term, in which case the memory is retained even after rehearsal stops. Long-term memories can be formed as a result of emotionally salient experiences even if the brain doesn't explicitly rehearse them. Long-term, memory-like effects can even occur in cases of priming (refer to "Preparing for priming," earlier in this chapter) where no conscious awareness exists of the initial, subliminal stimulus.

The kinds of long-term memory generated from short-term memory rehearsal are very different from implicit (non-declarative) memories, such as classical and operant conditioning. (Refer to "Conditioning classically and operantly," earlier in this chapter.) Long-term memory created by conscious effort produces what is called *explicit* or *declarative memory*. This means memory that you can talk about in words. Human explicit long-term memory has two major forms: semantic and episodic.

- ✔ **Semantic memory:** General world knowledge. Semantic memory is what you go to school to learn. It includes facts about the world in all subjects, and language usage including word definitions and grammar. Semantic memory is declarative because its contents can be accessed and reported verbally, such as knowing when was the Battle of Hastings, or the chemical formula for methane. You also have semantic memory for things you learn just by living.

- ✔ **Episodic memory:** Memories of specific events. Episodic memory contains source knowledge — knowledge of the time and context associated with an event that may also have a semantic component.

  Episodic memory is more complex than other memories because it is not primarily associational. It isn't generated by repetition and rehearsal; instead, it involves a reconstruction of the entire context in which an event took place. Episodic memory is dependent on frontal lobe activity, particularly the lateral prefrontal cortex that instantiates working memory.

  Loss of episodic memory ("Where did I leave my car keys?") is one of the first clinical signs of Alzheimer's disease.

The difference between semantic and episodic memory is the difference between knowing that Montgomery is the capital of Alabama (semantic) and knowing who taught you that fact and in what class (episodic).

Does your cat have episodic memory?

It's likely that humans greatly outstrip any other animals in episodic memory, if it can even be said that non-human animals even have episodic memory. Many animals can learn complex associations, and even exhibit single trial learning, but this is not the same as episodic memory, which is an internal reconstruction of prior experienced reality If any animals have episodic memory, it's unclear how this might be tested, given that animals can't verbally tell us the source aspects of what they've learned, as opposed to behaving in a way that demonstrates associative learning.

Memory Mechanisms and Brain Loci

Most short-term memory is disposable — like a grocery store list, you use it for the time you need it, and then you discard it. But some information rehearsed in short-term memory does become long-term. This happens because of the hippocampus, a medial temporal lobe structure.

Associating context with results in the hippocampus

Short-term memory typically involves initial activity in a sensory input system, such as vision and audition. High-level processing that leads to semantic item identification generates activity in the lateral prefrontal cortex. This brain area maintains an internal representation of the input after it's gone. The lateral prefrontal cortex also maintains other aspects of the current context after they're gone, such as your goals and what you were doing prior to that moment.

Remembering an episode, including your internal state and external input, involves reconstructing the salient reality of the event. This means taking a snapshot of all the relevant brain activity associated with the event so that the event and its context can be reproduced. The hippocampus takes this snapshot. Both the direct sensory representation of inputs and their internal representation in lateral prefrontal cortex project to the hippocampus. (This projection occurs through the parahippocampal cortices and the entorhinal cortex; refer to Chapter 7.)

The hippocampus gets inputs from the entire cortex because it represents what's going on in the current situation. Figure 12-2 shows that areas of visual cortex that code for color might project to a line of hippocampal coincidence detectors. Areas of sensory cortex that respond to types of animals (birds, frogs, and so forth) might project to a functionally orthogonal set of lines in the hippocampal matrix, such as shown in Figure 12-2. Some hippocampal coincidence detectors will respond to green frogs, for example. The matrix is actually elaborated in many dimensions to include inputs from the frontal lobe about the context in which you're seeing the green frog (while you were sitting in the park waiting for your friend). The result is some unique activation of hippocampal cells for all the elements of the episode, external and internal.

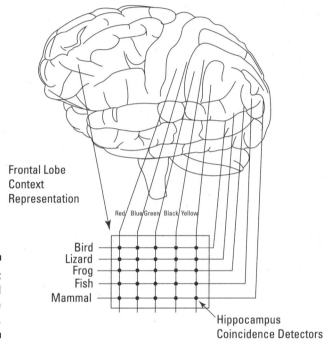

Figure 12-2: Cortical inputs to the hippocampus.

Strengthening synapses

Within the hippocampus is a set of modifiable neural AND gates (NMDA synapses, which I discuss in "Increasing response," a bit later on) that will be activated *if and only if* all their inputs are simultaneously active. A process called *long-term potentiation* strengthens these synapses, when several inputs are simultaneously active. A mirror process called *long-term depression,* reduces synaptic strength when synapses are not active simultaneously.

The strengthening of synapses in the hippocampus is not so important for the very short-term memory of your surroundings, which is the job of the lateral prefrontal cortex. Instead, the hippocampus transfers what is stored in short-term memory into long-term memory, which is actually stored in the neocortex itself. Neuroscientists know this because of Brenda Milner's studies of the famous patient HM (see the nearby sidebar).

Living for today: The case of HM

HM had both hippocampi surgically removed to try to stop intractable epileptic seizures. His long-term memory was intact after the surgery, and he functioned normally in situations lasting a few minutes. However, he could form no new long-term memories. Hospital staff could have extended conversations with HM, but when they left the room and returned, HM would have no recollection of ever having seen them. HM always thought that the date was the date on which he had had the surgery in 1953, and he lived the rest of his life existing only in the present, with past, but no new memories. He was able to learn new motor skills such as mirror writing, for example, that demonstrated the lack of dependence of procedural memories on the hippocampus.

The hippocampus participates in memory formation in the cortex because the hippocampal neurons — whose synapses have been activated by simultaneous inputs from the cortex — project reciprocally back to the same areas of the cortex. The cortical areas that represented the salient sensory situation and activated the neurons in the hippocampus can, therefore, be activated by the hippocampus, re-creating that representation.

Sleeping for better long-term memory

Thinking about or rehearsing the memory of some experience causes neural activity to reverberate between the hippocampus and cortex. This happens regularly during REM sleep. This reverberatory activity alters modifiable synapses in the cortex (which also contains NMDA receptors) so that the cortex itself can reproduce the neural activity associated with an experience.

Long-term memory is "stored" in the same cortical areas that represented the experience initially. The hippocampus is a scratchpad for linking a set of neurons that were active during an event to form the long-term memory of that event.

Multi-electrode recordings made in the hippocampus of rats running mazes showed that cells in the rat hippocampus and surrounding cortex — called *place cells* and *grid cells* — respond when the rat was in a particular place in the maze, with different cells activated by different places in the maze. When the rats slept after the maze training sessions and entered REM sleep, their hippocampi "played back" the correct maze traversal sequence by activating, in sequence, the place and grid cells and the cortical areas stimulated by the sequence of maze locations. Preventing the rats from having REM sleep resulted in their not consolidating the day's training well.

Remembering pain with the amygdala

The amygdala is a classic limbic system structure lying just anterior to the hippocampus. The amygdalae are involved in memory formation for emotionally salient events. Many parallels exist between the interaction of the hippocampus and lateral prefrontal cortex with the amygdala and ventromedial (orbitofrontal) cortex.

Like the hippocampus, while the amygdala is important for forming long-term memory, the memory is not located there. The amygdala is essential for emotionally salient learning, such as *fear conditioning* — a type of classical conditioning in which a neutral stimulus becomes paired with an aversive one, producing fear reactions. Most emotionally salient stimuli increase amygdalar activity. The representation of stimuli that activate the amygdala occurs primarily in orbitofrontal cortex. Neurons there are activated by situations that entail danger, such as a car heading toward you across the median.

Learning by Changing Synaptic Strengths

One of the most famous issues in the history of neurobiology is the "search for the memory engram" — what changes in the brain allow learning to occur and memory to exist. After the case of HM (refer to the sidebar "Living for today: The case of HM"), many laboratories sprang up in the 1970s and 1980s looking for synaptic strength modifications in the brains of mammals, like laboratory rats. Recordings were made in hippocampal brain slices — preparations involving taking a slice from a deceased animal's brain and keeping it alive by immersing it in artificial cerebrospinal fluid (like the normal extracellular fluid in the brain and spinal cord). Recordings were made of single neuron activity to monitor subtle synaptic alterations when cells were stimulated in patterns that duplicated simultaneously active, strong inputs from the neocortex.

Increasing response: NMDA receptor changes

A number of laboratories observed that learning-related changes in synaptic weights in the hippocampus involve an unusual receptor type for glutamate, which had properties that had been predicted for modifiable synapses. These were the *NMDA receptors.* (NMDA stands for n-methyl D-aspartate, the name of an exogenous chemical agonist that selectively activates this receptor.)

The NMDA receptor, which is abundant in the hippocampus, causes changes in the synaptic strength of nearby AMPA receptors as a function of simultaneously active or coincident inputs. The way this works is that the NMDA receptor ion channel is normally blocked by a magnesium ion in the mouth of the pore. This magnesium ion is removed if an adjacent non-NMDA glutamate ion channel is also activated and depolarizes the neural membrane. Activation of the NMDA receptor requires both its presynaptic terminal to release glutamate and another presynaptic terminal to release glutamate to an adjacent receptor.

The NMDA receptor channel passes sodium, like most excitatory receptor channels. However, it also allows calcium to pass through the channel as well as sodium. Calcium entry into neurons typically has second messenger effects (refer to Chapter 3). One of these effects seems to be to increase, under some circumstances, the potency of the synapse by increasing the receptor response to the glutamate input.

Making presynaptic strength changes

Synaptic modification depends on both presynaptic and postsynaptic mechanisms. When synapses are simultaneously activated on a postsynaptic cell in the hippocampus, opening its NMDA channels, the cell may send a message back to the presynaptic inputs, increasing their strength. One messenger substance proposed for this is nitric oxide (NO — not the same as the anesthetic nitrous oxide, N_2O). Another proposed messenger of this type is anandamide (an endocannabinoid).

This retrograde signaling process is sometimes called *retrograde neurotransmission*. Retrograde neurotransmitters are synthesized in the postsynaptic neuron and have effects on the axon terminal of presynaptic neurons, such as long-term potentiation. Of course, post-synaptic mechanisms are a fundamental part of both LTP and LTD.

Animal versus computer memory

Use of the term *memory* has created a fundamental confusion in neurobiology about how the brain adapts to experience during learning. In computers, memories are stored data strings without any intrinsic meaning, until the data strings are combined with information that allows them to be interpreted according to rules stored elsewhere.

Our brains don't work like computers. Memory in brains is a change in the neural architecture, such that the processing chain from stimulus to response operates differently. Memory in brains involves re-creating reality. The neural circuits that originally processed stimuli become active in this re-creation, which includes many stimuli, the state of the brain at the time, and aspects of the behavioral output.

Forgetting It: Amnesia and Other Memory Loss

We can lose a memory by two different processes: forgetting the memory or failing to retrieve the memory. Practically, distinguishing between these two processes is difficult.

In *forgetting*, the memory is lost because the synaptic modifications underlying the memory are altered, or the neurons that instantiate the memory die or become inactive. A memory may exist, however, but be temporarily irretrievable. You know this when the memory comes back to you later, under different circumstances. Often, you're able to retrieve the memory because of some property of your environment is similar to the initial situation in which the memory was created. This emphasizes the re-creational aspects of memory.

Losing yourself in amnesia

A common soap opera plot involves a character losing his or her memory and interacting with other characters in a completely new way. This sort of amnesia actually does occur, but it's typically temporary. The cause may be a brain *ischemia* (oxygen and nutrient deprivation) from a vascular incident or a blow to the head (which may secondarily cause an ischemia). This sort of memory loss may include complete loss of episodic information from the present back to some point in the past, as well as semantic loss over a similar period. Semantic and procedural information from early life — such as knowing the capital of Alabama or how to tie one's shoes — may remain intact.

Electroconvulsive therapy (ECT, or shock treatment) also produces memory loss. The pattern tends to involve a four- to six-month retrograde loss and a month or two of anterograde inabilities to form new memories. In many cases, most of the retrograde lost memories return. This gives a clue about the memory consolidation process, which must take place over several months.

Damaging the hippocampus

In the movie *Groundhog Day* starring Bill Murray, he wakes up every morning with memories intact, but doomed to repeat the same scenario. This is the opposite of HM (refer to the sidebar earlier in this chapter), who mentally relived every day anew without any memory of the people or events since his bilateral hippocampus removal. Damage to the hippocampus and nearby temporal lobe cortical structures interferes with memory formation, and can eventually compromise the ability to retain recently encountered items or semantic information.

Evidence increasingly suggests that learning in healthy brains is accompanied by multiplication of neurons in the hippocampus, not just changing synaptic weights of neurons that have existed since the first year of life. Stress, abuse, and neuropathologies can severely reduce the multiplication of neurons in the hippocampus, and prevent learned adaptation to new information.

Ignoring consequences: Frontal lobe damage

Damage to the part of the frontal lobe — the dorsolateral prefrontal cortex — disrupts working memory and, therefore, the ability to form episodic memories. The result of damage to ventromedial prefrontal cortex was made famous by the case of Phineas Gage, a railroad worker who suffered this kind of damage. The injury transformed Gage from a normal, reliable, and responsible crew foreman to an irresponsible gambler who swore constantly.

The key to understanding the role of the ventromedial prefrontal cortex is to remember its interaction with the amygdala. The amygdala is the cortical area that produces the representation of situations that are likely to have negative consequences, particularly social situations. The interaction between ventromedial prefrontal cortex and the amygdala allows learning of new contingencies that are predictive of negative consequences. So, damage to the ventromedial prefrontal cortex can cause people to do risky or inappropriate things, because they have no fear of negative consequences.

Examining Alzheimer's disease

The first symptom of Alzheimer's disease is memory loss, particularly episodic memory. The early biochemistry of Alzheimer's disease involves acetylcholine transmission in the brain, but cellular details remain poorly understood.

A leading candidate for the cause of Alzheimer's is abnormally folded amyloid beta protein in the brain. This protein is a byproduct of an amyloid precursor protein that is believed to be necessary during neuronal development. The misfolded amyloid beta proteins form amyloid plaques outside neurons — known as *senile plaques* or *neuritic plaques*.

Alzheimer's disease is also associated with abnormal collection of a protein called *tau* inside neurons. Tau's normal function is to stabilize microtubules in the cell cytoskeleton. Tau is normally regulated by phosphorylation, but in Alzheimer's it becomes over phosphorylated and accumulates as filamentous masses inside neurons. These *neurofibrillary tangles* are associated with amyloid plaques outside neurons.

Neurons that use the neurotransmitter acetylcholine are particularly susceptible to the damage from Alzheimer's. Some researchers believe that cholinergic transmission is causal in the formation of plaques and tangles. Many medications used to treat Alzheimer's symptoms seek to increase acetylcholine levels or efficacy by inhibiting acetylcholinesterases, which are the enzymes that break down acetylcholine in the synaptic cleft. Cholinergic input is a critical part of hippocampal physiology, and the loss of these inputs might compromise the hippocampus's ability to form episodic memories. No truly effective treatments for Alzheimer's are available, and these agents can only temporarily relieve symptoms; they don't slow the progress of the disease itself.

The course of Alzheimer's proceeds from episodic to semantic memory loss, and then finally to large-scale death of neurons throughout the brain. Death is usually caused by the disruption of body function regulation carried out by subcortical brain areas.

Improving Your Learning

Despite that fact that most college graduates spend at least 16 years in formal schooling, we don't know much about how learning takes place, or how it may be improved.

Classical learning theory shows that repetition, particularly when associated with reinforcement and punishments, causes behaviors to be retained, including the ability to recapitulate facts in semantic memory. Less well understood, because we have no real animal model to study, is the difference between *deep learning* and *shallow learning*. Deep learning is the linkage of new information to multiple levels of one's already-existing semantic network.

Studying hard versus studying well: Schedules

Repetition results in learning, but some ways of conducting repetition while studying are much more effective than others. Two major practices can improve learning for a given amount of time:

- ✓ **Deep association:** Deep content association refers to linking new facts to multiple aspects of your knowledge base. Suppose you're studying the Battle of Hastings. The shallow method would be to simply memorize facts about the locations, people, and timing. A deeper way to learn about it would be to simulate the battle in your mind or with tools such as a map or computer program. If you considered the situations the commanders faced and their resources and decisions, you would be much more likely to remember the progress of the battle, because you would understand *why* certain things happened, not just that they happened.

- ✓ **Distributed scheduling:** The second major factor affecting learning is its schedule. Cramming is bad. Learning is much more effective when spread out over time. Part of this probably has to do with context. Learning in one session tends to be linked to the context in which studying occurs. This makes recall difficult if any changes happen to your state of mind or environment. However, if you practice learning at multiple times, in multiple contexts, learning will be deeper and you'll be more likely to recall what you've learned.

Traveling the path to better memory

Since ancient times, we've known of specific techniques to help us memorize lists. The most well known is called the *journey method* or *method of loci.* In this method, the person imagines walking a familiar route and associating a word on the list to be remembered with specific landmarks on the route. This is an example of a deep association because the route the person uses is familiar, and she can remember the entire route. The technique creates a link between each landmark and an item on the list, so that the items to be remembered are embedded in the past, current, and future locations to be encountered that already exist in memory.

This technique appears to use regions of the brain that have to do with spatial learning, particularly the hippocampus. Multi-electrode recordings in rats have shown that much of their hippocampal resources are devoted to representation of place in spatial navigation. The journey method links a list to be learned to an already learned spatial representation. The hippocampus probably originally evolved primarily for learning in spatial navigation, and its role in episodic memory evolved later from that.

Chapter 13

The Frontal Lobes and Executive Brain

*I*nsects and invertebrates perform complex behaviors like flying without neocortex — and they get along just fine. They possess subcortical areas, which are good enough for controlling what they need to do. But for humans, that's not good enough.

In humans, almost all our brain matter serves the purpose of allowing us to act, and to decide how to act, intelligently — based on our previous experience. Without a neocortex, the number of possible behaviors we could perform, and the contingencies upon which we base our decisions to act, are very limited.

The frontal lobe is the brain area that controls the complex plans we need to make for doing all kinds of things, every day. Hitting tennis balls, driving cars, and climbing a ladder to paint the ceiling are all behaviors that require a frontal lobe to execute. And the human frontal lobe, particularly on the left side, allows us to have not only thoughts, but thoughts about thoughts, and thoughts about thoughts about thoughts. This chapter looks at how our brains allow us to act in complex ways depending on our experience and self-awareness.

Reflexes versus Conscious or Goal-Generated Action

Flight is one of the most complex animal behaviors. Wing movements must account for obstacles, wind and wind changes, air pressure, current altitude, and direction. Yet many primitive animals, such as insects, fly quite well. The intelligence necessary for flight in invertebrates is embedded in their genome, which "learned" or adapted over billions of years of evolution.

Insect flight demonstrates that complex behaviors do not necessarily require large brains. It has been suggested that large brains are required for complex planning, particularly for maintaining status and surviving in large social groups. But some insects — such as ants and bees — exist in large social groups with castes, but no social status within the caste. So, membership in large social groups also doesn't require a large brain.

The crucial difference between insect and mammalian social groups is that insect social groups are composed of a few castes. An insect's behavior is almost completely specified by a few types of responses to stimuli, as a function of its caste. But mammalian social groups consist of individuals, each of which has a specific identity and social rank. Interactions between mammals in a social group depend on things like their mutual rank, which other individuals are present and their ranks, and on the outcomes of previous encounter-experiences of all these individuals. This is particularly true for primates, who maintain separate, simultaneous male and female social hierarchies, with the male hierarchies in a constant status of flux due to dominance contests.

Large brains are associated with the need for complex representations of reality. A mammal can be in the exact same situation today — as represented by the senses — as yesterday; however, the appropriate behavior today could be quite different from what it was yesterday, depending on the memory of what was observed to happen yesterday between two other members of the troop.

The need for this type of situational intelligence drove hominid evolution far beyond the brain size needed for a complex behavior such as flight. It required the ability to enhance sensory processing to detect subtle facial expressions, posture changes, and cues from vocalization. It required episodic memory (refer to Chapter 12) for the outcomes of specific encounters, and subtle changes in vocalizations that conveyed, or sometime hid, information about status.

The neocortex, particularly the frontal lobes, allowed a much more nuanced control of behavior than was possible from limbic stimulus-response instinctive control. The representation of complex contingencies in the brain allowed complex planning and tool making. Producing subtle, experience-dependent vocalization led to language, sophisticated cooperation, and the explicit teaching of young. Our large contingency-representing brains also produced bluffing, lying, deceit, war, altruism, and all-encompassing spiritual explanations for reality.

Turning ideas and goals into action

The brain is not designed by engineers, but by evolution via natural selection. One thing obvious to any graduate student in neurobiology is that the nervous system consists of a lot of "hacks" — repairs or patches of a large system to deal with an unforeseen contingency, while causing the least amount of disruption to the system as possible.

 Hacks work best in modular hierarchical systems, because this structure limits the effects of the hack inserted to deal with the unforeseen contingency. For example, an ancient evolutionary hack is to use the reflex of stepping when falling forward to generate walking. Many brain functions are implemented by neural circuits no engineer would design, but that were adapted for new uses from existing circuits.

Non-mammalian vertebrates such as lizards and frogs can generate all their locomotive behaviors without a neocortex by using the basal ganglia, cerebellum, and spinal pattern generators and reflexes. When mammals evolved a neocortex, they didn't throw all this neural circuitry away and "redesign" the entire system. Instead, mammals co-opted the lower, yet competent systems they inherited by controlling them at a higher level, based on more complex contingencies and learning.

For example, monkey A might notice a rival coming into its area. Monkey A does not want to confront monkey B, because he has an ally who is not around now. Monkey A does not want to flee or give evidence of submission. Monkey A's best strategy is to use deceit and leave quickly, but without showing fear. Monkey A's frontal lobes are generating all these calculations, using the monkey's subcortical gait control systems to carry out the actions of its limbs moving it away from monkey B. The subcortical limbic systems might be prompting monkey A to flee hurriedly from the threat, but it does not.

Humans in particular among mammals have generated novel behaviors. Examples are odd gaits like skipping, or dexterous hand use for making and using tools. These behaviors have led to the development of a nearly complete cortical circuit for control of the limbs that largely bypasses more subcortical control than most other mammals. Abstract goals represented in the prefrontal cortex activate either the supplementary cortex and cerebellum or the premotor cortex and parietal lobe for generating action sequences. These areas, in turn, activate the primary motor cortex just anterior to the central sulcus to control muscles directly (refer to Chapter 8 for more details). These areas allow new and learned capabilities, such as hitting a tennis backhand.

Representing actions at multiple levels

Most goals can be reached in many ways. If you want ice cream, you can drive to the grocery store or to an ice cream parlor, or walk or cycle to those places; you can ask your neighbor if she has any; or you can make it yourself if you have an ice cream maker and the ingredients.

The goal of wanting ice cream is very abstract, probably represented in lateral prefrontal cortex with inputs from hunger mechanisms and memory. Evidence suggests that this goal may simultaneously activate many of the possible ways of achieving it. The activation of goal resolution paths generates the sub-goals required for each of them. Your frontal lobe has to sort out the requirements for the sub-goals as well.

The real hallmark of frontal lobe engagement is what happens when the planned procedure doesn't work. If you planned to cycle to the grocery store but your bike has a flat tire, is it now more appropriate to fix the tire or try to get to the store another way? Your frontal lobes are constantly doing all these calculations for all your goals. Much of this is unconscious, and much of it depends on learning and experience that could not have been programmed by evolution.

Deciding How to Do It: The Frontal Lobes and Action Execution

Play is a nearly universal behavior in young mammals. It's behavior practice. Predator mammals play at catching and knocking down prey, while prey animals practice escaping. Mammals also explore, establish, and defend territories. This requires complex spatial memory that includes visual, olfactory, and audio sensory processing. The complex associations between what is perceived in the environment, experience, and learned contingency-specific behaviors depend on processing in the frontal lobes.

Originating abstract plans

The frontal lobes are connected extensively with the limbic system. One way to think about limbic system control of behavior is to think about the limbic system as a device for switching states. Most animals have a finite number of goal states, such as seeking water, food, a mate, or shelter. The limbic system receives input from the body's homeostatic mechanisms, and, with limited sensory input dependency, selects the highest priority from a set of evolutionarily programmed behaviors, such as seeking a water hole or a mate.

Role of frontal lobes

The frontal lobes add the ability to represent reality in the context of past experience and current goals. Even if an animal is extremely thirsty, letting another member of the herd drink first may be a better idea, in case the crocodile the animals remembers has come back. The frontal lobes are overriding the highest-priority state selected by the limbic system based on something that is not detected now, but remembered.

Frontal lobes allow abstract decisions and planning not closely linked to current body state or observable environmental cues. A thirsty collection of animals may drink from a water hole until satisfied and then leave. A frontal lobe competent troupe may avoid the water hole at a particular time of day during which they remember that lions show up — allowing the other animals water access at a very bad time.

Complexity of contingency planning

This kind of abstract contingency planning doesn't require consciousness, but it does require very complex learning, memory, and nuanced representations of reality. Vocalizations that refer to internal representations of reality, rather than to what is actually there, can be the first underpinnings of language. For example, a monkey gives a call that signals the presence of a lion because the monkey remembers that lions show up at sunset, not because the monkey is actually looking at a lion now.

Converting plans to body control

The problem with abstract plans is that one can carry them out in many ways. Complex plans have multiple steps, each of which is contingent on the availability of certain resources, on having the prior steps completed, and on the ability to begin the next step in the sequence.

At one level, complex processing in the frontal lobes is necessary to execute a sequence of sub-goals necessary to accomplish an overall goal. At a higher level is vetoing the execution of the sequence if any of the sub-goals down the line is not accomplishable. For example, don't even start going to the water hole if the wind is blowing in such a direction that you won't be able to smell the lions.

In the frontal lobes, the activation of high-level goals in prefrontal cortex appears to activate all the neural circuit sub-goal chains that can satisfy the goal. Athletic coaches know that imagining hitting a tennis forehand activates the premotor sequence for doing so, and can improve a player's skill, even though the actual output to the muscles is suppressed. A similar thing occurs in movement dreams in REM sleep, where motor sequences are activated all the way to the spinal level, but the final output is suppressed so you don't actually move (except for cases where thrashing and sleepwalking occur).

Executing a goal requires that abstract plans be translated into specific motor sequences and then to muscle contractions. Neural activity starts with representations of high-level goals in prefrontal cortex, and moves to activate supplementary motor or premotor cortex, which then drives motor neuron outputs in primary motor cortex. This process involves interactions with subcortical structures such as the basal ganglia, which I discuss next.

Initiating Action in the Basal Ganglia

Earlier in this chapter, I talk about the frontal lobes overriding the limbic system and basal ganglia control of behavior (refer also to Chapter 8). The basal ganglia remain involved in executing the action, however. This fact is dramatically obvious from observations of patients with Parkinson's disease, which is associated with loss of dopaminergic transmission from the substantia nigra.

Parkinson's patients can certainly formulate abstract motor plans, but they have trouble initiating and executing them. This suggests that the instantiation of the motor sequence conceived in the frontal lobes still depends on subcortical structures to initiate, implement, and provide feedback control to deal with errors.

Preparing for action

The basal ganglia interact with the neocortex and thalamus for voluntary motor control. Their function is to select, among the simultaneously active frontal lobe motor programs, the one to execute at a particular time. The overall output of the basal ganglia inhibits all the motor sequences except the one selected via its release from inhibition. The basal ganglia operate in a loop through the thalamus with the frontal lobes, such that the particular frontal motor sequence that the basal ganglia selects is partly controlled by the frontal lobes.

One hypothesis of how this works is that the basal ganglia operate on a winner-takes-all selection among active frontal lobe motor program sequences. This selection may involve a threshold effect by which one program sequence in the frontal lobes that is slightly more active than the others is selected and reinforced through the thalamus. This selection process is important in procedural learning and learning routine behaviors in particular situations.

Patterning and oscillating

Many oscillatory rhythms occur in the brain that are evident in electro-encephalograph (EEG) recordings. Different frequency bands have been given different names, such as beta for 15 Hz to 30 Hz and theta for 3 Hz to 10 Hz. These rhythms are important in the normal functioning of the basal ganglia, with abnormally large, static, synchronized rhythms associated with Parkinson's disease limb tremor. Medications that release dopamine reduce these beta oscillations and increase oscillations above 60 Hertz (high-gamma band).

Activity in the subthalamic nucleus, a frequent target of electrical stimulation to relieve Parkinson's symptoms, is important for the preparation of voluntary movements. Synchronization of subthalamic nucleus activity in the beta band is associated with movement initiation. However, the static, beta frequency oscillations in the basal ganglia in Parkinson's disease patients interfere with the ability to initiate and execute selected movements, causing the *akinesia* (loss of voluntary movement) and *bradykinesia* (slow movement) of Parkinson's disease.

Also, between the basal ganglia and the cerebellum is an important neural loop (see Chapter 8). This loop regulates the selection and initiation of action via pattern classification operations in the *striatum* (the input layer of the basal ganglia, consisting of the caudate and putamen). Spiny neurons in the striatum disinhibit one particular thalamo-cortical loop activity pattern that increases at the expense of others. The loop with the cerebellum then amplifies and refines this pattern as it continues during the action sequence.

Coordinating through the Supplementary and Premotor Cortices

Just anterior to the primary motor cortex are two areas: The *supplementary motor area* (SMA) takes up the medial area anterior to the primary motor cortex, while the *premotor cortex* (PMC; Brodmann area 6) is lateral. These areas are between the abstract representation of goals and plans in the prefrontal cortex and the control of muscles or muscle groups in the primary motor cortex.

The SMA and PMC organize goals into muscle movement sequences. But they do this differently. Well-known, internally driven movement sequences activate the SMA, while sensory-guided movement — such as manipulating a novel object — activates the PMC.

Feeding back to guide movement

The PMC is involved in more complex movements than mediated by the primary motor cortex, which might by itself control simple actions like squeezing a ball with the hand. The lateral position of the PMC in each hemisphere places it near the primary motor cortex areas that control the body's trunk muscles.

The PMC receives sensory feedback from the parietal lobe through the thalamus. The PMC projects not only to primary motor cortex, but directly to the spinal cord, the *striatum* (the input nuclei of the basal ganglia), and the motor thalamus. The PMC is important for guiding our movement using sensory feedback. Complex movements, such as climbing, are associated with the PMC. (If, say, you're climbing a ladder, you need to move all four limbs in a coordinated way while being aware of the space around your body.) Because of the direct projections from PMC to the spinal cord, the hierarchy between the PMC and the primary motor cortex is not absolute, and the PMC can control movement bypassing the primary motor cortex.

Neurons in the PMC are active when you're learning motor sequences. Neurons in the dorsal PMC became active in response to a stimulus cue to act, and may remain active during any delay before the action occurs. Some evidence exists that entire action sequences are represented in the PMC as *behavioral repertoires,* such that different parts of the movement repertoire are represented in different PMC sub-regions. The sub-regions compute spatial trajectory and control the movements of joints and muscles.

Learning motor sequences: Supplementary motor cortex

The SMA is medial and anterior to the primary motor cortex leg representation. The SMA controls movements and movement sequences that are generated internally, rather than triggered by sensory events. It may also be involved in stabilizing the body, particularly in coordinating both sides of the body together. Like the PMC, neurons in the SMA also project directly to the spinal cord and may directly control movement.

The SMA receives strong inputs from most prefrontal cortex, but much less input from the parietal cortex. The SMA is strongly connected to the thalamus and striatum. The SMA is important for complex locomotion such as climbing, leaping, and other complex behavioral repertoires, particularly those that have been learned and internalized.

The supplementary eye field (SEF) is located anteriorly in the SMA. This area and the frontal eye field (FEF) anterior to that in the frontal cortex are involved in generating saccadic eye movements. Some evidence suggests that FEF represents saccades with respect to the target location on the retina, whereas saccades may be represented in the SEF with respect to their location relative to the head. The pattern of connections between these two areas suggests a mapping between them that converts the head-oriented saccade representation in SEF to a retina oriented saccade representation in FEF.

Learning motor sequences

Early behaviorists believed that sequence learning comprised a reflex chain in which the completion of each movement in the chain triggered the next. However, this cannot be the whole story because movements can occur even when sensory feedback, and some movement sequences occur too quickly to depend on sensory feedback. Learned motor sequences are efficiently represented in hierarchical plan organizations that combine lower-level sequences into larger units, called *chunking*. (Refer to Chapter 12 for more.)

Practicing mentally

Sequence learning can be explicit or implicit. *Explicit sequence learning* means being aware that you're practicing a skill, like hitting a tennis ball. Implicit learning means that, during practice, we get better at something without being aware of exactly how that is occurring. In a typical sequence when we're acquiring a skill, we're more attentive in the initial phase (explicit learning), but after repeated practice, the skill becomes almost automatic as we improve (implicit learning).

Even if it's raining outside, you can still practice your tennis serve — in your mind! Practice can be effective even if the activity is only imagined. This imagined activity is called *motor imagery,* and it has been shown to be effective in sports training and to rehabilitate motor deficits associated with some neurological disorders such as multiple sclerosis and motor deficits from strokes.

Motor imagery activates early and late stages of motor control, including the supplementary motor area, the primary motor cortex, parietal cortex, basal ganglia, and cerebellum. Activation of the primary motor cortex during motor imagery is, however, at a less intense level than during actual action execution. This is sufficient to increase muscular activity, and is specific to the muscles associated with the imagined action and proportional to the imagined effort.

Sequencing in the cerebellum and strengthening synaptic pathways

When a neural code or representation for a learned skill is created in the brain, it's called a *procedural memory*. The cerebellum plays an essential role in motor and other procedural learning, particularly where fine adjustments have to be made to the action sequence.

The cerebellum has several major cell types in a stereotypical, repeated circuit (see Figure 13-1). Purkinje cells in outer layers of the cerebellum inhibit deep cerebellar nuclei. The thin dendritic arbors of aligned Purkinje cells form stacks through which parallel fibers from the deeper layers pass. The parallel fibers (the axons of the granule cells) make excitatory (glutamatergic) but weak synapses onto Purkinje cell dendritic spines. Climbing fibers, which originate from the inferior olivary nucleus in the medulla, have a more potent excitatory input to the Purkinje cell that is nearer to dendrites and cell soma.

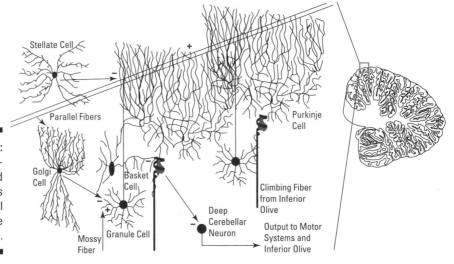

Figure 13-1:
The organization and connections of major cell types of the cerebellum.

Motor learning in the cerebellum is mediated primarily by long-term depression (LTD) of parallel fiber synapses onto Purkinje cells. Climbing fibers provide the teaching signal that induces synaptic modification in parallel fiber–Purkinje cell synapses. Climbing fiber activity represents an error signal.

Purkinje cells have two different types of action potentials. *Simple spikes* occur spontaneously and when Purkinje cells are activated by the parallel fibers. *Complex spikes* exhibit an initial large-amplitude potential followed by a burst of smaller-amplitude spikes induced by climbing fiber activation. Complex spikes can generate calcium-mediated action potentials in the Purkinje cell dendrites. This can shift Purkinje cell activity from a quiet state to a spontaneously active state. The complex spike, generated by the climbing fiber, serves as an error signal during learning — complex spike activity increases when a mismatch occurs between an intended movement and the movement actually executed.

Basket and stellate cells in the cerebellar molecular layer (refer to Figure 13-1) make GABAergic inhibitory inputs to the Purkinje cell. Stellate cells synapse onto Purkinje cell dendrites, but basket cells contact the Purkinje cell axon initial segment. Basket cells mediate feedforward inhibition (see Chapter 6) onto Purkinje cells as part of the process of sequence tuning.

Whereas *feedback* inhibition, such as in spinal cord reflexes, tends to maintain a limb in a particular position, *feedforward* inhibition is used to program actions such as slowing down a limb before it reaches the target, so that if you reach to grab an apple hanging from a tree limb, your hand doesn't go past the apple, but stops in the right place. This occurs prior to any sensory feedback coming from contact with the apple.

Activation of presynaptic NMDA receptors in stellate cells increases their GABA release and changes the composition of their glutamate receptor subunit. These long-lasting changes are one of the associative learning cellular mechanisms in the cerebellum.

Mirroring Others: Mirror Neurons

In primates, *mirror neurons* have been recorded in the premotor cortex, the supplementary motor area, the primary somatosensory cortex, and the inferior parietal cortex. These neurons fire when an animal performs a specific act and, interestingly, when the animal observes the same action performed by another animal or a human. The neurons are named *mirror neurons* because their activity reflects the behavior of another animal doing what would activate the neuron in the observer animal. Brain activity consistent with that of mirror neurons has been found in humans, and evidence exists for them even in birds.

Mirror neurons were discovered by the Italian researchers Giocomo Rizzolatti and colleagues in the 1980s while recording from neurons in the ventral premotor cortex of the macaque monkey that were involved in the control of hand and mouth actions during eating. Some of the neurons responded when the monkey saw a person pick up food, as well as when the monkey picked it up itself.

Defining mirroring behaviors

Mirror neurons appear to help us do many things:

- **Learn new skills by imitating others:** If mirror neurons simulate observed actions, their activity may be like a kind of mental practice for an action sequence.

- **Understand the actions and intentions of others:** In social situations, mirror neurons have also been suggested to help an animal understand others. This is consistent with suggestions that autism may involve some problem with the mirror neuron system. It has also been suggested that the human Broca's region is homologous to the area of the monkey ventral premotor cortex where mirror neurons have been recorded. A significant number of neurons in the macaque monkey inferior parietal cortex also have mirror properties, responding to direct hand gestures and observed ones.

- **Empathize:** Some evidence exists for the involvement of mirror neurons in empathy. The anterior cingulate cortex, anterior insula, and inferior frontal cortex are active when people experience emotions such as disgust, pain, and happiness, as well as when subjects see another person experiencing these emotions. People who score higher on self-report questionnaires for empathy show stronger activation of mirror neurons for emotions and hand gestures.

A more controversial idea is that mirror neurons may provide the neurological basis of self-awareness in humans by representing actions at an abstract level.

Imitating others as a function of mirroring

If mirror neurons mediate automatic imitation and motor mimicry, then the mirror neuron system may contribute to cognitive functions such as social awareness and other social behavior according to having what's called a *theory of mind.* Automatic imitation is where a person observing a body movement deliberately performs a similar one. This can mediate empathizing with the person we're observing and understanding his or her intentions.

Some researchers argue that human language evolved from a mirror neuron system for understanding gestures. Human brain areas homologous to those where mirror neurons have been found in monkeys are located in the inferior frontal cortex, close to Broca's area, a main language region of the brain. When people gesture to each other, as in the game of charades, fMRI activity increases in brain areas of human observers, consistent with being driven by mirror neurons.

Chapter 14

Language, Intelligence, Emotions, and Consciousness

*L*anguage, consciousness, and clear thought are uniquely human traits. (However, if your dog can ask for his dinner in full sentences, please post the video online and send me the link.) And they're impressive capabilities, considering the relatively small size of our brains. How a brain only about twice the size of a chimpanzee's, but smaller than that of an elephant developed these traits is unclear, although many theories exist. This chapter looks at the differences between human and non-human brains that may be responsible for the leap to consciousness. It also discusses the notion of intelligence and emotional intelligence, and considers that mysterious but important idea that is quite special to humanity — consciousness.

Adapting Our Brains for Language

Language requires a brain that can perform complex sensory processing, execute complex behavior, and communicate by utterances and postures (body language). Somewhere along the lines of evolution, our brains adapted language capabilities. In this section, I look at the major organizational features of the brain that adapted for language and consciousness.

Knowing how the brain is organized

If we look at the brain as a collection of 100 billion neurons with a thousand synapses each, the possibility of truly understanding it seems hopeless. However, knowing four principles of brain organization is a good start to understanding how the brain works:

- ✔ **Neurons are countable.** Usually less than 100 types of neurons are found in any particular region of the central nervous system.

- ✔ **Neuronal circuits tend to have similar structures even in different areas of the brain.** All of the neocortex is thought to contain essentially the same neural circuit, repeated in millions of minicolumns.

- ✔ **The brain works using a "small world" of connections.** Local connections are much denser than those over long distances. Having most processing happen over short distances means the brain is modular and compact. Results of connections are shipped over a relatively small numbers of output axons to other brain regions.

- ✔ **The brain is hierarchical** (although some modules do work in a reciprocal way, sending feedback between each other). High-level controllers control low-level controllers, like a home's thermostat that operates the furnace and air conditioner to maintain the temperature.

To understand the brain, you need to understand how a finite number of basic types of neurons work, how these neurons operate in a finite number of neural circuits, what the different processing modules are (a finite number), and how the overall control scheme is laid out. Of course, this sounds simpler than it actually is, but these principles are much easier to understand than trying to tackle the billions of neurons and their synapses.

Thinking thanks to the neocortex

Science generally believes (or assumes) that whatever differentiates human brains (which have consciousness) from non-conscious brains resides in the neocortex. This assumption is based on the fact that neocortex expansion differentiates mammals from non-mammals, primates from other mammals, and humans from primates. It's also based on the fact that, in the case of language — which enables consciousness — damage to specific brain areas (Wernicke's and Broca's areas) causes specific language problems.

Assuming that neocortex expansion alone is responsible for consciousness may not be entirely correct. The cerebellum, for example, expands considerably in primates and humans compared to other mammals. But even if unique human abilities originated in some changes in the neocortex, they cascaded into changes in subcortical structures as well.

The neocortex is the place to start looking for the basis of higher cognitive functions. Taking a top-down view of the brain starts with the four major lobes of the neocortex: frontal, parietal, temporal, and occipital. The frontal lobe organizes motor output, while the other three lobes process sensory information and interact with the frontal lobe to store long- and short-term memory. The parietal, temporal, and occipital lobes project to subcortical structures and to the frontal lobes as part of behavior generation.

One of the most baffling facts about the neocortex is that its structure is very similar in all parts of the brain in all mammals. Some differences, such as layer "granularity" or being "striate" do exist, but the fundamental minicolumn circuit is mostly the same. Therefore, something about this basic processing architecture very well may enable consciousness.

Processing in gray matter

The neocortex has six layers and is made up of gray and white matter (refer to Chapter 9). The 3- to 5-millimeter layer of gray matter is where the cell bodies and dendrites of the neurons do most of the processing. White matter beneath is composed of axons that mediate cortical–cortical and cortical–subcortical connections (in both directions).

Transmitting in white matter

Neocortex expanded in two major ways as mammals and primates evolved:

- **Increase in area:** Having an unchanging, canonical cortical minicolumn circuit as the neocortex expands means that the cortical area must increase to do more processing. This area increase eventually caused the cortex to become convoluted to fit inside the skull — like wadding up a piece of paper to cram it in a coffee cup.

- **Increase in white matter:** The brain needs more interconnections as the number of neurons goes up. Interconnections ultimately limit brain size. Each cortical neuron has a few thousand output synapses in a brain of 100 billion other neurons.

The physical limits of connectivity for 100 billion neurons results in the "small world" principle of neocortical connectivity. Most connections in a minicolumn are local and involve "interneurons" that are only connected in one minicolumn. A small percentage of pyramidal cells constitutes the output of the minicolumn, and even then most of their connections are within a few hundred micrometers. Only a small percentage of neocortical pyramidal cells projects centimeters or more. This occurs in a fairly limited number of major axon tracts, the identification of which is a goal of the currently much discussed "connectome" project.

Sensory processing in occipital, parietal, and temporal lobes

The five senses are processed in the parietal, temporal, and occipital lobes. However, research shows that these areas are not purely sensory.

Throughout this book I often refer to these lobes as "sensory," but that's an oversimplification. (When it comes to the brain, nothing is every simple.) Remember that sensory processing is part of executing motor behavior, or taking action.

For example, blind people, who have no retinal output to drive the occipital lobe, activate this lobe when identifying objects by touch, which requires internally representing the object's shape and layout. It has also been shown that the firing of neurons in V1 (visual area 1 — refer to Chapter 10) depends on what an animal, such as a monkey, does depending on the visual information. That is, V1 responses are dependent on different actions being executed.

One remarkable aspect of cortical connectivity is that areas that project "upstream" in the processing hierarchy, such as V1 to V2, typically receive an almost equal reciprocal connection. Primary sensory areas (such as V1, S1, and A1) that receive inputs from the thalamus also project back to the thalamus. Reticular and higher-order thalamic areas can modulate activity in all primary projection pathways.

High-level sensory areas can drive lower-level sensory areas. High-level sensory areas can themselves be driven by the frontal lobe, a motor control lobe. So, motor behavior possibilities can modulate sensory processing. This means that you see what you need to see and hear what you need to hear to carry out the task you're doing.

Specializing for memory

A common misconception is that memory in the human brain works like the memory of a computer. In computers, memory is a data string stored in a specific location. It has an address so the data can be stored and retrieved when needed. But in our brains, memory involves modification of the synapses of neurons that were active when the memory was created. This allows us to, in a way, re-create and reestablish the original brain configuration associated with the memory. (I discuss memory in Chapter 12.)

Many animals, including invertebrates, have long-term memories that last for days, months, or years. Mammals use the hippocampus to transfer memory from short term to long term.

Neurons in the hippocampus project back to the neocortical areas that activated them. Interplay between hippocampal and neocortical activity reproduces important aspects of the state to be remembered in the neocortex that initially represented that state. Synapses in the neocortex (including NMDA receptors) are modified so that the cortex can re-create the to-be-remembered state, even if the hippocampus is removed.

The "sensory" areas of the neocortex, then, process sensory information not only contingent on its motor use, but also based on prior experience. This whole process is very different from the way standard computers work, and it's poorly understood by neurobiologists today.

Following Thought through Sensory Pathways and Hierarchies

To better understand the neocortex, we need to look at its relation to and dependence on the thalamus. Virtually all sensory input — except for a major olfactory pathway — relays through the thalamus to reach the cortex. Thalamic relays also control motor programs in the front lobes.

The thalamus also integrates activities in various cortical areas. Considerable evidence indicates that awareness in humans and animals depends on the circuit by which the prefrontal sensory neocortices interact through the thalamus. To understand this circuit, we have to consider how the thalamus controls neocortical function.

Relaying to the thalamus and cortex

Although, as I say earlier in this chapter, human memory and computer memory work quite differently, you can use another computer metaphor to understand the interaction between the thalamus and neocortex. This is called the *subroutine*.

In a well-organized computer program, a "main" program sequences the major steps in the computation. This main program *calls* subroutines or functions for more detailed calculations, and the results are returned to the main routine sequence. Of course, the subroutines themselves may call other, even lower-level, routines.

Taking the visual system as an example, we know that about 1 million retinal ganglion cell axons reach the lateral geniculate nucleus of the thalamus on each side of the brain. About the same number of thalamic relay neurons project to the neocortex, where they directly drive 100 to 200 times that many neurons in V1 alone. V1 projects to higher visual areas like V2, but also back to thalamus, as do the higher areas. The projection and return from the thalamus to the neocortex works like a computer program's subroutine call with the thalamus running the main program and the neocortex computing details.

Projecting back to the thalamus

Thalamic neurons are often called *relay cells* because their receptive fields are similar to those of the inputs they receive from sensory areas. But neocortical sensory areas contain neurons with complex and specific response properties, which are in primary, thalamic recipient areas — and even more so in higher-order sensory processing areas.

The reciprocal projection from cortex to thalamus modulates the thalamic output. For example, say a linear feature in a visual image is weak. Then line or edge detectors in the cortex may activate and enhance the firing of the center surround cells along that line to increase its "neural contrast."

One way that neural contrast is increased in the thalamic output appears to be by *correlated firing*. The tendency for neurons to fire at the same time for some visual input to which they are responding.

Figure 14-1 shows how correlated firing works. On the left are the responses of a retinal ganglion cell to repetitions of a flash of a small spot. This is called a *raster plot*. Each vertical hash mark represents an action potential that occurred during the one-second recording time after the spot was turned on.

Like virtually all sensory neurons in all brains, the responses elicited by repetitions of an identical stimulus are similar, but not identical for each repetition. At the bottom of the raster plots is the peri- (or post-) stimulus time histogram (PSTH). It's the sum or average of all spikes for all stimuli in a sequence of time bins (typically 20 milliseconds).

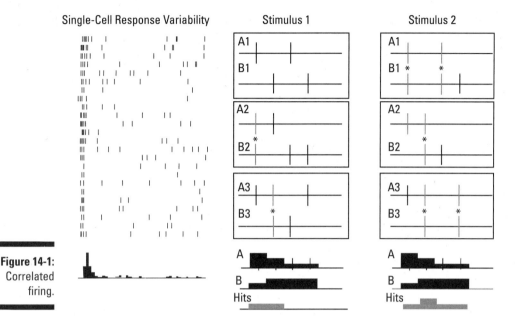

Figure 14-1:
Correlated
firing.

The idea that the spike pattern doesn't convey information has been overturned in the last decades. This is illustrated for a hypothetical set of rasters and PSTHs on the right of Figure 14-1. In the left column (Stimulus 1), two cells, A and B, show typical response variability. Their PSTHs are shown at the bottom. The asterisks in the second and third stimuli rasters show occasions where spikes in the two cells happened to occur at the same time.

In the right column (Stimulus 2), I have rearranged the spikes slightly among the stimuli so that the PSTHs remain unchanged. However, now the number of "hits," denoted by the asterisks is much higher. Recording from one cell at a time would not reveal the differences between the firing correlation differences between stimulus sequence 1 and 2. But in stimulus sequence 2 there is much higher correlated firing.

The importance of correlated firing is that cells A and B would be much more likely to produce a spike on a postsynaptic target when the spikes occurred at nearly exactly the same time, as in sequence 2, versus not so, as in sequence 1. Correlated firing can elevate a small percentage of activity in the brain above the background of all the rest of the neural activity. Numerous mechanisms exist by which neurons can adjust spike timing in development and real time to select some activity for general brain awareness above the background activity.

An important function of feedback between cortical areas and between cortical and subcortical structures (such as the thalamus) is to increase correlated firing for sensory input that is important. Correlated firing is a major mechanism of attention. It can integrate and select neural activity across the entire brain. Considerable evidence exists that correlated firing underlies all brain activity we're conscious of.

Gating and integrating functions

The other major modulator of thalamic activity is through reticular zones. These may change activity in one area of the thalamus within one sense (for example, enhancing the neural activity coding for red things if you're looking for something red), or between senses (enhancing vision at the expense of audition).

The thalamus does not drastically change the character of the sensory and motor information relayed through it. But it does modulate that activity through correlated firing and other mechanisms to enhance some information at the expense of the rest. In other words, it mediates attention.

This attention mechanism depends on processing in the cortex itself, which includes long-term memory changes in the cortex that are induced by experience, and frontal lobe representations of current goals and contingencies.

Speaking Your Mind: Language, Vision, and the Brain Hemispheres

Language sets humans apart from all other animals, and it's more than communication. *Language* is a symbolic system that uses rule-based grammar to enable almost infinite expressivity. Specialized brain regions — on the left side in most people — mediate the understanding and production of language. Damage to these areas can result in language-specific dysfunctions. The right hemisphere of the brain also has special capabilities for certain types of holistic processing, notably visual representations of images. Different processing styles of the left and right hemispheres of the brain lead to our unique human capabilities.

Comparing communication and language

One of the most persistent sources of debate in neuroscience and related fields — such as psychology, anthropology, sociology, and even philosophy — is the relation between animal communication, human language, and consciousness. Why is language so special?

Animals communicate. Insects communicate via pheromones, and birds and monkeys carry on extensive and elaborate verbal communication. Some dogs have been shown to recognize over 100 words. And some chimpanzees have coined novel multi-word utterances such as "water bird" for duck.

The difference between language and other communication is grammar. Think of the difference between arithmetic and algebra: Arithmetic allows you to count things and put them in order. But algebra allows you to represent abstract relationships and to manipulate those abstract relationships using equations.

Communication systems based on hundreds of verbalizations have only as much power as the number of words. A grammatical language, however, can represent relationships between what the words stand for, and relationships between relationships, such as the relationship between the self and another relationship. As caveman Og might say, "We avoid path with hungry tiger."

Internal vocalizing enables consciousness. Thoughts consist of symbolic representations of reality through words and grammar. Thoughts form specific memories that can be retrieved and related to one's current situation. This does not mean that nonverbal thought does not exist, but only that its power to guide behavior is very limited unless the thought is embedded in the complex verbally based representation of the world.

Locating language in the brain

The primary language areas (Wernicke's area and Broca's area) are located in the left hemisphere in 95 percent of all right-handed people and the majority of left-handed people. The language hemisphere is also usually the dominant hemisphere for eye dominance, as well as hand dominance.

Figure 14-2 shows the left hemisphere of a human brain from the side. Wernicke's area is at the junction of the temporal and parietal lobes at the posterior section of the superior temporal gyrus, typically associated with Brodmann area 22. This is a high-order auditory processing area necessary for understanding language and producing language that is coherent.

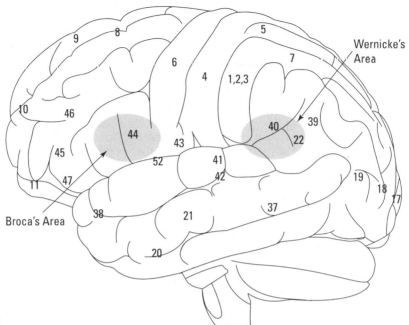

Figure 14-2:
Language
areas of the
brain.

Broca's area (and Brodmann area 44) contains the neural machinery for producing language. This frontal lobe area is part of the premotor cortex area, which is near the primary motor cortex areas that control the tongue, lips, and vocal cords — all necessary for producing language.

Losing language from neural dysfunction

Brain damage to Wernicke's area causes a specific language loss called *Wernicke's aphasia*. An aphasia is a loss of ability to either understand or produce speech, or both, due to some brain damage. Wernicke's aphasia is associated with impaired language comprehension and production. People with damage to this area have great difficulty understanding speech. They can produce speech that has a normal-sounding rhythm, but the speech itself is almost meaningless (also called *fluent aphasia*). They also have difficulty identifying complex nonverbal sounds like jangling keys, machine noises, and animal vocalizations.

Damage to Broca's area reduces speech production, depending on the extent of the damage. Extensive damage to areas 44 and 45 may almost totally eliminate speech, such as Broca's famous patient who could only utter one word, *tan*. Less extensive damage results in people being able to utter only short sentences with simple words. Broca's patients also have difficulty understanding longer, multisyllabic words, and sentences in passive voice, such as "The apple was eaten by the boy."

Examining visual processing asymmetries

The right hemisphere of the brain has specializations for visual processing, and these are well documented. The ability to recognize faces, for example, is highly dependent on the fusiform face area, which is in the right medial temporal lobe. This is a high-order visual processing area in the "what" pathway (refer to Chapter 10).

Damage to the right parietal lobe results in *hemi-neglect,* in which patients ignore objects in the left visual field. Men with such damage may not shave the left sides of their faces, for example, or they may hit the left side of the garage when driving a car into it.

The left hemisphere represents knowledge based on rules, and the right hemisphere represents knowledge based on examples. The left hemisphere representation of a room would consist of relationships that can be put in words, such as "The lamp is in the right-rear corner, and the table is in the front middle." The right hemisphere representation would be more like a literal image, not something you could actually verbalize. Expressing this inner image in language requires sending the right-brain image to the left, language-capable hemisphere. Other differences between the "style" of processing between the two cerebral hemispheres is discussed in Chapter 9.

Considering where consciousness lives

Helen Keller had a brain infection that caused her to lose her vision and hearing when she was just 19 months old. She gained the ability to communicate with sign language at around age 7. By her own accounts, Keller was largely unconscious before she was able to communicate.

Many people suffering from epilepsy have had their corpus callosum sectioned to prevent seizures from spreading from one hemisphere to the other. In these people, when stimuli are presented to the right visual field (left brain hemisphere), they can verbally identify and discuss the stimuli quite normally. However, they have little ability to identify or understand objects when stimuli are presented to the left visual field (right brain hemisphere).

The reason for these differences in consciousness is clearly linked to language, but not any specific part of the left hemisphere. Forty percent of left-handers and a small percentage of right-handers who have language in the right hemisphere are as conscious as people with left-hemisphere language. Severe damage to the right hemisphere or even its removal in infants can result in normal language in the right hemisphere as well.

Consciousness sits on top of a great deal of brain processing of which we're normally not conscious. Awareness, like animals can have, can exist without consciousness, as is the case in animals. But unique human consciousness goes beyond awareness. It is a symbolic representation system. Consciousness allows us to express and manipulate complex thoughts, both externally (through verbal language) and internally (by thinking). Consciousness is a *process,* not a place.

Defining Intelligence

We generally think of consciousness (as I discuss in the preceding section) as being unique to humans. But intelligence — like awareness — is something that we also attribute to animals. People say their dogs are intelligent, and robots are said to be intelligent machines. (Heck, we even have smartphones!) One way to figure out intelligence is to look at examples of what's considered intelligent, which is typically intelligent *behavior.*

Intelligence is nearly always identified with *adaptive behavior.* This means optimizing what one does in a complex, changing environment. *Reflexive behavior,* however complex, is built into the genes. This behavior generally happens without our thinking about it and isn't thought of as intelligent — although you could make a case that evolutionarily adapted behavior, such as refusing to eat something that tastes good but has produced illness in the past, is intelligent. A similar comparison could be between machines that are programmed to do things, versus those that learn to do things.

Math, language, and social intelligence

A fundamental problem in assessing intelligence is that there are different types of intelligence. The tendency for an individual's intelligence score in different domains to be correlated across a variety of tests is represented by Spearman's g factor (IQ) and its derivatives.

Language intelligence, including vocabulary and the ability to understand written passages, is a left-brain-dominant skill. While executing rules-based tasks and mathematical procedures may also be a left-brain skill, translating real-world situations into mathematical form requires visualization and other right-brain abilities. Virtually all assessments of intelligence recognize these kinds of differences.

Other types of intelligence, such as musical and athletic, have been assessed in schemes such as Gardner's multi-intelligence list of eight basic components.

Social or interpersonal intelligence has gotten a lot of attention recently. *Social intelligence* is the adaptive ability to understand the intentions of others, and alter our own behavior to acknowledge and use social situations to our advantage. Social intelligence may have a neurobiological basis in the orbitofrontal cortex and amygdala system. Social intelligence can be low in people who otherwise have high verbal and math intelligence. Social, but not IQ test, intelligence may also be lost with orbitofrontal damage.

People who have vastly high intelligence in one domain as compared to other domains are called *savants*. A defining characteristic of autism, for example, is having poor language skills, but very high performance skill in some other specific domain.

Intelligence components for decisions, abstract thinking, problem solving

Many people who study intelligence consider what's called *meta-intelligence* to be its highest form. *Meta-intelligence* is an executive function that refers to self-reflective capabilities, knowing one's own strengths and weaknesses, and being able to predict one's reactions to situations. R. J. Sternberg, among others, has championed meta-intelligence.

Meta-intelligence is composed of meta-components used in problem solving and decision making. These meta-components use what are called *performance components* to carry out cognition. *Performance components* are like IQ domains, basic skills and processes for adaptive modification of behavior, including perception, long-term memory, language, and spatial abilities.

For example, Gardner's bodily kinesthetic intelligence domain entails the ability to control body motions skillfully. Clearly many animals have the ability to do this — in many cases, far better than humans. However, animals don't have the meta-cognitive ability to reflect on and reason about body movements, or invent entirely new ones by reasoning. Only humans do.

Meta-intelligence capabilities are associated with the human prefrontal cortex. This area of the brain develops relatively late, with axons not being fully myelinated until the late teenage years. Much of what IQ researchers mean by meta-cognition is embodied in the common idea of wisdom.

Investigating intelligence factors

Two factors that may indicate intelligence are the size of the brain and the speed at which the brain can process information.

Brain size

The brain is a lot of work for the body to maintain. In humans the brain consumes about 20 percent of our total metabolism, but it accounts for only about 2 percent of our body weight. Brains, like other organs, scale up with body weight. The brains of whales can reach 18 pounds, elephants 11 pounds, and dolphins 3.5 pounds, while human brains average just over 3 pounds.

However, some very large animals, such as dinosaurs, lizards, and alligators, have relatively small brains compared to mammals. Across species, brains got generally bigger in mammals than non-mammals, and in primates compared to other mammals, and, now, in humans compared to other primates.

Most of the increase in primate and human brain size is in the neocortex. For a given size, species that appear to behave in an intelligent way tend to have larger brains than those that don't. But, within a species, the correlation is weak between intelligence and brain size.

Processing speed

The other brain characteristic frequently mentioned as a foundation for intelligence is processing speed or processing efficiency. This is particularly true for processing perceptually complex stimuli. *Processing speed* is related to how fast a person can execute a sequence of mental operations to accomplish some task.

Neural processing speed as it relates to IQ differences appears to be due to a variety of genetic factors. High processing speed may be a cause of high IQ, or partly a result of it.

Emotional Intelligence

Some of the emotion-processing areas of the brain are ancient. They include subcortical structures, such as the limbic system. Mammals, particularly primates, added large areas of the neocortex, such as the orbito-frontal cortex. These areas interact with the older emotion systems, giving us more complex emotional detection and responses.

Some people think of emotions as the opposite of reason. But emotions are a useful and necessary part of cognition. Emotions not only mediate our instinctual behaviors, but also allow us to learn and adapt important new behaviors that are not rules-based.

Damage to particular parts of the brain, such as the orbito-frontal cortex, can result in individuals who have normal IQs but who are deficient in emotional processing. These people are severely dysfunctional in normal life situations.

Feeling the basic emotions

Emotions tend to arise in situations linked to physical or social survival. They can be positive or negative, weak or strong. The research of the American psychologist Paul Ekman suggests that six emotions are physiologically distinct, measurable, and universally recognized across cultures:

- ✔ Anger
- ✔ Disgust
- ✔ Fear
- ✔ Happiness
- ✔ Sadness
- ✔ Surprise

Mixtures of the basic emotions can produce more complex emotions, such as contempt, which is a mixture of disgust and anger.

In his book *The Expression of the Emotions in Man and Animals,* Charles Darwin argued that emotions serve a communication purpose in humans that helps us to survive and is, thus, selected for. This idea implies that emotions should have universal cross-cultural expression. It also implies that emotions are connected to basic needs that are necessary for survival.

Engaging basic drives (hunger, thirst, anger fear, sex) as emotions

The idea that emotions are universal is consistent with the idea that emotions are concerned with the basic drives and homeostatic needs that existed before humans. When we experience an emotion, we're experiencing a brain state associated with the current highest-priority goal. If we're dehydrated, the desire for water becomes intense and consuming, for example.

Emotion is typically linked to the activation of the autonomic nervous system (refer to Chapter 6). Fear, for example, activates the sympathetic branch of the autonomic nervous system to produce elevated heart rate, faster breathing, and sweating. Extreme hunger can active the parasympathetic autonomic nervous system to lower metabolism and conserve resources, but this activation may abruptly switch to sympathetic if obtainable food appears. Autonomic modulation operates via the release of hormones.

Expressing emotions to communicate

Humans have developed a complex communication system around emotions that includes both displaying emotions and perceiving them. Basic emotions have consistent expression patterns. Emotional expression includes verbal and nonverbal behaviors that communicate an internal state.

Facial expressions are particularly important in expressing emotions, for example, when crying, smiling, and laughing. These facial emotional expressions communicate what we're feeling quite clearly. Emotional facial expressions can come on quickly, before or even without our being consciously aware of our emotional state.

However, people can obviously control emotional expressions — that's how professional actors make their living! Ordinary people consciously control their emotional expressions to communicate with others and to manipulate the emotions of others, which are essential social skills in all primate groups.

Realistic emotional displays, as in method acting, activate similar areas of the brain that normal emotional experience activates. Artificially activating these brain areas by purposely controlling an emotion can still cause the actor to experience the real emotional state.

Reacting quickly

The amygdala is one of the most important areas of the limbic system responsible for emotions. In the "low road" theory of the American neuroscientist Joseph LeDoux, some sensory information that reaches the thalamus is projected directly along a fast pathway to the amygdala. The olfactory system contains direct projections to the amygdala that do not even pass through the thalamus (refer to Chapter 11). This fast pathway is important for being able to react quickly in response to fear in the face of a threat. These are the fast reactions that occur first, before we have time to think about what's really happening and the slower but more sophisticated cortical analysis can happen. The amygdala functions as a memory organizer for the orbitofrontal cortex, which embodies a more sophisticated representation of threats and non-threats. A normal person might be very afraid of all snakes, but an experienced forester might learn to have no fear of garter snakes.

Applying instincts to new situations

An important aspect of emotional intelligence is using *educated instincts*. Learning to fly an airplane involves unlearning a fear of heights. But it also involves learning to be afraid of specific sensory stimuli such as gauges that show low gas or an overheated engine.

Dangerous situations, whether physical or social, strongly activate the amygdala-orbitofrontal system. This system communicates with the rest of the brain by inducing feelings. Normal people with intact amygdala-orbitofrontal systems become very nervous about placing gambling bets as large as their mortgage payments, walking through certain parts of town at night, or telling dirty jokes in front of their boss. These are all situations we've learned are dangerous, and which generate limbic system–like emotional reactions, including activating the autonomic nervous system. Emotional intelligence involves listening to these types of feelings, even if we can't readily put into words why we feel uneasy.

Storing memories of strong emotional reactions

Some researchers believe the amygdala never forgets. That is, the contingencies of any situation that has predicted a threat will always activate the amygdala, even after the situation is over. The job of the orbitofrontal cortex, then, is to override the amygdala's activation of the autonomic fight-or-flight response.

When you first started driving, you were probably a bit nervous every time an oncoming car passed within a few feet of you in the opposite lane. After you had driven a few months, the autonomic reaction went away, but your amygdala is probably still activated. The reaction may be translated into gripping the steering wheel a bit more tightly, just in case. But the conscious fear is almost gone.

Understanding Consciousness

Consciousness is the 800-pound gorilla in the room of neuroscience. Most neuroscientists carry on their research without acknowledging consciousness directly, but it's always there. Only one species on earth has consciousness, and virtually every "normal" member of that species has it fully. What can today's neurobiology say about it?

Without denying the existence of visual, auditory, and other sensory imagery that is nonverbal, most human consciousness is associated with internal verbalization. All humans conduct a running internal dialog that explains current reality, recalls past situations, and plans for future ones. Did language cause consciousness?

Learning language instinctually

Prior to the age of about two years, human infants not only behave much differently from our closest relatives, chimpanzees, but they're also less competent in motor activities such as moving and climbing. Then the language explosion begins! When we're exposed to language, it generally develops in the same ordered progression. We apply labels and sentences to objects in the world, to their relations, and to actions involving these objects — all without really getting clear instruction. This is what the American linguist Steven Pinker called "the language instinct."

We know that the language instinct is ubiquitous in human brains and has only evolved in one species. Imagine how strong the selection pressure must have been to master speech. Neuroscientists believe that the brain that evolved such a strong language instinct must have been compelled to classify and name objects, relationships, and actions.

Developing internal language and consciousness

We can assume that the need to name things was first used for person-to-person communication. What must have been invented next was *subvocalization* (talking to yourself in an inner voice without actually speaking). This may have occurred when an early hominid was about to speak, but was interrupted. A brain that has the need to name objects and see object relations and actions in sentences has an internal monologue — that internal monologue is consciousness.

Inner-speech consciousness was mankind's first digital invention. Speech is digital because it's made up of a finite number of sounds (in each language) that are put together in groups to make words, with a small number of words forming sentences. Although you can modify the meaning of speech with your tone or style, the digital nature of speech means that every person can agree on a finite set of definitions and arrangements that we can all understand. Internal speech is a running narrative explanation of reality — past, present, and future.

Part IV

Developmental, Neurological, and Mental Disorders and Treatments

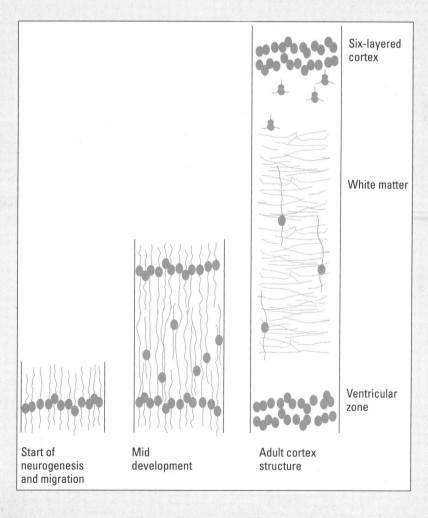

Six-layered cortex

White matter

Ventricular zone

Start of neurogenesis and migration

Mid development

Adult cortex structure

Find out whether depression is "all in the mind" in a free article at www.dummies.com/extras/neurobiology.

In this part . . .

- ✓ See how your brain develops discrete structures from a small ball of cells.

- ✓ Identify things that can go wrong in the brain and muscles, impairing a person's ability to move.

- ✓ See why and how broken brains produce broken minds.

- ✓ Consider whether the brain can be repaired, or even replaced.

Chapter 15

Developing the Brain and Nervous System

In This Chapter

▶ Seeing how cells divide and develop

▶ Focusing on the brain development

▶ Going through the layers of the neocortex

▶ Examining birth defects and neural disorders

A new life starts with a single fertilized zygote cell formed when two gamete cells are joined by means of sexual reproduction. The word *zygote* is actually derived from the Greek word meaning "joined." This zygote cell and its daughter cells and their daughter cells then divide many times to produce the entire organism, including the brain.

In this chapter, I take you through how the brain, particularly the neocortex, develops from simple cells into its final six-layered structure. I also discuss how neurons and parts of the brain are organized. Finally, I cover some common neural problems — some that start before birth and some that occur in old age.

Dividing and Differentiating after Conception

In *eukaryotes* (organisms whose cells have nuclei in their DNA), chromosomes exist in pairs — one member of the pair from the father and one from the mother. In the normal process of cell division (called *mitosis;* refer to Chapter 2), the cell replicates its chromosomes and then separates them into two identical sets that are divided into two nuclei. Next, cytokinesis occurs, which is the process that divides the entire cell into two.

Humans have 46 chromosomes in 23 pairs. In all but the XX and XY sex chromosomes, both chromosomes are typically similar in DNA sequence and length. Each chromosome itself consists of double-stranded DNA (refer to Chapter 2), so human cells have a total of 92 DNA strands.

In sexual reproduction, a different kind of cell division occurs. This cell division is called *meiosis* and it produces *haploid cells* (cells with a single set of unpaired chromosomes) called *gametes* or *germ cells.* The union of two gametes is the beginning of the new organism's development.

Meiosis, gametes, and zygotes

During meiosis, each gamete gets half of the DNA of "normal" diploid somatic cells. Figure 15-1 illustrates the meiosis process.

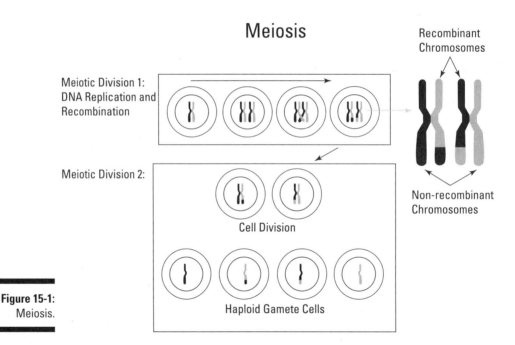

Figure 15-1: Meiosis.

Crossover

As haploid gametes are produced in meiosis, a process called *crossover* results in some daughter cells getting a DNA strand that is a mixture of both strands of the parent *duplex cell* (a cell with double-stranded DNA).

Crossover produces a new daughter cell chromosome. This new chromosome contains pieces of both chromosomes in the parental cell. If the crossover occurs within a DNA section that codes for a protein, instead of at a gene border or in a non-coding section, a new gene can be produced.

Without crossover, the genes between the mother and father would be mixed by the process of randomly getting one or the other member of each parent's pair of chromosomes. But all the genes in that parental chromosome would remain intact and unaltered, a mutation or some post-replication mechanism occurs (refer to Chapter 2).

Each egg and sperm the parent produces is unique, both in the mixture of which chromosome of the pair it receives from each parent, and by the crossover production of new hybrid DNA sequences within a chromosome.

Degeneracy

DNA consists of one of four possible bases at each location: adenine (A), cytosine (C), thymine (T), and guanine (G). A triplet of three consecutive bases is called a *codon*. The number of uniquely possible codons is 64 (four possible bases at each of three positions), although only 61 of the 64 possible codons code for amino acids.

Actually, however, only 47 *distinct* amino acids are generated by DNA, so some amino acids are coded by more than one codon. For example, GAA and GAG both specify the same amino acid (glutamic acid). This redundancy is called *degeneracy.*

Because some amino acids are coded by more than one codon, mutations can change some bases in the DNA with no effect on the amino acid. Also, some amino acids in some proteins can be switched without significantly affecting how the protein folds or its function.

Genetic disorders

When scientists are searching for a disorder's genetic basis, it helps if the unknown disease-causing gene is close on the same chromosome to a gene that specifies an easily observable trait, such as hair color, with a known genetic base. Because crossover more infrequently cleaves between genes that are close together rather than farther apart, scientists can examine the chromosomes of people who have the observable trait and look for the nearby chromosome location with the disease mutation.

Scientists now understand something about the function of about 50 percent of the 20,000 human genes. Human genes average about 3,000 base pairs (with considerable variation). Some genes consist of several million base pairs. Finding the genetic mutation that causes a developmental disorder means finding one genetic mutation out of about 3 billion base pairs in the human genome, amid variation from person to person of about 0.1 percent, or approximately 1 million base pairs.

Partitioning the body: Endoderm, mesoderm, ectoderm

When the sperm fertilizes the egg, it produces a cell called a *zygote*. A zygote has paired chromosomes like the parent organisms, but with a mixture of the parents' genes, plus some unique gene mixtures from crossover (see the "Crossover" section, earlier in this chapter). The zygote divides by mitosis and creates a sphere of cells called the *blastula*. The cells in the blastula are *totipotent* stem cells, which means they can give rise to all body cell types for several divisions. For example, a single fertilized zygote cell can divide once and separate, with each daughter forming an identical twin.

After a few divisions (about four days), the daughter cells are no longer totipotent. They become committed to specialized cell lines comprising the three germ layers: endoderm, mesoderm, and ectoderm. The nervous system is derived from the ectoderm line. The first stages of neural development are based on the processes of specialization and migration.

The purpose of junk DNA

Many molecular biologists were shocked when it was originally reported that approximately 98 percent of human DNA is never translated into any protein. The term *junk DNA* was applied to such sequences, implying that this DNA was in some sense vestigial, having once had a function that is now no longer needed. The situation turns out to be more complicated than this. Much of the genome is regulatory, coding for translational and transcriptional regulation of protein-coding sequences, rather than coding for protein directly. Some of the DNA once termed "junk" may be performing this function.

Non-coding introns also exist within DNA coding exons. The gene for a protein may have multiple coding regions (exons) interrupted by regions that are not coded (introns). Both introns and exons are initially produced in the messenger RNA that's used to make the final protein, but the intron segments are removed by RNA splicing processes in the cell before the protein gets manufactured. Nevertheless, much of the genome really is "junk" in that it consists of repeats of one to three base pairs over and over again that is never transcribed into a protein.

Specialization

As cells within the major endoderm, mesoderm, and ectoderm cell lines continue to divide, they become even more differentiated or specialized. Cell potency works on a continuum, starting with totipotency, then pluripotency, multipotency, oligopotency, and finally unipotency. Pluripotent neural stem cells can give rise to any nervous system cell. As more divisions lower potency, neural stem cells can only differentiate into more specific neuronal lines. At the end of development, unipotent neuronal stem cells produce only specific neuronal cell types in specific nervous system areas.

The specialization process involves restricting what DNA is expressed in particular cell lines using mechanisms such as DNA methylation and histone acetylation (see Chapter 2). During developmental cell division, not only is the parent cell DNA replicated, but also its epigenetic methylation and acetylation pattern are replicated. This pattern is altered or supplemented in divisions in which the potency is reduced as the cell line becomes more specialized.

Migration

The other major early developmental mechanism is *migration*. Neural precursor cells migrate to different parts of the developing brain to self-organize into different brain structures. When the neurons have reached their final positions, they extend axons and dendrites, which allow them to communicate with other neurons via synapses. Synaptic communication between neurons establishes functional neural circuits.

Before an embryo's nervous system is formed, cells at the dorsal and ventral poles of the embryo and at other key locations release chemical messengers that establish gradients across the embryo. Developing cells sense the multiple chemical gradients and use this information to determine where they should be and what sort of tissue they should become. Glial cells also express surface markers that receptors on migrating cells recognize to guide their movement. These markers are sometimes called *trophic substances*.

Later these markers attract and guide axonal growth. The chemical gradients specified by the genome encode both the production of trophic and adhesion factor, and the responses of particular cells to them. During development, these factors guide developing cells, such that some cell types in nucleus A send their axons to nucleus B and, when they get there, synapse on dendrites bearing cell surface marker C.

Neural migration is controlled by glial cells and trophic factors. Early in development, some ectoderm cells stop dividing and differentiate into glial cells, which form the "scaffolding" of the nervous system. Neurons migrate along the processes of glial cells guided by cell adhesion molecules.

Descending from the ectoderm into the nervous system

In humans, the period from fertilization until the end of the tenth week of gestation is called the *embryonic period*. The embryo spends its first few days traveling down the Fallopian tube.

After the zygote has divided several times it is called a *morula*.

After the seventh cell division, the 128-cell embryo is called a *blastula*. The blastula consists of a spherical layer of cells called the *blastoderm* that surrounds the *blastocoel* — a fluid-filled cavity. In mammals, at this stage, an inner cell mass (the *blastocyst*) exists that is distinct from the surrounding blastula. Through this stage, the size of the embryo remains nearly constant, because each division produces successively smaller cells. The blastocyst reaches the uterus around the fifth day after fertilization.

The blastula becomes disk shaped and then egg shaped. At about day 15 the narrow end, a structure called the *primitive streak* appears that extends along the middle of the blastula for about half its length. Later, this forms a shallow groove, called the *primitive groove*. The mesoderm then forms between the ectoderm and endoderm, with the ectoderm as the outermost layer and the endoderm the innermost.

Blastulating into the neural groove and tube

In the next phase, the embryo is called a *gastrula*. During gastrulation, cells begin to differentiate and are no longer totipotent (refer to "Partitioning the body: Endoderm, mesoderm, ectoderm," earlier in this chapter).

Two longitudinal folds in the ectoderm arise in front of the primitive streak. The neural groove lies between these folds. The neural groove continues to deepen and ultimately the tops of the folds come together and make a closed tube called the *neural tube*. The ectodermal wall of this tube becomes the nervous system.

The first place where the neural folds meet to produce the neural tube is where the hindbrain forms. This region has a rhomboidal shape, which is why it's called the *rhombencephalon*. A ridge of ectodermal cells along the prominent margin of each neural fold becomes the neural crest. The spinal nerve, cranial nerve, and autonomic system ganglia are derived from the neural crest.

Embryos in evolution

High school biology teachers usually point out that the stages of embryonic development *(ontogeny)* do not repeat the stages of evolution *(phylogeny)*, although it looks that way. Early human embryos resemble similar stages in our evolutionary ancestors such as lizards. Later stages are similar to many other mammals, particularly primates. This idea clearly isn't literally true because some stages in the human embryo aren't present in any ancestor species. However, because mammals evolved from cold-blooded vertebrates but have a longer embryonic gestation, they share the same overall body plan and many of mammals' early gestational forms are similar to their cold-blooded ancestors. Later-stage human embryos resemble those of other primates because most of the differentiation between humans and primates occurs late in embryonic development.

Differentiating along the anterior posterior axis

At the cephalic (top) end of the neural groove, three vesicles form that comprise the three cerebral vesicles. The three main structures are the forebrain, midbrain, and hindbrain. I go into more detail about these structures later in this chapter under "Cephalizing the hindbrain, midbrain, and forebrain." In Figure 15-2, you can see these main vesicles and the embryonic nervous system at several key stages.

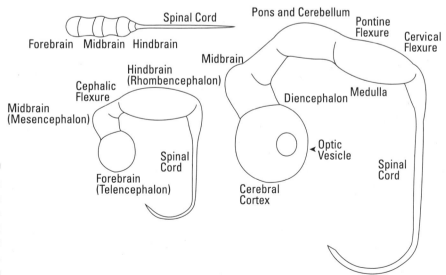

Figure 15-2: Structures of the developing nervous system.

The walls of these vesicles develop into various parts of the brain, whereas the remaining cavities become the brain's ventricles. The posterior part of the neural tube forms the medulla and spinal cord. The cavity becomes the spinal cord central canal.

Covering the brain with meninges: Dura, arachnoid, and pia

The central nervous system — brain and spinal cord — is protected by the meninges, which consist of three layers:

- ✔ **The dura mater:** This is the outermost layer, which is composed of dense fibrous tissue. The dura mater around the brain is usually attached to the skull. The dura around the spinal cord is attached to the bones of the spinal vertebral canal. It contains a few large blood vessels that divide into the capillaries in the pia (see later in this list).

- ✔ **The arachnoid mater:** This middle layer is the arachnoid. The name comes from its spider web–like appearance. It consists of a thin, transparent membrane of fibrous tissue.

  Neither the dura nor the arachnoid descend into the sulci.

- ✔ **The pia mater:** This is the innermost layer and it follows the brain surface (and that of the spinal cord). It's a fibrous, thin membrane. Blood vessels pass through the pia mater to the brain and spinal cord. Space between the arachnoid and the pia mater is filled with cerebrospinal fluid.

The dura is attached to the arachnoid, while the pia is attached to the underlying central nervous system tissue. The dura and arachnoid can separate in an injury, with the space between them called *subdural space* where bleeding may occur.

The meninges may play a role in the development of the nervous system. They release diffusible factors that modulate neural progenitor cells. They also help set up the pial basement membrane that forms a base for radial fibers of neuroepithelial stem cells.

Polarizing the Brain: Ganglia versus Brains

In animals, nervous systems first evolved using action potentials for distant cells to signal between each other. Early invertebrates — such as jellyfish — have diffuse nerve nets but not a central nervous system. Here I discuss the basic body plan from millions of years ago, and the three-segment brain structure we have today.

Basic body plan

Most animals descended from a common wormlike ancestor (form 550 to 600 million years ago) that was basically symmetric on both sides *(bilaterian)*. Its body consisted of the following components, which make up the basic structure we see in worms — the simplest bilaterian animals of today:

- ✔ A gut cavity running from mouth to anus
- ✔ A nerve cord with an enlarged specialized area called a *ganglion,* for each body segment
- ✔ A single large anterior ganglion, the brain, typically associated with the mouth and unique sensory organs such as eyes

The segmental spinal ganglia in mammals are part of the general bilaterian body plan. These ganglia project sensory and motor nerves that innervate the associated surface of the body and its muscles. In this scheme, the top three segments are the forebrain, midbrain, and hindbrain.

Differentiating the spinal cord from the brain proper

The three segments forming the brain — the hindbrain, midbrain, and forebrain — are unique because of the location of the mouth and major sensory organs such as eye, ears, vestibular system, taste, and smell. The brain processes sensory information and organizes motor behavior in accordance with this information.

Differentiating into the hindbrain, midbrain, and forebrain

All vertebrates have the following enlarged anterior three-segment specialization made up of the following structures:

- ✔ **The forebrain (prosencephalon):** This area differentiates into the diencephalon (primarily thalamus, hypothalamus, and pretectum) and the telencephalon (cerebrum). The telencephalon consists of the cerebral cortex and underlying white matter (derived from the dorsal telencephalon, or pallium) and the basal ganglia (derived from the ventral telencephalon, or subpallium). The telencephalon also divides at the midline to develop into the left and right cerebral hemispheres.

- ✔ **The midbrain (mesencephalon):** This area arises from the middle brain segment, the mesencephalon. The midbrain mesencephalon does not divide further into distinct brain areas, though there are a number of very specialized areas within it. The midbrain consists of the tectum, tegmentum, and cerebral peduncles, among other structures. At its caudal (tail) border are the pons and cerebellum, while above it rostrally are the diencephalonic structures such as the thalamus and hypothalamus.

- ✔ **The hindbrain (rhombencephalon):** This area develops into the medulla (from the myelencephalon), pons, and cerebellum. During development, the human rhombencephalon is composed of eight swellings called *rhombomeres.* The metencephalon, which forms the pons and cerebellum, develops from rhombomeres Rh3 through Rh1.

Genetically, the hindbrain appears to be homologous to a structure called the *sub-oesophageal ganglion* in arthropods (spiders and ticks). If so, then the hindbrain evolved at least as far back as the last common ancestor of chordates and arthropods, over 500 million years ago.

In cold-blooded vertebrates such as lizards, these segments are approximately equal in size, as they are in early mammalian ontogeny. However, in mammals, the forebrain becomes increasingly enlarged, becoming by far the dominant percentage of total brain mass, especially in primates and large mammalian species.

Layering the Neocortex

The neocortex has a uniform, six-layer cellular circuit organization. This structure suggests that the entire neocortex develops, at least initially, using a common set of general layout rules. This set of circuit development rules generates a structure that serves to process inputs from all five senses, as well as execute programs for motor control. In the follow sections, I take you through the development of the neocortex and how it is organized.

Migrating along radial glia and other glial roles

The neocortex and underlying white matter develop from a specialized layer of neural stem cells in the *ventricular zone,* which is located at the outer wall of the prosencephalon, and later telencephalon. (Refer to "Descending from the ectoderm into the nervous system," earlier in this chapter.)

Specialized glial cells, called *radial glia,* take the first step in neocortex development. Radial glia are extended cells whose processes reach from the ventricular zone to the cortical plate just below the pia, which will become the surface of the cortex.

After this scaffolding of radial glial fibers is in place, progenitor cells divide asymmetrically in the ventricular zone. One daughter of the division remains a neural stem cell, but the other daughter becomes an intermediate progenitor cell. This cell will divide symmetrically in the subventricular zone to generate neurons that will migrate to a particular neocortical layer and differentiate into a specific cell type, such as a pyramidal cell. The migrating neural progenitor cell is called a *migratory precursor cell.*

Neural precursor cells migrate up the radial glial processes to form the six-layered gray matter of the neocortex that sits on top of the white matter axons. These six layers are built from the bottom up. The first neural precursor cells leaving the ventricular zone travel just a short distance up the radial glial processes where they stop and begin differentiating. Precursor cells born later in the ventricular zone migrate up through cells in the first layer to form another layer on top. This process continues until the last layer, 6, is formed, which is the most superficial cell layer of the cortex.

Evidence suggests that each radial glial cell, and the precursor neurons that migrate along it, form a fundamental unit of cortical organization called the *minicolumn.* A minicolumn is a "unit circuit" consisting of about 100 cells dispersed vertically across the six cortical layers. Minicolumns are made up of a number of standard cell types interconnected in a standard way. Several hundred million minicolumns constitute the neocortex in humans. Figure 15-3 depicts minicolumns at various stages of the development of the neocortex.

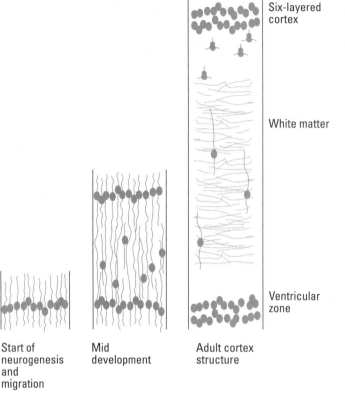

Six-layered cortex

White matter

Ventricular zone

Figure 15-3: Radial glia and neural migration form neocortex minicolumns.

Start of neurogenesis and migration

Mid development

Adult cortex structure

In sensory cortex, for example, all cells in a given minicolumn have approximately the same receptive field location (although they may respond to stimuli differently). Subtle errors in minicolumn layout may underlie mental disorders such as autism.

The neural precursor cells are born "knowing" the layer to which they should migrate. If you transplant precursor cells from a donor to a recipient animal at a different developmental stage, the donor cells go to the layer they would have migrated to in the donor, not the layer to which other cells are migrating in the recipient.

Cells differentiate into cell types according to what part of the DNA is *expressed,* or read out, by messenger RNA and converted into proteins. This process is controlled by sections of DNA that make RNA sequences that regulate the expression of other DNA segments. DNA expression is affected by the past and present environment of the cell. As development proceeds, cells become increasingly specialized until they differentiate into a final cell type and remain so for the life of the organism.

Differentiating at journey's end

Most neural circuits consist of excitatory integrating and output neurons. These neurons are embedded in a network of inhibitory interneurons that transform inputs to the brain that are relayed by the excitatory output neurons. In the neocortex, the major excitatory integrative and relay cells are the pyramidal cells.

Pyramidal cells

The major fully differentiated neuron type in the neocortex is the *pyramidal cell.* Pyramidal neurons are typically the largest neocortical neurons. Their name comes from their triangularly shaped somas. Pyramidal cells have a large ascending apical dendrite, multiple basal dendrites at the level of the cell body, and a large number of dendritic spines. (This neuronal morphology also found in cells in the hippocampus and amygdala.) Pyramidal cells typically have a single axon that releases glutamate at its terminal. Pyramidal cells are the primary output units of the neocortex.

Most of the excitatory input of pyramidal cells is from glutamate onto the spines, while inhibitory inputs (primarily GABA, and some glycine) occur on dendritic shafts (particularly large dendrites), the cell soma, and occasionally on the axon. A typical pyramidal cell receives tens of thousands of excitatory inputs and several thousand inhibitory inputs.

Thousands of excitatory and inhibitory inputs activate a variety of voltage-gated ion channels. These include Na+, Ca2+, and K+ channels in the dendrites that can amplify inputs. It has also been shown that action potentials generated in the soma or initial segment of the axon can back-propagate into the dendritic tree. This process may trigger synaptic plasticity by mechanisms such as Hebbian learning, where inputs active when the cell fires an action potential are strengthened. This makes the cell increasingly sensitive to that effective combination of inputs.

Three major physiological subclasses of pyramidal neurons exist: RSad, RSna, and IB.

- ✔ **RSad (regular spiking adapting):** RSad pyramidal neurons fire single action potentials that are followed by a hyperpolarizing after-potential. This after-potential mediates what is called *spike frequency adaptation* (SFA), a change in response properties after a short period of high firing rate.

- ✔ **RSna (regular spiking non-adapting):** RSna pyramidal cells tend to fire a train of action potentials (more than five) after an EPSP, but do not adapt as a result of this spike train.

- ✔ **IB (intrinsically bursting):** IB pyramidal cells respond to EPSPs with a burst of a few action potentials and do not show SFA.

Cortical interneurons

Interneurons have dense, local inhibitory connections. Neurochemically, three groups of cortical inhibitory interneurons have been defined:

- Parvalbumin expressing
- Somatostatin, calbindin, and/or NPY (neuropeptide Y) expressing
- Calretinin, VIP (vasoactive intestinal polypeptide), and/or CCK (cholecystokinin) expressing

Anatomically, morphological classes of interneurons include the following:

- **Chandelier cells:** These cells have an extensive local axonal arbour with large boutons that innervate the axon initial segments of pyramidal cells. Cortical layers 2 through 6 contain numerous chandelier cells. Their axon terminals are typically parvalbumin immunopositive.

- **Basket cells:** These cells have varying morphologies and tend to innervate the proximal dendrites and somas of pyramidal cells. One neurochemical type of basket cell contains parvalbumin and is fast-spiking. Another type is regular-spiking and contain CCK and/or VIP.

Some parvalbumin-containing cells exist that are neither basket nor chandelier cells.

- **Double bouquet cells:** These cells have unmyelinated, vertical descending axons that split into multiple output branches called *collaterals*. They form a very dense, local axonal arbour that innervates dendritic spines and fine dendrites of spiny cells and the somas and dendrites of smooth cells (see the end of this list). They are typically located in layers 2 through 4 and immunoreactive for calbindin, calretinin, and/or VIP.

- **Martinotti cells:** Located in layer 5, martinotti cells have a dendritic morphology with two zones of branching (called *bitufted*) and are calbindin and/or somatostatin-immunoreactive. Their axons project to cortical layer 1 with a large number of small unmyelinated collaterals that synapse on cortical neurons in intermediate layers as they ascend.

- **Spider web:** These neurogliaform cells have dense local dendritic and axonal arbours. Their physiology is characterized as "late-spiking," meaning their responses are delayed relative to other cortical neurons.

- **Spiny:** These are interneurons with sparse dendritic and axonal arbors and innervate distal pyramidal dendrites. They're calbindin or somatostatin immunoreactive, and have a burst-firing physiology.

- **Stellate, smooth cells:** These interneurons have few spines on their dendrites and are often found in layer IV.

What's so magic about six layers?

The neocortex is characteristic of mammals derived embryonically from the dorsal telencephalon. It is the newest part of the cerebral cortex to evolve. The neocortex generally consists of six layers of gray matter, with the most superficial layer 1 at the surface, to layer 6 at the border with the underlying white matter. Older types of cortex include the archicortex and paleocortex (together referred to as *allocortex*) in the limbic system.

The neocortex appears to have allowed the brain to evolve to be larger because of its ability to represent different types of inputs, process those inputs, and communicate the results of processing to other areas of cortex in a standard way. Cognitive enhancements in multiple senses and motor control evolved by devoting more area at a given stage of processing for higher acuity, and more areas for greater sophistication of processing.

Excitatory pyramidal neurons constitute about 80 percent of neocortical neurons, while inhibitory interneurons account for the remaining 20 percent. Different cell types in different layers have specific functions and connections. The layers of the neocortex have the following functions:

- **Layer 1,** the molecular layer, consists mainly of apical dendritic arborizations of pyramidal cells and cortical–cortical axons.

- **Layer 2,** the external granular layer, contains stellate and small pyramidal cells.

- **Layer 3,** the external pyramidal layer, contains mostly small pyramidal neurons and vertically oriented interneurons. This layer is the main source of projections from one column to other cortical columns.

    Layers 1 through 3 process cortico-cortical connections.

- **Layer 4,** called the internal granular layer in some areas of the cortex, receives thalamic input and inputs from the opposite hemisphere. It contains pyramidal and stellate cells. Some cortical areas lack a layer IV and are called *agranular.*

- **Layer 5** is called the internal pyramidal layer. Large pyramidal cells there project to subcortical structures, such as the basal ganglia, brainstem, and spinal cord.

- **Layer 6** is referred to as the polymorphic or multiform layer. Much of its large pyramidal cell output goes to the thalamus to mediate feedback and gating of input coming to the cortex. This layer also has small, spindle-like pyramidal and multiform cells.

Forming neurons: Dendrites and axons

After the neocortical six-layered structure is set, axonal wiring takes place. Axons from the thalamus reach the cortex, and cortical neurons project to subcortical areas, including the thalamus, and to other areas of neocortex. These axonal projections form the white matter, guided by chemical affinities and cell surface markers on glial cells (refer to Chapter 14).

The term *genetic blueprint* gives the impression that the genetic code has a structural "plan" for the organism. But what it really specifies is a set of cellular responses that comprise "rules" or procedures that cells follow when responding to their environments by manufacturing proteins. During development, the relevant responses include manufacturing cell surface markers and knowing when (and whether) to move or differentiate when they come into contact with other cells' surface markers.

The last part of development involves elaborating neurons' dendritic trees and axonal projections. This process is controlled by a number of mechanisms. One is competition between projecting neurons for target synapses. This process depends on activity in the neurons both during and after embryonic development.

As neurons differentiate, they tend to produce particular types of dendritic trees. These trees bear specific cell surface markers that attract the terminal boutons of axons of other, specific cells. In invertebrates, this wiring process is almost completely specified, with several thousand identically laid neurons with almost the same synapses from animal to animal. In vertebrates, however, and mammals, in particular, things are much more complicated, as I discuss next.

Cortical maps

Sensory projections to the neocortex often are organized as maps, which typically reflect how primary sensory areas — such as the retina for seeing, skin for sensing touch, or cochlea for hearing — are organized. These maps facilitate neural computation. (Refer to Chapters 10 and 11 for more about how the brain processes sensory information.)

Competing for cortical space

Within any given sense, and between senses, there is competition for cortical area. Experiments have shown that if some area of a cortical map is deprived of its input, other, usually adjacent, inputs will begin to activate it. Important research today is asking the question of whether this new activation comes from inputs that were always there, but silent, or whether new inputs grow into a denervated area. The answer depends on whether the deprivation occurs during development before critical periods, or afterward.

Critical periods: Failure to interact with the environment

The normal primary visual cortex contains a map in which retinal ganglion cells project to adjacent cortical cells. Similarly, the somatosensory system has an orderly, although distorted, map of the skin on the neocortex. Early in development, projections are produced from different sensory nuclei in the thalamus to the appropriate part of the neocortex.

This genetically specified map is later refined by other, activity-dependent mechanisms. Many of these mechanisms have what are called *critical periods*. During critical periods, neuroplasticity is enabled so neural activity can change or maintain connectivity. After critical periods, the same input may have little or no effect on connectivity.

Neuroplasticity modifies the nervous system during development at many levels in many ways, from changes in cellular responses due to learning, to large-scale cortical remapping from injury.

Correlating firing and wiring

The nervous system grows by altering the strength of connections between neurons, and pruning neurons that don't end up with significant connections. We don't know exactly how the brain determines what is "significant" in the connectivity of individual neurons. It may be the total number of connections compared to neighbors.

In humans, after infancy, most neural changes involve changes in synapses rather than numbers of neurons, although myelination of axon tracts also has a significant developmental timescale that extends through adolescence.

The critical period in vision

David Hubel and Torsten Wiesel, from the Harvard University School of Medicine, studied the idea of neuroplasticity during critical periods. Their work showed that depriving the cortex of visual input from one eye through a critical period caused a permanent loss of that eye's ability to drive cortical cells in area V1. Afterward, no amount of visual input from that eye restored these connections, so that even though the eye was functioning normally, the animal could not use it for sight.

Hebb's law

An important aspect of synaptic plasticity is called *Hebb's law.* In the developing nervous system, cells are competing for synaptic space. In the retina, for example, bipolar and amacrine cells compete for synaptic input to ganglion cell dendritic trees, while at the same time ganglion cell axons are competing for synaptic space on the dendrites of relay cells in the thalamus. Higher-order cells need a way to keep synapses driven by the "winners" and to discard those of the "losers."

In 1949, Donald O. Hebb, a Canadian psychologist, postulated a principle by which synapses could be modified according to activity that was local to the synapse and not dependent on any information or process not directly associated with the synapse itself. In Hebb's words, "When an axon of cell A is near enough to excite cell B and repeatedly or persistently takes part in firing it, some growth process or metabolic change takes place in one or both cells such that A's efficiency, as one of the cells firing B, is increased." Typically, when both pre- and post-synaptic sides of the synapse were frequently activated together, each side could release a complementary metabolic substance that together would strengthen the synapse.

Hebb's law, as it became known, hypothesized that synaptic modification occurs according to correlated activity in the pre- and post-synaptic elements of synapses. In the case of cortical maps, consider two ganglion cells that are adjacent to each other in the retina with receptive fields that overlap to some degree. Objects projected onto this area of the retina will tend to affect both nearby ganglion cells and produce similar light distributions in their receptive fields, so that the firing of adjacent retinal ganglion cells tends to be correlated.

When the axons of these ganglion cells reach the thalamus, they initially branch extensively and try to innervate many targets. But over time, because the axons of adjacent ganglion cells tend to be correlated with each other and with target cells they both innervate, their synaptic weights onto those target cells are increased. Meanwhile, the weights of distant uncorrelated ganglion cells do not get weight increases when they innervate the same target.

As long as the initial projection from the retina to the thalamus is approximately ordered by chemical gradients (refer to: Partitioning the body: Endoderm, mesoderm, ectoderm," earlier in this chapter), Hebb's law guarantees that the final wiring will form a good map. During development of the visual system — before the retina even has photoreceptors — waves of organized self-induced spontaneous firing move across the retina constantly to produce a position-dependent internally generated correlated firing. This process repeats itself at every level of the nervous system, through many stages of neocortical processing.

Birth defects through teratogens

During embryonic development, activity-dependent modification of synapses help to prune synapses. As part of this process, neurons are first overproduced; then, later, the Hebbian "losers" die off.

One unique aspect of human development is that the production of neurons in humans continues for months after birth. Then, after about a year, plasticity effects are mostly limited to changing synaptic weights in an anatomically established system. However, in some places, notably the hippocampus, generation of new neurons occurs in adults.

Environmental insults can have large effects on development of the human brain. The embryo is particularly susceptible to foreign chemicals because its cells are responding to chemical gradients and cell surface markers. Environmental substances that have little effect on adults can have profound effects on embryonic development. The general term for a substance that causes birth defects is *teratogen*. The following are all teratogens:

- ✔ Environmental toxins, such as lead from paint and organic mercury, that cause mental retardation

- ✔ Ionizing radiation, such as from atomic test fallout and X-rays

- ✔ Infections, such as rubella, herpes virus, cytomegalovirus (CMV), and syphilis

- ✔ Prescription drugs such as the tranquilizer thalidomide (which produced gross limb deformities in fetuses) and methotrexate (an anticancer drug)

- ✔ Overexposure to non-prescription substances not regarded as toxic, like alcohol (fetal alcohol syndrome) and caffeine

- ✔ Metabolic imbalances and deficiencies, such as diabetes and folic acid deficiency

Developmental Neural Disorders

The developing nervous system is building itself by chemical gradients and affinities, and it's fragile. Changes in just one amino acid in some proteins can wreak havoc on the developing system.

Each human genome is like an experiment because it is a new, unique combination of genes derived from two parents. The first stage of this experiment is whether this new genome can successfully control the development of a viable fetus. Some proteins produced by crossover or mutation will not function properly, often with disastrous effects. One important way of studying the developing nervous system is looking at the effects of known or deliberate mutations in animals, particularly mice.

Tracing genetic development using mice

The mouse genome was sequenced in about 2002. These small, rapidly multiplying animals grow to adulthood in a few months, making them a model for genetic studies in mammals. Mice share many genes in common with humans, and because they breed and mature quickly, the effect of *DNA mutations* (a change in the genotype) can be tested rapidly on large numbers of animals.

In mice, some mutations spontaneously occur that may mimic a similar mutation in humans. Researchers can also deliberately induce specific mutations by inserting a new DNA segment in the mouse embryo, or silencing an intrinsic gene. The technique called *knockout* involves removing or suppressing a particular gene or gene sequence. If a mutation in a particular protein is suspected to underlie a human genetic effect, researchers can selectively make specific amino acid substitutions at particular positions in the protein in different lines of mice to reveal which amino acid substitutions are likely to have caused the human genetic defect.

A well-known case of a spontaneous mutation was the reeler mouse (so-called because of its tendency to spin around unevenly while moving), reported in the early 1950s. This mouse had an abnormally small cerebellum and disrupted neocortical organization due to a defect in reelin, an extracellular matrix protein used to guide cell migration.

In knockout, mice genes are turned off by changing their premotor regions so they aren't transcribed. This mimics a mutation that either silences transcription or alters the genetic sequence to produce an ineffective protein in humans. Knockouts have been generated to study human disorders such as diabetes, cancer, heart disease, arthritis, aging, obesity, Parkinson's disease, and even substance abuse.

Known single mutation disorders

Well-known single mutation genetic disorders are sickle cell anemia, cystic fibrosis, Tay–Sachs disease, and hemophilia, for example. All these disorders are *autosomal recessive,* meaning that the inheritor must receive a defective gene from both parents to have the disorder. In *autosomal dominant* genetic disorders, such as Huntington's disease, a single dominant gene inherited from either parent produces the disorder.

Multi-locus mutation disorders

In many genetic disorders, no single gene has been identified or multiple mutations occur to produce the disorder. Some genetic disorders have multiple genetic causes with different levels of severity and susceptibility to environmental effects.

Autism and schizophrenia show high inheritance and tend to run in families. However, both of these disorders do not show 100 percent *concordance* (expression of the dysfunction in both individuals) even in identical twins with the same genome. This means that the genetic constellations that under-lie these disorders must create (in some cases, very high) susceptibilities to the disorder, but there still must be an environmental factor, such as slight differences in diet or social factors. Also, both of these disorders appear with widely varying severity and susceptibility to environmental influences, suggesting that they have multiple genetic causes.

These variations suggest that positive feedback mechanisms may be at work, allowing some people to break or never enter the disease spiral, while others do. Different people clearly handle the genetic "deck" they are dealt differ-ently and end up with very different outcomes. This is a major mystery for 21st-century neurobiology to explore.

Birth defects

Two well-known birth defects of the brain are spina bifida and hydrocephalus.

Spina bifida

One of the most common birth defects worldwide is spina bifida (myelomenin-gocele), with an incidence of about 1 in every 1,000 births. This developmental disorder is characterized by the incomplete closing of the embryonic neural tube (refer to "Descending from the ectoderm into the nervous system," earlier in this chapter) because some vertebrae overlying the spinal cord do not fuse and remain open. The most common location of spina bifida is in the lumbar and sacral areas.

Although spina bifida can be alleviated surgically, but the surgery does not usually restore normal function. The incidence of spina bifida can be decreased by up to 70 percent when the mother takes daily folic acid supplements prior to conception.

Hydrocephalus

Hydrocephalus, often colloquially referred to as "water on the brain," is caused by an abnormal accumulation of cerebrospinal fluid in the brain's ventricles. This leads to high intracranial pressure, which causes the head to get progressively larger. Hydrocephalus is caused by congenital malformations that block normal drainage of the fluid from the ventricles, or from an overproduction of cerebrospinal fluid. It can also result from complications of head injuries or brain infections.

Hydrocephalus is associated with mental disability, convulsions, and in severe cases, death, usually from brainstem compression. Symptoms in less severe cases include nausea, vomiting, and sleepiness.

Aging effects over the lifespan

The process of *axon myelination,* in which axons are wrapped with myelin sheaths to make action potential conduction faster and more reliable, continues until nearly the end of adolescence. The last parts of the brain to be fully myelinated are the frontal lobes, the areas of the brain most needed for abstract thought and judgment.

The aging process

During normal adulthood, cell numbers and structure are generally stable. Learning primarily modifies synaptic strengths, although neurons in areas such as the olfactory lobe and hippocampus continue to be replaced. The number of neurons starts to decline at middle age, due to additional neural pruning, the accumulation of toxins and metabolic errors, and possibly genetic factors that program cell life.

Aging is a complex process. It involves mechanisms that range from the sub-cellular level to the whole organism. The telomeres at the end of chromosomes inside the nucleus of cells appear to be capable of only a finite number of divisions. Each time a cell divides, the telomeres shorten until they become too short for the cell to divide any more. The cell then may become inactive or die. Joints wear out and blood vessels harden or get clogged with deposits at the whole organism level. Tissues and organs of the body can malfunction, which can adversely affect other parts of the body.

Theories of aging

Some theories of aging say that death is the result of the accumulation of random degeneration in multiple tissues. Other theories point to specific phenomena, such as telomere shortening, that suggest that cell life and, therefore, aging are actually programmed. In any case, most athletic and raw cognitive ability functions peak in the mid- to late 20s. Cognitive capabilities, such as those associated with wisdom, continue to increase beyond this age, however.

Aging and brain dysfunctions

Aging is a major risk factor for neurodegenerative diseases, such as Alzheimer's disease, Parkinson's disease, and vascular disease that affects the brain. Both genetic factors and environmental triggers appear to be involved in these disorders.

Alzheimer's disease

Alzheimer's disease, which used to be called "senile dementia," was once thought to be a more or less inevitable consequence of aging. Now we know that it's a specific disease associated with the accumulation of tau proteins and neurofibrillary tangles. The probability of having this disorder increases greatly with aging, but it is not inevitable. Very few young people have Alzheimer's, and some very old people do not have Alzheimer's.

The neurons that die in the initial stages of Alzheimer's disease are mostly those that use acetylcholine as a neurotransmitter, particularly in the hippocampus. After that, other neurons die as well. Alzheimer's typically progresses with the loss of episodic memory ("I can't remember where I put my keys"), followed by loss of semantic memory ("I don't know where I am, and I don't recognize anything"). Later, the person has almost complete loss of cognitive function. Death occurs from massive neuronal loss that eventually gets in the way of bodily maintenance functions.

Parkinson's disease

Parkinson's disease is associated with the death of dopaminergic cells in the substantia nigra (a basal ganglia nucleus). The death of these cells interferes with a person's ability to make voluntary movements or voluntary corrections as he walks, such as stepping over an obstacle. Complex evidence suggests that this disease is due to a genetic deficiency plus an environmental trigger. (I discuss Parkinson's disease in more detail in Chapter 16.)

Autoimmune disorders

Several neuronal degeneration disorders that are more common during aging are believed to be *autoimmune disorders*. These disorders arise when antibodies are made that attack body tissues rather than foreign invaders.

Autoimmune disorders may result from viral infections in which some part of the viral protein coat is similar to (or evolved to mimic) a tissue in the body, which develops antibodies to it and, therefore, to itself.

Multiple sclerosis (MS) is one of the most common nervous system autoimmune diseases. In MS, the myelin sheaths that wrap the axons of the brain and spinal cord are attacked. This leads to reduced conduction speed and reliability and eventually to failure to conduct action potentials along these axons. The first sign of the disease is often muscular weakness. This may proceed to total paralysis and cognitive disability, although the course of the disease is highly variable. MS usually appears first in early adulthood, and it's more common in women than in men.

Vascular disease and stroke

Aging increases the risk of vascular disease and stroke. A *stroke* is an interruption of the normal blood supply to the brain. Strokes can be *ischemic,* in which vessel blockages produce loss of nutrient and waste transport, or *hemorrhagic,* in which blood vessels leak blood into the brain. Strokes are associated with a temporary disruption of brain function in the affected region due to neuronal injury. Recovery can happen through plasticity and relearning, often aided by specific rehabilitation.

Mini or "silent" strokes may go unnoticed because they produce few noticeable symptoms. Sometimes people will experience a series of small strokes over several years that slowly compromise brain function, followed by a much larger stroke.

Tumors

Tumors *(neoplasms)* can occur in the brain, with initial symptoms ranging from nausea to muscular weakness to vision problems. A relatively common brain tumor type with a poor prognosis is a *glioma,* a tumor derived from glial cells in the brain. Gliomas are rarely curable, in part because the strong blood–brain barrier isolates the brain from the immune system so that a few cancerous cells can initiate tumors and spread to multiple brain areas.

Secondary tumors of the brain are tumors that have invaded the brain from cancers that originated in other organs through the lymphatic system and blood vessels. These secondary brain tumors occur often in the terminal phases of patients with incurable cancer that originated elsewhere in the body, which is the most common cause of brain tumors.

Chapter 16

Movement Disorders

. . . .

. . . .

*N*eurological illnesses are among the most costly health problems in the United States, and movement disorders are an important consequence of many neurological disorders. With other diseases, such as Parkinson's disease and Huntington's disease, the main symptoms are movement problems. Movement disorders can stem from a variety of genetic causes, be a consequence of an infectious disease, or be brought on by environmental factors that involve damage to muscles, motor neurons, the spinal cord, or the central nervous system. These disorders account for a significant percentage of all disability.

In this chapter, I discuss the causes (when known) and symptoms of various movement disorders and how they affect the brain and body.

When the Wheels Come Off: Motor Disorders

Motor disorders are physical disabilities in which sufferers have either some significant limit in the physical function of one or more limbs or a disability in learning or making skilled movements. Motor disabilities can manifest in the lower limbs as mobility impairment, in the upper limbs as poor manual dexterity, or as a general loss of coordination or strength.

Conditions that lead to poor respiratory function can limit endurance and thereby compromise motor activity. Epilepsy causes intermittent loss of movement control. Motor disabilities may also be associated with impairment of motor functions of the autonomic nervous system or damage to the heart, respiratory system, or digestive system.

Major early developmental disorders

Prenatal disabilities can occur from genetic disorders, infectious disease, or fetal developmental accidents. Premature birth and problems during the birth process can produce motor disorders from nervous system damage due to trauma or oxygen deprivation. Accidents and infections can occur before, during, and after birth that produce motor disabilities early in life.

Motor and other dysfunctions that exist at birth or manifest shortly after are called *congenital disorders.* Congenital disorders may result from genetic abnormalities, infectious disease, injuries, or exposure to substances that cause birth defects (*teratogens;* see Chapter 15). A well-known example of teratogens is the tranquilizer thalidomide, which appeared to be beneficial and harmless to adults, but ended up causing severe limb malformations in the developing fetuses of mothers who took the drug.

About 5 percent of young children have poor motor coordination that interferes with their performance in school and social interactions.

Cerebral palsy is one of the most commonly occurring neurological motor impairments (about 2 per 1,000 children). The term *cerebral palsy* (which means paralysis or tremors from brain damage) refers to the symptoms of the disease because it may be caused by numerous factors, many of which are not well understood. It's usually associated with a brain lesion that occurs before the brain is fully developed. Different types of brain injury cause many different manifestations of cerebral palsy.

Injuries and diseases

Infectious diseases and prenatal, birth, and early childhood injuries cause many motor disorders:

- ✔ **TORCH complex:** Infections that cause congenital abnormalities that can include motor deficits are referred to as the *TORCH complex:*

    • **Toxoplasmosis.**

- **Other infections:** This group includes coxsackie virus, syphilis, varicella-zoster virus (commonly known as chicken pox), HIV, and parvovirus B19. These agents are capable of crossing the placenta when the mother is infected.

- **Rubella.**

- **Cytomegalovirus (CMV):** It is now clear that maternal CMV infections can lead to complications such as low birth weight, microcephaly, and seizures. This results in varying degrees of mental disability, hearing, and coordination problems.

- **Herpes simplex virus.**

✔ **Acquired brain injuries:** Injuries that occur after the neonatal period but during childhood are referred to as *acquired brain injuries.* This includes traumatic injuries such as blows to the head, weapon injuries, and injuries from shaking, as well as non-traumatic injuries such as tumors and infections.

Developmental brain plasticity (refer to Chapter 15) may partially alleviate symptoms from these injuries over time, but some motor deficits, such as poor coordination, may never fully recover.

Lifespan motor disorders

Although injuries and infections can compromise motor function at any age, certain risks for dysfunction increase with age. This list includes cumulative exposure to environmental toxins, decline in vascular function, nervous system tumors, and some genetic diseases with effects that manifest late in life. (I discuss these diseases more fully in Chapter 15.)

Some genetic diseases manifest in adulthood without any known environmental trigger, such as Huntington's disease. Other genetic diseases may produce a susceptibility to develop motor dysfunctions that will manifest depending on unknown environmental factors.

The most well-known lifespan neurological disorder is Alzheimer's disease (refer to Chapter 15). Although its earliest symptoms are not motor problems, later symptoms include loss of motor control and even compromise of the autonomic nervous system.

Failing Forces: Muscle Diseases

Neuromuscular diseases can impair muscle functioning because of pathologies in the muscle, motor neurons, or neuromuscular junction. These diseases usually manifest initially as weakness, and then proceed to *paresis* (partial paralysis) and full paralysis. Many of these disease are typically not associated with cognitive dysfunction until end-stage phases, when the autonomic nervous system is compromised and organs are affected.

Diseases that affect the muscle directly are called primary *myopathic* (muscular) disorders. The myopathies called dystrophies are characterized by progressive muscle degeneration due to the muscle's inability to regenerate as part of the normal process of use-damage and repair. Severe dystrophies begin with weakness, progress to paralysis, and eventually end in death from respiratory failure. These diseases can be congenital, usually from genetic abnormalities, or inflammatory, from infections or from the immune system attacking the muscle. Well-known examples include muscular dystrophies and infection-related myopathies such as polymyositis.

Muscular dystrophy

Muscular dystrophy (MD) is characterized by progressive skeletal muscle weakness and the death of muscle tissue. The most severe and common form of MD, Duchenne muscular dystrophy, is named after the French neurologist Guillaume Duchenne.

Duchenne MD occurs in about 1 in 3,600 boys. It is due to a recessive gene on the X-linked chromosome. Because girls have two X chromosomes and the gene is recessive, they don't suffer from the disease with a single Duchenne MD gene, whereas a boy would have no overriding dominant gene on his Y chromosome. The Duchenne mutation is in the dystrophin gene that codes for the protein dystrophin, a structural component of muscle tissue.

Duchenne MD symptoms usually appear (in males) by age 6. These symptoms include progressive weakness of the legs that later includes the arms and neck. In the course of the disease, muscle tissue degenerates and is replaced by fibrotic tissue and fat. Most sufferers are wheelchair dependent by age 12. The average life expectancy for these patients is about 25.

There are other types of muscular dystrophy such as Becker MD, myotonic MD, and Emery-Dreifuss MD. All types of MD predominantly affect males, but females typically carry the disease gene. MD also is associated with disorders in the autonomic system such as the heart, gastrointestinal system, and endocrine glands.

Inflammatory myopathies

Chronic inflammation of the muscles can occur due to infection, resulting in polymyositis. This produces an inflammatory myopathy associated with weakness in the musculature of the shoulder and hips due to loss of muscle mass. Polymyositic can also be associated with a characteristic smooth or scaly skin rash. This can lead to an autoimmune connective tissue disorder. Polymyositis is often treated with steroids and other anti-inflammatories.

Inflammation of the muscles is generally called a *myositis.* Most myositis is caused by an autoimmune reaction. Autoimmune reactions are thought to occur in many cases where part of the protein of an infectious agent (virus or bacteria), is similar to proteins in the body (for example, in the muscle), such that mounting an immune reaction to the invader causes an autoimmune attack on the body's own protein. The invading microorganisms have presumably evolved proteins like their hosts to evade initial immune detection.

Neuromuscular Junction Disorders

Neuromuscular junction disorders are disorders that affect transmissions from motor neurons to the acetylcholine receptors on the muscle end plate, which is responsible for contracting the muscle on neural command (refer to Chapters 3, 4, and 5). Myasthenia gravis and Lambert–Eaton syndrome are examples of neuromuscular junction disorders.

Myasthenia gravis

Myasthenia gravis (MG) is an autoimmune disorder having an incidence of up to 30 new cases per million people per year. It's caused by the production of antibodies that block acetylcholine receptors at the neuromuscular junction motor end plate.

MG's initial symptoms include muscles that are weak and easily fatigued — the hallmarks of the disease. During activity, muscles weaken excessively compared to normal fatigue, but they improve again after rest. Typical initial symptoms are usually associated with muscles in the head that control eye and eyelid movement, facial expressions, chewing, swallowing, and speech generation. Respiratory muscles and those that control limb and neck movements can also be affected.

MG can have a sudden onset, and afterward symptoms can appear intermittently. A common initial symptom is *ptosis* (a drooping of the eyelids). In what's called a *myasthenic crisis,* the respiratory muscles can be paralyzed, which is life threatening and may require assisted ventilation. These crises may be triggered in MG sufferers by infection, fever, adverse reactions to medication, or emotional stress.

Although MG is an autoimmune disease, the pathogen that causes it is not known. A genetic predisposition exists for getting the disease for particular HLA types. (HLA is human leukocyte antigen, a component of the major histocompatibility complex, which is the unique set of cell surface markers expressed in each individual person.) It's also associated with abnormalities of the thymus or thymus tumors, and is sometimes stabilized by removal of the thymus, which is involved in the production of the autoimmune antibodies.

MG symptoms can be alleviated with acetylcholinesterase inhibitors that prolong the lifetime of acetylcholine in the synaptic cleft to make up for reduced receptor numbers or function. This treats only the symptoms and does not deal with the immunological cause of the disease.

Immunosuppressants are sometimes used to reduce the immune response. A positive response to immunosuppressants distinguishes MG from other myasthenic syndromes that do not respond to immunosuppressive treatments. In some MG cases, removal of the thymus gland alleviates symptoms by reducing the immune response.

Lambert–Eaton syndrome

Another notable neuromuscular junction disorder is *Lambert–Eaton myasthenic syndrome.* This autoimmune disease occurs when antibodies are made to the voltage-dependent calcium channel necessary for presynaptic neurotransmitter release (refer to Chapter 4), as well as muscle cell contraction (refer to Chapter 5). In Lambert–Eaton myasthenic syndrome, the primary problem is decreased release of acetylcholine at the motor neuron presynaptic terminal.

Toxins

A number of naturally occurring toxins produced by microorganisms, snakes, and spiders affect the neuromuscular junction. Botulinum toxin prevents the release of acetylcholine from the presynaptic motor terminal, resulting in muscle paralysis. Toxins in cobra snake venom bind to the acetylcholine receptor, blocking its activation by acetylcholine from the motor neuron. Black widow spider venom contains the neurotoxin latrotoxin that depletes acetylcholine from the presynaptic terminal also producing paralysis. The toxin does this by artificially stimulating the fusion of acetylcholine synaptic vesicles with the presynaptic membrane producing massive release, followed by depletion.

Motor Neuron Damage

Damage to motor neurons occurs in injuries, strokes, and diseases that lead to either spasticity or paralysis. Damage can occur in lower alpha motor neurons or in upper motor neurons originating in the frontal lobe (refer to Chapters 5, 6, and 8). Damage to sensory neurons in the skin, muscles, and tendons can produce paralysis by eliminating feedback to the spinal cord and brain about limb position and force.

Amyotrophic lateral sclerosis

Amyotrophic lateral sclerosis (ALS; also known as Lou Gehrig's disease) is a debilitating motor neuron disease characterized by the death of motor neurons in the brain, brainstem, and spinal cord. It produces progressive weakness via muscle atrophy. Symptoms include limb weakness and muscle spasticity, as well as difficulty swallowing, speaking, and breathing. The near end stage of the disease is characterized by loss of all voluntary movement except for eye movement. At the terminal stage, eye movement and control over the bladder and bowel are lost, and cognitive decline such as dementia may occur.

Susceptibility to ALS has a clear genetic component. In about one-quarter of ALS cases, chromosome 21 has an autosomal-dominant defect where it codes for superoxide dismutase enzymes that catalyze the breakdown of the super-oxide radical ($O2-$) into oxygen and hydrogen peroxide. These enzymes are important in the antioxidant defense of cells exposed to oxygen.

ALS is the most common of the five motor neuron diseases that affect upper motor neurons (in the frontal lobe or cranial nerves) and/or lower motor neurons (such as alpha motor neurons of the spinal cord that synapse on muscles): ALS, primary lateral sclerosis, progressive muscular atrophy, progressive bulbar palsy, and pseudobulbar palsy.

Multiple sclerosis

Multiple sclerosis (MS) is not strictly a motor neuron disease. Instead, MS is a disease of the myelin sheaths around axons of the brain and spinal cord that does not primarily affect motor neurons until late in its course.

Myelin wrappings by glial cells — called *oligodendrocytes* — in the central nervous system, and Schwann cells in the peripheral nervous system, permit rapid and reliable conduction of action potentials along axons. In MS, these glial axon wrappings are damaged by inflammation. This disease starts with unreliable and slow neural conduction, and can lead to complete conduction loss in some axon tracts.

MS is an autoimmune disease whose underlying trigger for the production of autoantibodies is unknown. Risk factors include genetics, infections, and some environmental factors. The disease occurs more frequently in women than in men, and its onset is typically in early adulthood. It occurs in about 1 in 1,000 people. For unknown reasons, MS is more common in non-equatorial latitudes than near the equator. Following onset, symptoms can occur either intermittently in attacks that mitigate somewhat afterward, or in a progressive form. Although early symptoms are primarily loss of muscle strength in the limbs, the disease can progress to include cognitive and psychiatric difficulties. MS has no known cure.

Viral infections

Not only can viruses attack the nervous system, but, in many cases, the nervous system is the way they enter the body.

Polio

Polio (poliomyelitis) is an infectious viral disease that characteristically attacks the nervous system. When the virus enters the central nervous system, it preferentially destroys motor neurons, causing muscle weakness and paralysis. Rehabilitation may be able to alleviate some of the paralysis by inducing the reduced number of remaining motor neurons to sprout more axon terminals to innervate more muscle cells for enhanced contraction force. A downside of this, however, is that the random death of motor neurons that occurs during aging is particularly disabling for polio survivors because each motor neuron that dies is doing a large part of the muscle contraction work.

Rabies

Rabies is another viral infection that affects the nervous system, typically leading to massive brain damage and death within days of entering the central nervous system. After an infected animal bites a person (or another animal), the rabies virus gets to the brain through the axons of peripheral nerves by binding to the acetylcholine receptor.

Hijacking pinocytosis

In neurotransmission, vesicles filled with the neurotransmitter fuse with the cell membrane to dump their contents into the synaptic cleft. If the procedures were to keep going forever, the result would be an unsustainable increase in the cell membrane. Recycling counteracts this, when the axon terminals of motor neurons pinch off a bit of membrane and recycle it to make more synaptic vesicles, a process called *pinocytosis.*

During pinocytosis, as the cell membrane folds back in on itself and pinches off to release the vesicle (called an *endosome*) inside the cell, whatever is in the interior of the vesicle as it forms gets taken up by the cell. This makes axon terminals such as those of motor neurons vulnerable to viruses, which they take up in the recycling process. Polio and rabies viruses enter motor neuron axons terminals during this process and then travel to the central nervous system. Rabies viruses massively attack other neurons, and the disease is typically fatal unless the infected person (or animal) receives a vaccine that can stimulate the production of antibodies.

Basal Ganglia and Other Diseases

Sources of upper motor neuron dysfunction include strokes, Parkinson's Huntington's, and Creutzfeldt–Jakob diseases. These dysfunctions may affect primary motor neurons in cortical area M1 that project to lower motor neurons that are connected to muscles. Effects may also occur in other frontal areas, such as the supplementary and premotor cortices, and in the basal ganglia.

Parkinson's disease

Parkinson's disease is named after the English physician James Parkinson who published a description of it in 1817. Its cause is unknown, although it can be produced experimentally by ingestion of the synthetic opioid MPTP.

Early symptoms include rigidity, tremor (shaking), slow movement, and difficulty with initiating movement or stepping over obstacles. In late stages of the disease, cognitive compromise and dementia may occur. The onset of Parkinson's disease typically occurs after age 50. The disease has no known cause, though it involves genetic factors.

Although Parkinson' disease isn't usually associated with marked cognitive impairment in early stages, it can cause mood problems including depression, apathy, anxiety, and poor impulse control. These can lead to medication overuse, binge eating, hypersexuality, and excessive gambling. Some of these symptoms may be related to treatments that attempt to increase dopamine levels rather than primarily from the disease itself.

At the cellular level, Parkinson's is characterized by inclusions called Lewy bodies in dopaminergic neurons in the substantia nigra. These contain a protein called alpha-synuclein whose normal function is not currently well understood, but is believed to be involved in the regulation of membrane stability. Mutations in the genes that code for synucleins are known to cause some forms of the disease. Lewy bodies are aggregates (aggresome) of alpha-synuclein and other proteins such as ubiquitin and sometimes Tau proteins.

Dopamine released by neurons in the substantia nigra amplifies activity in the basal ganglia direct pathway from the striatum that disinhibits the thalamic projection to the motor cortex (refer to Chapter 8). This increases activation of the motor pathway that will be executed. This dopamine release also reduces the effect of inhibition through an indirect pathway. The reduction of dopamine release in Parkinson's disease reduces the ability to initiate movement via both direct and indirect pathways via a reduction of the drive to the motor thalamus that gates the cortical excitatory projections to the corticospinal tract and brainstem.

Parkinson's has some known risk and protective factors. Some insecticides (such as rotenone) are associated with an increased risk of Parkinson's, while cigarette smoking is associated with a reduced risk for unknown reasons. Early attempts to treat Parkinson symptoms with injections of dopamine were ineffective because it does not cross the blood–brain barrier. However, a metabolic precursor in dopamine synthesis, L-dopa, does cross this barrier and can relieve symptoms for some period of time. However, as the disease progresses, dopaminergic neurons are depleted so that supplying dopamine precursors is no longer effective. Additionally, artificially increasing dopamine levels produces a complication called *dyskinesia,* in which involuntary writhing movements, similar to those in Huntington's disease, occur. The treatment can also produce hallucinations and delusions.

Huntington's disease

Huntington's disease is a neurodegenerative genetic disorder that initially affects neurons in the striatum, producing an effect that is in some ways the opposite of Parkinson's disease. The major symptom is involuntary writhing movements called *chorea*. It may also produce subtle cognitive or mood problems. Later symptoms include compromise of muscle coordination, cognitive impairment, and psychiatric problems, including dementia and memory loss similar to Alzheimer's disease. Commonly noted diagnostic symptoms beyond the writhing include physical instability, abnormal facial expression, and difficulties chewing, swallowing, and speaking.

Huntington's disease is caused by an autosomal dominant mutation (if either gene is mutated, the disease will appear) in the gene called Huntingtin. The function of the normal Huntingtin protein is not well understood, but it interacts with over 100 other proteins. The onset of Huntington's is typically in middle age. Its incidence is higher among people of Western European ancestry than in those of Asian or African descent. It strikes men and women about equally.

We can now determine if a person has the mutation that will develop into Huntington's disease in childhood, before the onset of symptoms. Ethical debates about using the test and its results in minors and insurance screening issues do exist. This disease has no cure, though its symptoms can be partly relieved through pharmacological treatment.

Neuropathies: Losing peripheral sensation

Peripheral neuropathy is a dysfunction of the peripheral nerves, either motor neurons that innervate the muscles from the spinal cord or brainstem, or sensory neurons that convey touch, temperature, pain, and position information to the spinal cord or brain. Neuropathies may also involve the autonomic nervous innervations of internal organs and blood vessels. Peripheral neuropathies may be caused either by systemic illness or trauma to the nerve.

Symptoms of neuropathy depend on which motor or sensory nerves are affected. Motor neuropathies can produce muscle weakness, spasms, and loss of balance or coordination. Sensory neuropathy can manifest as insensitivity to pain, numbness, tingling, or burning sensations. Autonomic neuropathy is associated with involuntary function problems such as high or low heart rate and blood pressure, bladder dysfunction such as incontinence, and sexual dysfunction.

Peripheral neuropathies are often classified in the following two ways:

- **Mononeuropathy (only one nerve involved):** Common mononeuropathies resulting from nerve compression include carpal tunnel syndrome. Mononeuritis multiplex involves several noncontiguous nerves, often as a result of diabetes mellitus.

- **Polyneuropathy (many nerves involved):** This term is often synonymous with peripheral neuropathy. Its most frequent cause is diabetic neuropathy. Other causes include Lyme disease, toxins, vitamin deficiencies, and side effects of some prescribed drugs.

Another term for peripheral nerve dysfunction is *neuritis,* a general term for nerve inflammation. Neuritis can develop from physical injury or overuse, or from infections such as herpes simplex virus, shingles (from chickenpox virus), and Lyme disease. Chemical injuries and radiation can also cause neuritis.

A well-known paralysis can result from pure sensory peripheral neuropathy. *Afferent sensory nerves* (sensory nerves projecting toward the brain) convey information about limb position to the spine and the brain (refer to Chapter 6). Diseases such as diabetes can cause peripheral neuropathies in which the sensory nerves do not function. In these cases, as in strokes that affect the somatosensory areas of the neocortex, patients refuse to use the deafferented limbs, even though the neural motor command structure may be totally intact. Therapies such as constraint-induced therapy are often successful in allowing patients to regain function of sensory deafferented limbs — essentially forcing them to do so by restraining the non-affected limb.

Strokes and Injuries

Strokes are vascular incidents that have neurological effects via a cascade of events that leads to nerve death. Accidents, such as head trauma, can have similar effects.

Suffering a stroke

A *stroke* (also called a *cerebrovascular accident*) involves the loss of brain function from a disturbance in the brain's blood supply. Strokes are the second leading cause of death worldwide. Stroke can cause permanent neurological damage and death. High blood pressure, age, diabetes, and atrial fibrillation are risk factors for stroke.

The two major types of stroke are as follows:

- ✔ **Ischemic strokes:** Ischemic strokes are due to a lack of blood flow caused by blockage, such as *thrombosis* (a blood clot in a brain blood vessel), *embolism* (an embolus or clot arriving through the vasculature from elsewhere in the body), or *systemic hypoperfusion* (loss of adequate blood supply, such as during shock). Strokes deprive the brain tissue of adequate oxygen and glucose for metabolism and allow waste products normally removed by the vasculature to build up to toxic levels.

- ✔ **Hemorrhagic strokes:** Hemorrhagic strokes involve bleeding into the brain, which leads to ischemic effects and toxic alteration of the regulated concentrations of ions and other substances in the extracellular space. Hemorrhagic strokes are often associated with the loss of consciousness, headache, and vomiting due to the increased intracranial pressure from the leaking blood physically compressing brain tissue.

Stroke symptoms typically have a sudden onset and depend on the area of the brain affected. Strokes affecting the nervous system can affect any part of the brain or major nerve tracts such as the spinothalamic and corticospinal tracts. A major indicator of stroke is asymmetry in symptoms. A stroke on the left side of the brain will affect the right side of the body, and vice versa. Strokes on the left side of the brain often produce *aphasia* (speech difficulties) along with right-side paresis or paralysis. Visual field defects are typically associated with occipital lobe damage, while memory deficits occur with strokes that affect the temporal lobe. Parietal lobe lesions, particularly on the right side, produce left visual field *hemi-neglect* (failure to notice or attend to objects in the left visual field). Frontal lobe strokes impair cognitive functions and produce confusion and incoherent thinking.

Stroke without symptoms

In recent years, the phenomenon of "silent strokes" has been recognized via neuroimaging such as MRI. These strokes lack any outward symptoms, and patients are typically unaware they have suffered a stroke. However, these strokes still damage the brain. A sequence of silent strokes often eventually accumulates damage that crosses a threshold for neural dysfunction. They also tend to precede major strokes.

Injuring the brain

Brain injuries can produce similar kinds of damage to brain tissue from trauma as from strokes; they also produce similar symptoms. A brain injury from external forces is typically called a *traumatic brain injury* (TBI). The most common causes of adult TBI are violence, motorcycle and auto accidents, construction accidents, and sports. In children, falls, auto accidents, and abuse account for most cases. Worldwide, TBI is a major cause of disability.

Recent imaging techniques have enhanced the ability to detect brain injuries that were not evident by using early imaging modalities like X-rays such as *edema* (swelling) and diffuse axonal injury to cortical white matter.

Areas of the brain that are particularly susceptible to injury include the orbitofrontal cortex and the anterior temporal lobes. As would be predicted from damage to these areas, such lesions can compromise decision making, social behavior, and emotional regulation. Damage to motor control areas can produce *hemiparesis* (partial paralysis on one side), while damage to the left side of the brain specifically can produce aphasia.

Damage to the brain from physical force is also often accompanied by a *hematoma* (bleeding into the brain), with similar effects as from hemorrhagic strokes. A common symptom of brain injury is unequal pupil size. Moderate or severe TBIs may produce persistent headaches, vomiting, convulsions, slurred speech, and aphasia, among other symptoms.

It is now clear from sports studies that any brain injury that is associated with even momentary loss of consciousness carries a significant risk of brain damage. In normal, healthy children and young adults the brain may compensate well for such injuries, but their effects may accumulate past a threshold that exceeds the ability of the brain to compensate. Even heading the ball in soccer appears to be statistically associated with brain tissue loss without ever being accompanied by loss of consciousness.

Spinal cord injuries

Although tumors can originate in the spinal cord, injury is the cause of most spinal cord dysfunction. The effects of the injury depend on the "completeness" of the trauma and the level of the spinal cord at which it occurs. The most common causes of these injuries are motor vehicle accidents, falls, sports injuries, and violence. More than 80 percent of spinal cord injuries are in men.

At the cellular level, the main effects of such injuries are death of cells whose somas are within the spinal cord, and transection of sensory and motor axons. The death of neurons at the level of the injury primarily affects only the dermatome and *myotome* (the set of muscles innervated from a specific spinal segment) of that spinal segment. The transection of axon tracts at a segment, however, interrupts all sensory information passing up from below that segment, and all motor commands from above going down through that segment. These long axon tracts are also particularly susceptible to injury, and do not regenerate in the central nervous system. Severe spinal cord injuries are very disabling, and the higher they are, the more of the body is affected.

In a very severe spinal injury, termed *complete,* a person loses all sensory and motor function below the injured area. *Incomplete* injuries have less total effects in the same regions. In what is called *sacral sparing,* there remains some cutaneous sensation in sacral dermatomes for injuries above that level, even though sensation is lost in the thoracic and lumbar dermatomes at higher levels, but below the level of the lesion. Sacral sparing may be due to the fibers going to and from the sacral dermatomes and myotomes being less likely to be destroyed by injury compression for mechanical reasons such as protection via the lamination of sacral fibers within the spinal cord.

Severe injuries to the high cervical (neck) segments can produce quadriplegia and loss of respiratory control. Lower cervical injuries or incomplete high injuries may allow some respiratory control and limited hand and arm use. Cervical injuries are also associated with poor regulation of heart rate, blood pressure, and body temperature.

Complete thoracic spinal-level injuries typically result in paraplegia of the legs but hand, arm, neck, and breathing functions are retained. Lumbosacral injuries decrease control of the legs, urinary system, and anus. Sacral spinal segment injuries compromise sexual function.

A persistent mystery about spinal cord and other central nervous system injuries is the fact that the peripheral nervous system, but not the central nervous system, in mammals, regenerates axon pathways after transection. Also, cold-blooded vertebrates like fish can regenerate even central nervous system tracts like the optic nerve. One idea has to do with the fact that peripheral nervous system axons are wrapped by Schwann cells, whereas central axons are wrapped by oligodendrocytes.

Treatments for spinal cord injuries have involved transplanting Schwann cells and stem cells into the damaged spinal cord area. Other treatments involve immediate suppression of inflammation after the injury. Many of these treatment approaches offer hope for effective rehabilitation, if not immediately, perhaps within the next 10 to 20 years. There are also prosthetic approaches, which I discuss next.

Substituting machines: Motor prostheses

Damage to any motor control areas in the central nervous system from strokes or head injuries can produce paralysis, *paresis* (weakness), or *apraxia* (lack of motor skill or dexterity). Falls and other injuries can damage spinal pathways. Many cell biological approaches attempted to promote regrowth of transected sensory and motor axons in the spinal cord. Several recent approaches attempted to reduce scar tissue formation that may block regrowth by injecting anti-inflammatory agents into the damaged spinal area immediately after the injury.

Engineering-oriented, artificial approaches also exist. For example, implanting arrays of recording electrodes in primary motor cortex to "intercept" the commands to move the muscles, relaying these signals through wires past the spinal cord transection, and electronically driving the muscle itself by direct electrical stimulation or stimulating the alpha motor neurons (refer to Chapter 5).

One little-appreciated possible outcome of the artificial approaches is their potential effect on the nervous system. In many incomplete spinal injuries, intact sensory and motor fibers may remain, but just not enough to allow the person to move his or her limb. Artificial limb movement may keep these neural pathways from degenerating and generates plasticity that, like rehab, allows these remaining pathways to take over enough target neurons to permit movement without the artificial aid, eventually. In the absence of any movement, the entire neural system degenerates from lack of activity.

Chapter 17

Brain Dysfunction and Mental Illness

Mental illness is a disease of the mind that causes severe cognitive, emotional, or behavioral problems. Mental illnesses are probably the most costly and challenging health problems in the United States and worldwide.

But what causes mental illness? Mental disease is not caused by an infection (usually), nor is it always associated with a genetic abnormality (although it can be). Mental illnesses are of many kinds with many causes, both genetic and environmental. Known genetic abnormalities produce neurological deficits such as Down syndrome. Child abuse and substance abuse can produce mental illness in people without genetic abnormalities.

In this chapter, I cover the mental illnesses known to be brain dysfunctions from genetic problems and environmental factors, such as toxic chemicals and social causes.

Understanding Mental Illness as Neural Dysfunction

The genetic code used to build the brain (as well as the rest of the body) is often called a "blueprint," but it's really more like a computer program. Many of the nucleotide sequences specify RNA, whose function is to regulate the expression of other nucleotide sequences, rather than produce proteins that become part of the body. As the fertilized zygote divides repeatedly, the daughter cells differentiate into different tissue types that are determined by what subset of the cell DNA is expressed (refer to Chapter 15).

Several factors affect cell differentiation:

✔ Environmental factors that enter the cell and affect DNA expression

✔ Substances outside the cell but within the organism, such as diffusible messengers and membrane cell adhesion markers

✔ Substances and energy from outside the organism, from the environment, such as chemical teratogens like thalidomide that penetrate in utero to the fetus and affect the development of visual and auditory sensory systems

Organisms, particularly the brains of organisms, are products of both genetics and environmental factors.

Building brains

Given that the brain is a product of genetics and environmental factors (including in utero experience), we can propose a model in which a genetically "normal" DNA sequence interacts with "normal" experience to produce a normal outcome — a functional brain without neurological defect or mental illness. An "abnormal" DNA sequence with normal experience or a normal DNA sequence with abnormal experience may lead to neurological defects.

Having the outcome of brain development depend on environmental factors in a hostile and uncertain world may not seem like the best development strategy from an evolutionary standpoint. However, it actually makes sense. This strategy exists because it's possible to build a more complicated and competent organism for a particular environment if the environment affects the developmental process. But if the entire development is hard-coded in the genome, as may be the case with some invertebrates, the organism is not as adaptable. The environment affects organisms differently in the embryological period, childhood, and adulthood.

Developing while growing

During fetal growth, the brain increases in size and lays down its major structures and axon tracts. This process is highly susceptible to genetic defects, environmental toxins, and nutritional deficiencies. These problems may cause entire brain regions to be missing, malformed, or improperly connected.

Toxins, nutritional deficiencies, and drugs that have no serious long-term ill effects in adults can have devastating effects on brain development in utero.

Early childhood presents another important vulnerability. During childhood, the processes of modulating synapses and myelinating axon tracts in the brain are continuing. Experience from sensory input and the outcome of behavior that is guided by that input affect these processes directly. Attempting behavior to accomplish goals, like trying to walk, produces its own sensory input in a feedback loop that helps wire the brain to allow sensory control of behavior. Skills like language and swimming, for example, which children learn easily, are much harder for adults to learn. The lack of social engagement in autistic children — which may be based on sensory deficiencies such as poor visual processing of facial expressions — may lead, through a kind of deprivation, to permanent social incompetence in adulthood.

Turning thoughts into synapses

Scientists used to believe that in adulthood, synaptic strengths may be tweaked by experience, but producing new neurons or neural connections was not possible. In this model, the brain produced memory and learning through only subtle changes in neural connectivity.

We now know that new neurons can arise in some parts of the adult brain, like the hippocampus; new synapses can be formed in many parts of the brain; and changes in synaptic weights may dynamically reconfigure the brain's functional architecture.

The idea of "use it or lose it" may apply to many cognitive capabilities. Because many cognitive capabilities enable other ones, a small positive or negative change in cognitive function can have far-reaching effects on the operation of the brain that can change the brain's structure for better or worse. Thoughts, inspirations, near-death experiences, and other strong emotional experiences can rewire the brain.

Exploring the Genetic Causes of Brain Dysfunction

Brain damage can cause mental dysfunction, and genetic abnormalities can cause structural brain dysfunction. A number of long-known syndromes have a genetic basis that we understand fairly well today. Many of these syndromes are due to mutations at a single DNA nucleotide, which changes the protein coded by one amino acid.

Mutations occur by many mechanisms, such as ionizing radiation, replication, and transcription errors. Down syndrome is caused by *trisomy,* the extra duplication of part of chromosome 21.

Mutations at single locations

Mutations of a single DNA nucleotide can change the amino acid within the protein coded by the DNA sequence. This can change the way the protein folds, which is dependent on the different charges on different amino acid side chains. A misfolded protein may not only fail to perform a necessary function in the brain, but may itself be toxic. In this section, I discuss several well-known brain dysfunctions based on mutations.

Fragile X syndrome

Fragile X syndrome results from a mutation on the X chromosome at a locus that appears to be prone to mutation (hence, the name "Fragile X"). It is the most common inherited cause of mental disability. The symptoms of the disability are similar to autism.

Those with Fragile X syndrome exhibit mental retardation and several characteristic features:

- ✔ The physical features of Fragile X include an elongated face, large protruding ears, flat feet, and low muscle tone.
- ✔ The behavioral traits include social anxiety, and an aversion to looking at faces (called *gaze aversion*). The behavior traits are associated with reduced function in the prefrontal areas of the brain.

Rett syndrome

Rett syndrome is a developmental brain disorder characterized by a tendency toward *microcephaly* (small head) and reduced levels of the neurotransmitters norepinephrine and dopamine. It is caused by a mutation of a gene called (MECP2). The syndrome affects females almost exclusively because affected males typically die in utero. People with this mutation tend to have small hands and feet and are prone to scoliosis. Behavior traits include poor verbal skills and repetitive hand wringing.

Williams syndrome

Williams syndrome is a relatively rare neuro-developmental disorder that is characterized by mental retardation, but strong language skills. It can be caused by a deletion of a number of different genes on chromosome 7.

Individuals with Williams syndrome tend to be overly sociable and highly verbal. The physical traits of this syndrome include an "elfin" facial appearance with a low nasal bridge.

Down syndrome

Down syndrome (also called trisomy 21) is caused by an extra chromosome 21 (or part of it). It occurs in more than 1 in 1,000 births, and is more common in children born of older parents due to the statistically greater chance of this particular random chromosome damage with aging. Down syndrome is associated with moderate to severe mental retardation. It also comes with frequent complications in other organ systems that reduce life expectancy. People with Down syndrome who do live into their 50s have a significantly increased risk of early Alzheimer's disease.

Autism

Autism has many genetic causes. It is referred to as a "spectrum disorder" because those with autism can have symptoms ranging from barely noticeable to severe mental retardation. Severe autism is debilitating, characterized by an almost total inability to engage in social interactions, extremely poor language abilities, and continuous repetitive behaviors, such as rocking.

Asperger's syndrome is typically included in the autism spectrum as autism without significant language delay or dysfunction. Some autistic individuals may have above-average intelligence and excel in certain technical or artistic areas. Many *savants* (people with extraordinary mathematical, memorization, or artistic skills) are autistic.

Although we know that the many causes of autism are genetic because it tends to be inherited, we do not know the genetic locations of the mutations that cause autism.

Knowing How the Nervous System Can Be Damaged in Utero

Mental illness can occur in a genetically normal brain if it suffers organic damage during development. Trauma, stress, toxins, and nutritional deficiencies can all generate brain dysfunction. These injuries can be severe and irreversible if they happen to the fetus.

Fetal alcohol syndrome

Fetal alcohol syndrome develops from excessive alcohol consumption by the mother during pregnancy. Fetal alcohol exposure is a significant cause of intellectual disability, occurring in about 1 per 1,000 live births.

Alcohol readily crosses the placental barrier. In the developing fetus, alcohol can damage neurons and brain structures and is associated with varying degrees of cognitive and functional disability, such as attention and memory deficits, impulsive behavior, and stunted overall growth. High fetal alcohol exposure is associated with distinctive facial features such as a short nose, thin upper lip, and skin folds at the corner of the eyes.

Several substances have the potential to compromise the neurological and physical health of developing babies if a mother abuses these substances. Besides alcohol, cocaine and methamphetamine are statistically associated with mental and behavioral problems. Even excessive caffeine and nicotine (from cigarettes) may lead to fetal problems. Poor diets can produce vitamin and nutrient deficiencies.

Maternal stress and infections

If a pregnant woman is chronically stressed, her child is more likely to have neurological or behavioral problems such as attention deficits, hyperactivity, anxiety, and language delay. Maternal stress changes the mother's hormone profile through the hypothalamic-pituitary-adrenal (HPA) axis via the secretion of *cortisol,* a stress hormone that can harm the developing nervous system. Some of these effects may be long lasting, such as effects on hippocampal function.

Maternal infections, such as from rubella (see the information on the TORCH complex in Chapter 15), can produce neurological dysfunction in the fetus. Viral infections such as HIV can be passed to the fetus.

Mixing Genetic and Developmental Components

The most well-known types of mental illness, such as depression and schizophrenia, have complex relationships between genetic factors and environmental triggers. These neurological dysfunctions have multiple causes, and the severity of symptoms varies greatly. Significant progress has been made in this century using brain imaging, genetics, and systems neuroscience to understand what goes wrong in various kinds of mental illness.

Depression and mania

Depression affects nearly 15 percent of the U.S. population. It is by far the most serious form of mental illness worldwide in terms of total expense, costing somewhere over $50 billion annually in the United States alone. Depression can be *monopolar,* characterized by depression only, or *bipolar,* with short episodes of *mania* (extreme mood elevation) alternating with longer depressive states.

Depression has multiple causes. Some have a strong genetic basis. For example, someone may live into adulthood without any significant depression until a single traumatic experience, such as the death of a child or spouse. Depression also can result from chronic lower-level stress. On the other hand, depression also runs in families and is highly inheritable without any known environmental triggers. When depression is caused by environmental factors in what was before a "non-depressed" brain, clearly the environmental incident must have changed adult brain function in some way.

Monoamine hypothesis

Monoamines are neurotransmitters and neuromodulators that contain one amino group that is connected to an aromatic ring by a two-carbon chain. The monoamine transmitter group includes serotonin, dopamine, epinephrine, and norepinephrine. Neural receptors for monoamine neurotransmitters affect phospholipase C and adenylyl cyclase, signaling cascades inside neurons that can turn genes in the nucleus on or off.

The monoamine hypothesis of depression suggests that specific monoamine deficits cause particular features of depression. In particular, norepinephrine deficiency reduces alertness and energy; serotonin deficiency produces anxiety, obsessions, and compulsions; and low dopamine levels lead to lowered attention, motivation, and *anhedonia* (reduced feelings of pleasure and reward).

Most antidepressants such as Prozac (a type of selective serotonin reuptake inhibitor, or SSRI) elevate levels of the neurotransmitter serotonin. Many antidepressants also elevate the levels of norepinephrine and dopamine and are prescribed according to the patient's symptoms and the symptoms' match with the monoamine hypothesis.

Depression that is treatable with SSRIs may be associated with a genetic link between different forms of the serotonin transporter (5-HTT) gene and the tendency for stressful life events to produce depression. People with short alleles of the 5-HTT gene are more prone to depression after stress, perhaps because of unusually severe negative feelings that stress triggers in such people. Normally, the release of serotonin is associated with feelings of satisfaction, such as after eating or orgasm. Dominant animals in hierarchical social structures have higher serotonin levels than lower-status animals.

However, a problem for the serotonin hypothesis is that depressed people do not have abnormally low serotonin levels. Also, artificially lowering these levels in people without depression doesn't cause depression. Elevating serotonin levels with drugs to alleviate depressive symptoms probably does not work by restoring an intrinsic serotonin deficiency.

Another hypothesis is that the enzyme that metabolizes monoamines (monoamine oxidase A, or MAO-A) may be overly active in depressed people, reducing monoamine levels to abnormally low levels. Some imaging studies have found elevated MAO-A activity in the brains of depressed people. However, lower, not elevated MAO-A activity is found in depressed youth. Pharmacological agents that deplete monoamines do not cause depression in healthy people nor do they worsen depressive symptoms in depressed people.

Several antidepressants do *not* act through the monoamine system. Here are two examples:

- **Opipramol:** This drug is a member of the tricyclic antidepressants, and acts primarily as an agonist at sigma receptors. These receptors were originally thought to be a type of opioid receptor; however, sigma receptors are activated by non-opioid drugs such as phencyclidine (PCP) and haloperidol. Other sigma agonists include cocaine, morphine, fluvoxamine, methamphetamine, and dextromethorphan. Opipramol also acts as a low to moderate affinity antagonist for the D2, 5-HT2, H1, H2, and muscarinic acetylcholine receptors.

- **Tianeptine:** This medication is a selective serotonin reuptake enhancer (SSRE), whose action is opposite that of SSRIs like Prozac. Tianeptine increases the concentration of dopamine in the nucleus accumbens, the brain area important for reward and motivation. It also modulates the D2 and D3 dopamine receptors and affects A1 (alpha 1 adrenergic) receptors.

Brain dysfunction theories of depression

The monoamine hypothesis and other similar drug therapies are based on the underlying idea that different neurotransmitters in the brain have different functions, and that dysfunction is associated with reduced or elevated levels of the neurotransmitter.

In many ways, this idea is almost too simple. The brain is an immensely complicated organ with thousands of distinct regions that all use a limited number of neurotransmitters. These neurotransmitters have completely different functions in different brain areas, but many pharmacological treatments reduce or elevate their concentrations everywhere.

A different view of the brain regards it as a system in which most functions are locally organized in specific areas in order to reduce the total volume of axon tracts. This approach means looking at differences in brain area operation, rather than neurotransmitter concentration, as the underlying problem in some mental illnesses.

Network theories

In a dynamic system constantly rewiring itself by learning, serious problems arise if the rewiring mechanism goes awry. This would be evident in changes in synaptic plasticity and dynamic neural connectivity. Chronic stress and depression appear to reduce plasticity and neural complexity, and antidepressants appear to increase this function. This suggests that the underlying cause of depression may be a network wiring problem.

The *network hypothesis* suggests that multiple brain regions involving multiple neurotransmitter systems are likely to be involved in depression disorders. Imaging studies have suggested the existence of several "main" brain networks based on connectivity and mutual activity:

- **Central executive network:** This network is located primarily in fronto-parietal cortical regions such as the dorsolateral prefrontal cortex and lateral posterior parietal cortex. These brain areas mediate working memory and are involved in decision making. Many psychiatric and neurological disorders are associated with central executive network dysfunction.

- **Default mode network:** The default mode network is a set of brain areas active when the brain is not highly engaged in any particular task. This network includes the prefrontal cortex, posterior cingulate, medial temporal lobe, and angular gyrus. The default mode network is more activated when depressed patients engage in self-focused, negative thinking than when non-depressed people do so.

- **Salience network:** This network is active when someone is detecting and orienting to salient external stimuli or events. This network includes the cingulate-frontal operculum, anterior cingulate, and anterior insula, particularly the right anterior insula. Excessive activation of this area may color all experience negatively, leading to depression.

Brain regions involved in depression

Certain regions of the brain may also play a role in depression:

- ✔ **Anterior cingulate cortex (ACC):** Some brain imaging studies have suggested that the ACC has an important function in depression. The ACC is activated by pain, the anticipation of pain, and negative experiences. Imaging studies show that it exhibits higher activity levels in depressed people than in non-depressed people.

- ✔ **Raphe nuclei:** Located in the upper brainstem, raphe nuclei are the primary source of serotonin-releasing axons in the brain. Depression is often associated with abnormally low activity in the dorsal raphe nuclei.

- ✔ **Ventral tegmental area (ventral tegmentum):** Located in the ventral midbrain, this area is a major part of the brain's reward system. Dopaminergic neurons in this area project to the nucleus accumbens. Many addictive drugs such as cocaine, increase the effects of dopamine in this network, while dopamine antagonists produce anhedonia. Long-term stress decreases dopamine release in the nucleus accumbens.

- ✔ **Subgenual cingulate (Brodmann area 25):** This area appears to be overactive in some types of depression. It may keep the sufferer stuck in a feedback loop in which negative, self-focused thoughts reinforce themselves through its interaction with the default mode network, the hypothalamus, amygdala, and brainstem. Serotoninergic drugs may have effects on this structure. Deep brain stimulation (which I discuss later in this chapter) in this area has had success in alleviating depression.

The disruption of circadian rhythms, mediated by the suprachiasmatic nucleus, may also underlie depression. A type of depression called seasonal affective disorder may be associated with decreased activity in the serotonergic or adenosine systems.

Non-pharmacological depression therapies

Several treatments for depression do not involve using medication.

- ✔ *Network theories* for depression target brain areas or circuits for therapy rather than neurotransmitters. Many non-pharmacological therapies target the ACC:

  - • **Partial ablation:** This is one therapy directed at the ACC. It is based on the accidental finding from clinical trials in which parts of the ACC such as area 25 were lesioned to relieve intolerable pain in some terminally ill patients. A significant percentage of these patients reported that they could still physically sense pain, but the sensation was no longer distressing — similar to the effects of some analgesics — and experience mood elevation.

- **Deep brain stimulation (DBS):** DBS involves placing electrodes in neural structures such as the ACC. Current pulses of certain frequencies partially inactivate the ACC in severely depressed patients who experienced immediate relief from pain as soon as the stimulation current was turned on.

    The use of DBS for depression followed a much more common use of DBS in the *subthalamic* nucleus for people with Parkinson's disease. DBS stimulation has produced immediate symptom relief in thousands of such Parkinson's patients without the side effects that occur with pharmacological therapies.

- *Downward spiral theories* consider that people tend to interpret experience more negatively when they're depressed. Downward spiral theories postulate a positive feedback process in which negative feelings or emotions create negative memories, creating further negative feelings or emotions, spiraling into inescapable depression. The therapeutic strategy is to break this feedback cycle.

- *Neuronal-modulation therapy* has also been used to treat depression:

    - **Electroconvulsive therapy (ECT):** ECT involves passing electric currents through the brain via scalp electrodes to induce a transient seizure that temporarily interrupts brain activity and causes retrograde memory loss. The memory loss typically spans the previous several months, some of which is recovered over the next days and weeks. There can also be some reduced ability to form new long-term memories for several weeks. ECT fell out of favor because of a general dislike of inducing seizures in patients, and other cognitive-loss side effects.

    - **Transcranial magnetic stimulation (TMS):** This therapy has been used in recent decades in a somewhat similar manner to ECT. TMS involves creating a millisecond, high-field magnetic pulse over a particular brain area via an external coil that produces currents inside the brain underneath the coil. These currents shut down brain activity in the affected area transiently without inducing a seizure, so the technique appears to be much more benign than ECT. Some clinical success has been achieved in treating depression with TMS.

Schizophrenia

Schizophrenia is a mental disorder characterized by disordered thought, paranoia, and delusional beliefs. It occurs in about 1 percent of the population worldwide, and is associated with significant social dysfunction and disability. People with severe cases of schizophrenia are often hospitalized.

People often confuse the two, but schizophrenia is *not* the same as split or multiple personality disorder.

Symptoms

Symptoms of schizophrenia typically appear in young adulthood, and they fall into two general categories:

- ✓ **Positive symptoms:** These are active processes such as hearing voices or trying to escape people the schizophrenic person imagines is following her. The schizophrenic person often believes these voices command her to commit inappropriate acts. Brain scans of schizophrenic people show activity in their auditory cortex during such auditory hallucinations. This suggests that an internal source in the brain is generating activity in auditory areas that the schizophrenic person cannot distinguish from something she actually hears.

- ✓ **Negative symptoms:** Mostly these symptoms are withdrawal and an inability to engage in social interactions, characterized by flat affect and emotion, anhedonia, loss of motivation, social withdrawal, and lack of attention to hygiene and routine activities of life. Although positive symptoms are harder to manage when patients act out delusional ideas, negative symptoms tend to contribute more to poor quality of life.

The genetic basis for schizophrenia

The typical age of schizophrenia onset is young adulthood, when myelination in the frontal lobe is being completed. This is the last major stage of axonal myelination during development. Schizophrenia appears to be dysfunction of the frontal lobe that has strong heritability.

The genetic basis of schizophrenia is apparent in the fact that if one identical twin has schizophrenia, the other twin has a 40 percent chance of developing the illness, even if he was raised separately. Moreover, there are known subclinical schizophrenic traits, like a particular kind of abnormal eye tracking, that occur frequently in non-schizophrenic close relatives of schizophrenic people.

Treatment options

Pharmacological treatments for alleviating positive symptoms of schizophrenia have improved in the last decades. Negative symptoms still do not respond well to most current medications. It is unclear why some drugs work better in some schizophrenic patients than others for positive symptoms, and why none of them alleviates negative symptoms well.

For positive symptoms most schizophrenic people are treated with antipsychotic medications such as clozapine, quetiapine, and risperidone. Unfortunately, many of these drugs have serious side effects. Many of the drugs that alleviate positive symptoms are agents that increase acetylcholine levels in the brain.

Nicotine, as from cigarettes, is a nicotinic agonist, and cigarette smoking, as a form of self-medication, is prevalent among people with schizophrenia. Research suggests a specific defect in the alpha-7 nicotinic acetylcholine receptor as the major molecular cause of schizophrenia.

Other antipsychotics suppress dopamine or serotonin receptor activity. An early theory of schizophrenia was that it was caused by excessive activation of a particular type of dopamine receptor, the D2. Drugs that block the D2 receptor reduced psychotic symptoms, while amphetamines, which enhance dopamine release, worsened symptoms. D2 agents are the typical antipsychotic medications such as chlorpromazine, haloperidol, and trifluoperazine.

Some newer antipsychotic medications, called *atypical antipsychotic medications,* enhance serotonin function with much less blocking effect on dopamine. Atypical drugs include clozapine, quetiapine, risperidone, and perphenazine.

Recent evidence suggests that abnormally low numbers of NMDA glutamate receptors are involved in schizophrenia. Postmortem analysis of the brains of schizophrenics show reduced receptor numbers compared to normal. NMDA receptor blocking drugs such as phencyclidine and ketamine mimic schizophrenic symptoms (the hallucinogen LSD has similar effects to ketamine).

Obsessive compulsive disorder

Obsessive compulsive disorder (OCD) is an anxiety disorder that is characterized by intrusive thoughts that generate repetitive behaviors to alleviate the anxiety related to the thought. About 2 percent of the population suffers from OCD.

Typical symptoms of OCD include washing excessively (particularly hand washing), repeatedly checking for something undone or missing, and performing everyday activities — such as dining or washing — in a ritualistic way. OCD is also associated with traits such as hoarding, preoccupation with sexual or religious thoughts, and irrational aversions, such as extreme fear of germs. Extreme cases of OCD are associated with paranoia and psychosis.

Unlike schizophrenics, however, OCD sufferers are typically aware of their obsessions and usually find them distressing, although they're unable to stop.

Some OCD has been linked to an abnormal serotonin neurotransmission, sometimes successfully treated with SSRIs. Mutations in genes linked to serotonin have been identified in some groups of OCD sufferers, but a strong genetic basis for its occurrence has not been identified. The genetic basis may be a susceptibility that environmental factors act on to produce the disorder.

Post traumatic stress disorder

Post-traumatic stress disorder (PTSD) is a severe anxiety disorder that develops after psychological trauma — such as experiencing a war or sexual abuse — that overwhelms the person's coping ability. Traumatic psychological events cause an overactive adrenaline response that persists after the event, making a person hyper-responsive to future fearful situations.

PTSD is associated with low basal cortisol levels and high catecholamine secretion characteristic of the classic fight-or-flight response. It may have a genetic susceptibility associated with differences in the GABA receptor, and is associated with having a smaller than normal hippocampus.

People prone to PTSD are also statistically more likely to have generalized anxiety disorders; a tendency toward alcohol, nicotine, and drug dependence; and a history of abuse as children.

Desensitization therapies, in which the PTSD sufferer re-experiences aspects of the stressor in a controlled environment, can sometimes mitigate some of its effects.

Epilepsy

Epilepsy is when seizures occur in the brain. *Seizures* are incidents of hypersynchronous neural activity during which normal brain function is severely compromised. The underlying cause of epilepsy is usually a dysfunctional brain area where the seizures originate and then spread to the rest of the brain. These seizure-originating areas are called *epileptic foci.* They occur commonly in the temporal lobe but can exist anywhere in the brain.

Most initial treatment for epilepsy uses drugs called *anticonvulsants.* Most of the 20 or so anticonvulsants approved by the Food and Drug Administration (FDA) are aimed at increasing GABA transmission in the brain. About 70 percent of patients experience a reduction of seizures with one or more of these drugs.

For epileptic sufferers in which anticonvulsants do *not* work, or those who cannot tolerate the negative drug side effects, surgery is an option. In epilepsy surgery, the surgical team try to locate the focus of the seizure and remove it without damaging important nearby brain areas, particularly those associated with language.

Eating and Drinking for Brain Function

The foods we eat and the liquids we drink contain many substances that can affect brain activity and function. Well-known substances include caffeine, alcohol, and nicotine. Nutritional supplements and even the balance of fat versus meat versus vegetables in the diet can affect neurotransmitter balances in the brain with cognitive and behavioral results.

Naturally occurring psychoactive substances

Nutrition, neuro-active substances, and drugs can have significant effects on brain function, for good or bad. These substances can be ingested from plants or pills. Many drugs and supplements act by mimicking neurotransmitters, while others modulate cell metabolism or membrane function.

Feeding the brain properly

Healthy brain activity depends on a healthy body, including its cardiovascular system. Nutrition and exercise that promote general health tend to promote brain health.

Some vitamins are thought to enhance brain function or slow its decline with aging. These include the B vitamins, vitamin D, omega-3 fatty acids, and isoflavones.

Certain agents, sometimes called *nootropics,* are thought to specifically enhance some brain functions such as cognition, memory, intelligence, motivation, attention, and concentration. These are variously called *smart drugs, memory enhancers, neuro-enhancers, cognitive enhancers,* and *intelligence enhancers.*

Psychoactive substances in nature

Naturally occurring psychoactive substances have been used in religious rituals for thousands of years. Notable examples include peyote (mescaline) and psilocybin, which activate serotonin receptors to produce hallucinations and euphoria. Cannabinoids in marijuana activate receptors called CB1 and CB2 in the brain's pain and immune control systems. There are also naturally occurring cholinergic antagonists from plants, such as the deadly nightshade and mandrake, which are hallucinogenic.

Most so-called smart drugs work by mimicking neurotransmitters, altering their endogenous levels, or antagonizing receptors. Many are derived from drugs used to treat neurological conditions like Alzheimer's disease or Parkinson's disease, such as L-dopa, the precursor to dopamine. Other dopamine agents include modafinil, L-phenylalanine L-tyrosine, biopterin, and pyridoxal-phosphate.

Some psychiatric drugs such as methylphenidate (Ritalin, used for ADHD) are taken in the belief that they increase productivity without producing euphoria or psychosis. Some common supplements include resveratrol (an MAO-A inhibitor), St. John's wort (an herbal supplement used for mild depression), ginseng, kava, co-enzyme Q-10 (an antioxidant), creatine (which modulates ATP levels), and ginkgo biloba and vincamine (which are vasodilators).

Needless to say, mucking around with your brain and nervous system without a thorough knowledge of the effects of these agents and without being able to monitor neurotransmitter and receptor levels is potentially very dangerous. Many of the agents I describe here have been used as herbal medication in other countries for some time, so at least they have a history of use to look at. If you take any supplement, do so carefully and under the advice of a physician.

Looking at commonly abused drugs

People abuse drugs that affect the brain for many different reasons. Often, taking drugs is a way to self-medicate that is habit forming. Here are some commonly abused substances:

- **Stimulants:** Some stimulants, such as amphetamines and methamphetamines, are initially taken to enhance productivity but end up causing addiction and psychosis.

- **Nicotine:** Taken in from cigarette smoking, nicotine can have short-term positive effects on alertness, attention, memory, and fine motor control. It seems to reduce some schizophrenic symptoms. However, cigarettes produce scores of toxic byproducts that lead to lung cancer, emphysema, and vascular system damage.

- **Caffeine:** Commonly ingested in coffee and tea, caffeine increases energy and alertness. It has a marginal paradoxical protective effect against Parkinson's disease, for unknown reasons.

- **Other substances:** Some drugs are taken only for euphoria, of course. These include dopaminergic agents such as cocaine, heroin, ecstasy (MDMA), and to a lesser extent marijuana, a cannabinoid. These drugs and alcohol are frequently abused, although the abuse potential varies among individuals.

Chapter 18

Making Better Brains

Since ancient times people have tried to fix broken brains and enhance normal ones. The ancient Egyptians practiced brain surgery by drilling holes through the skull, presumably to relieve some perceived pressure inside. Brain surgery has, thankfully, evolved since then, and less invasive brain manipulations are being used as research tools and as treatments for conditions like depression.

Although most brain research has been directed toward conquering mental illness and brain dysfunction, or enhancing function in normal brains, some modern brain research is directed toward building artificial brains, or artificial brain subsystems.

This chapter takes up various kinds of brain manipulations and the future of enhancing the workings of the brain.

Fixing the Brain with Surgery, Electricity, and Magnetism

Various drugs affect the brain in different ways (refer to Chapter 17). Most do so by mimicking neurotransmitters either as agonists or antagonists. However, other methods, such as surgery, electrical currents, and magnetic stimulation, have been or are being used to treat brain disease and mental illness.

Lobotomies and other brain surgery

Surgical techniques aimed to cure organic brain disease include removing tumors and excising brain areas thought to be the origin foci of epileptic seizures. A completely different class of brain surgery, however, is *psychosurgery,* which attempts to remove brain areas or transect fiber tracts to relieve cognitive or behavioral problems. One of the most infamous of these was the *prefrontal lobotomy,* which removes areas of the prefrontal lobe and was developed in Europe in the early 20th century. The theory behind this procedure was that mental illness was caused by too much activity in the prefrontal cortex, producing excessive emotion, stress, and even violent behavior.

Although many prefrontal lobotomies did lessen violent behavior and extreme emotional stress in patients, they also lost a great deal of cognitive function and motivation. This type of surgery is now extremely rare and generally considered unethical by most of the medical community. Prefrontal lobotomy causes irreversible cognitive loss and is not founded on a neurologically sound basis. Today, drugs are available that produce similar symptom relief without permanent, large-scale brain damage.

Electroconvulsive therapy

Electroconvulsive therapy (ECT, also formerly called *electroshock therapy*) passes an electrical current through the brain to produce an artificial seizure. It has been used as a psychiatric treatment for severe depression (and, originally, schizophrenia — refer to Chapter *17*). The direct mechanisms by which ECT relieves depression are poorly known, but it's clear that the seizure it produces disrupts memory, presumably by disrupting activity in brain circuits involving the hippocampus. Memory loss is both *retrograde* — for several months — and *anterograde* (poor consolidation of new memories) for perhaps a month or more. Often, some memory returns during the years after treatment.

Why should disrupting memory relieve depression? One hypothesis is that if the depression is "caused" by some traumatic incident, eliminating the memory of the incident should relieve the depression. This does appear to be the case in some instances. Outside of depression caused by a single traumatic incident is the idea that depression may involve a downward spiral of negative affect, which tends to enhance negative memories, causing more negative affect. By this hypothesis, disrupting general memory should break this cycle, which appears to be the case in some patients.

For reasons somewhat similar to those for psychosurgery, ECT is much rarer today than it was in the 20th century. It is still sometimes used to treat clinical depression or mania that has not responded to other treatment.

The unpleasantness of inducing a general seizure and general memory loss are considered too high a price in all but the most severe cases. Today, alternative therapies, such as drugs, and deep brain stimulation (which I discuss next), are used.

Deep brain stimulation

Deep brain stimulation (DBS) is an exciting recent development in the treatment of Parkinson's disease that has been extended to other conditions, including depression. In DBS, one or more electrodes are permanently inserted into a target region of the brain, and an implanted electronic device — similar to a cardiac pacemaker — passes current pulses through the electrode(s).

In Parkinson's disease the basal ganglia were the original target areas. The assumption was that artificial stimulation could restore subnormal neural activity from dopamine loss. However, despite the fact that the treatment often works (but with the electrodes implanted in the subthalamic nucleus rather than the substantia nigra), the situation is more complicated than this simple hypothesis suggests. It isn't clear whether the main effect of the stimulation is general excitation, general inhibition, or the production of some beneficial pacemaking activity that causes neurons to fire synchronously.

Regardless of how it works, the results of DBS in many patients have been dramatic. Parkinson's patients who exhibit the typical stooped posture and shuffling gate with the stimulator turned off are able to walk and engage in sports almost immediately when the current pulses are turned on.

Recently, the Food and Drug Administration (FDA) has also approved the use of DBS to treat pain and major depression because side effects of the DBS treatment for Parkinson's have sometimes alleviated these problems as well. There are also new experimental DBS treatments for obsessive-compulsive disorder (OCD) and Tourette's syndrome. In many patients, the symptom relief has been far better than any drug treatment with considerably less side effects.

Transcranial magnetic stimulation

Another noninvasive type of brain stimulation is *transcranial magnetic stimulation* (TMS), in which a special wire coil is placed outside the head over the brain area to be stimulated. A short, high-amplitude current pulse in the coil produces a brief, high magnetic field that is relatively localized under the coil. The TMS magnetic pulse appears to produce transient electrical currents in the brain that disrupt neural activity.

The effects of TMS resemble the effects of ECT. However, TMS stimulation is more localized, and TMS tries to avoid inducing a seizure. Instead, it produces only a transient disruption of local brain activity. TMS applied over most areas of the neocortex often has no conscious effect on the subject. In research studies, the subject's performance or behavior may be altered, however, indicating the involvement of that part of the brain and its timing on the subject's behavior.

The subject is aware that TMS is happening when primary motor cortex is stimulated, because it produces muscle activity by generating action potentials there. TMS pulses over occipital cortex can generate *phosphenes* (flashes of light).

Originally, TMS used single pulses; however, a new paradigm involving pulse trains is now being explored — *repetitive TMS* (rTMS). rTMS can have long-lasting effects. Some evidence suggests that rTMS may help alleviate certain types of depression, perhaps by disrupting memory like ECT, but with fewer side effects.

Transcranial direct current stimulation

Transcranial direct current stimulation (tDCS) involves injecting a small direct current between two electrodes on the scalp, typically about 2 milliamps. Often, subjects barely detect the onset of this current, and it produces no seizures, motor activity, or phosphenes. tDCS appears to stimulate brain activity in some general manner by lowering thresholds or elevating maintained activity. Areas of the brain near the anode appear to be stimulated and areas near the cathode depressed.

According to reports, tDCS has a wide range of effects, from improving math scores on standard tests to alleviating schizophrenic symptoms. tDCS holds the potential to be a powerful, yet simple tool for minimally invasive modulation of brain activity.

New paradigms are appearing in the scientific literature involving alternating or random currents that are not detectable by the subject, but have similar effects.

Meditation, lighting, and soothing sounds

The brain is a dynamic system — experience can change its internal connectivity. Thoughts and thought processes can change the state of the brain, which changes in frequency bands in the electroencephalography (EEG; refer to Chapter 4) show. Persistent brain states may cause long-lasting changes in the way the brain processes information.

Biofeedback, popular in the late 20th century, attempted to allow a person to control the level of EEG waves, such as the alpha rhythm (brain oscillations in the 8 Hz to 13 Hz range), by displaying the EEG or some index of alpha rhythm activity to the subject for feedback.

Meditation, prayer, and relaxation exercises clearly change brain rhythms and can produce effects lasting longer than the session. Mechanisms may include raising neurotransmitter levels of *endorphins* (internal pain reduction neurotransmitters) or oxytocin, or reducing levels of stress hormones, such as cortisol. High light levels at certain times of the day may alleviate seasonal affective disorder — a type of depression.

The mechanisms of these effects are poorly understood and highly variable, which has, unfortunately, led to some therapists selling their services to produce such effects without any evidence. Nevertheless, the power of thoughts to change the brain should not be underestimated, but it should be tested and investigated.

Repairing Brain Damage

We are beginning a revolution in the treatment of brain diseases. Genetic modifications that replace dysfunctional genes may prevent Alzheimer's disease, slow the effects of aging, and reverse brain dysfunctions from strokes. Stem cell transplants may regenerate damaged brain tissue. Growth factors may help to form new neural circuits or repair old ones. Drugs may reinstitute learning capacity in the adult brain so it's like that of a newborn.

Genes and growth factors

Genetic dysfunctions such as those associated with Down syndrome, Rett syndrome, and Fragile X syndrome (refer to Chapter 17) produce profound neurological disorders. The sequencing of the genome and understanding of its function may allow treatments that silence "bad" genes or add new "good" ones.

Genes and gene expression can be altered with *retroviruses* (RNA viruses that produce DNA in the host cell after they enter). The virally coded DNA is then incorporated into the host's genome, after which it replicates with the rest of the host cell's DNA and produces more viruses. Retroviruses can be engineered with sequences that knock out host genes or insert new genes into the host to substitute for a mutated or defective one, instead of producing more viruses. Early-phase clinical trials are underway that use gene therapy for one form of hereditary retinal degeneration.

Growth factors are hormones, proteins, and other substances that exist naturally in the brain to stimulate or regulate cell growth. The brain has many growth factors, such as the following:

- ✔ Brain-derived neurotrophic factor (BDNF)
- ✔ Epidermal growth factor (EGF)
- ✔ Fibroblast growth factor (FGF)
- ✔ Glial cell line-derived neurotrophic factor (GDNF)
- ✔ Insulin-like growth factor (IGF)
- ✔ Nerve growth factor (NGF)

These and other growth factors mediate signaling between cells, usually by binding to receptors on their surfaces, to induce cell differentiation and maturation.

In some cases, it has been observed that placing growth factor substances in wounds speeds healing after an injury. Manipulating growth factor levels in some brain regions may induce non-dividing cells in an adult to return to a juvenile state, and either divide or extend processes to restore function. Some research aims to manipulate growth factor levels with drugs, or by introducing special stem cells, which I discuss next.

Stem cells

Stem cells are plentiful during development (and exist afterward but are hard to find). They're *undifferentiated*, which means they can turn into specialized cells such as neurons, kidney cells, or blood vessel wall cells. Research has shown that injecting appropriate stem cells into damaged tissues like the brain or heart can cause the stem cells to differentiate appropriately in the host environment, sometimes repairing damage there.

Obtaining the stem cells is difficult for several reasons, including their rarity in adults, and ethical and rejection problems associated with harvesting embryos to get stem cells for transplants.

New techniques are allowing scientists to reverse the differentiation of some adult cells into particular types of stem cells for *autologous transplants* (transplantation of tissue generated from the person who receives the transplant). Some laboratories are attempting to restore vision caused by photoreceptor death by using stem cells to replace the photoreceptors. Stem cells that will release dopamine have been injected into the substantia nigra of Parkinson's patients with mixed success.

Brain–Machine Interfaces

Technology allows us to do things in better and easier ways. Physical machines lift more than we can lift and move us faster than we can run. Writing is a kind of sensory enhancement that externalizes memory, while phones and televisions allow us to see and hear across the planet and into space. What augmentation devices have rarely done until the last few decades is interact with the brain directly. We control vehicles with our hands, and we receive artificially generated sensory input through our eyes and ears.

Now we're entering an era in which sensory input can conceivably be put directly into the brain, and external devices may be controlled by motor centers in the brain. These ultimately may augment normal human capabilities, but most of the first applications are prosthetic.

On the input side, the goal is to restore the highly disabling loss of major senses such as vision and hearing. On the output side, the goal is to circumvent paralysis from spinal cord and brain injuries. Can vision signals be put directly into the nervous system, and motor signals taken out effectively for prosthetic devices? What needs to happen for these things to be possible?

Inputting information to the brain

Hearing and vision are major inputs to the brain that can be lost through damage to the peripheral sensory apparatus — the inner ear in the case of hearing and the retina in the case of vision. (Refer to Chapter 10 for more about vision, hearing, and the brain.)

Hearing

The *artificial cochlear stimulator* is one of the most successful applications of neuroprostheses. Cochlear stimulators consist of a microphone, frequency analyzer, and transmitter worn outside the head, and a receiver and cochlear stimulator implanted in the head. The stimulator is a linear array of 20 to 30 electrodes threaded into the cochlea. Pulses on these electrodes stimulate auditory fibers to fire, which the brain interprets as sound. Many of the 200,000 cochlear implants worldwide allow the people who wear them to converse normally, face to face or over the phone.

Vision

The situation for a visual prosthesis is much more difficult than for hearing. The visual system is a more complex system involving one million ganglion cell axons versus 30,000 auditory nerve fibers. It isn't clear where to put stimulators for the visual system and what signals to put on them.

Seeing progress in visual prostheses

Some of the first visual prostheses were implanted in visual cortex, notably by American biomedical researcher Dr. William H. Dobelle and colleagues. Some of his patients were able to read Braille via the phosphemes generated by direct electrical stimulation, but they were not in general able to identify complex objects.

Most current research is concentrated on stimulating retinal ganglion cells either by current pulses or by genetically modifying ganglion cells to express light-sensitive channels so they become intrinsically photosensitive and can act without any photoreceptors when these have died.

Artificial vision devices have been implanted in either the retina or visual cortex. Signals from a small camera are used to drive neural stimulators. Devices located in the retina have been used when the vision loss is caused by photoreceptor death but the rest of the retina, including the output retinal ganglion cells, is intact. Current devices have allowed some blind patients to see a few blobs of light by direct ganglion cell stimulation, but they haven't yielded high enough acuity for reading or driving.

Reading the brain's output code

Spinal cord injuries and strokes have resulted in incurable paralysis for millions of Americans. And in most of these cases, the damaged cells and axons cannot be regrown to restore movement.

Research is being done to electronically bypass spinal cord injuries. The strategy is to record the activity of command neurons in the primary motor cortex, relay them past the injury, and use them to control the muscles via the alpha motor neurons in the spinal cord, or directly by electrically stimulating the muscle. Microelectrode arrays, similar to those that might stimulate cells in a retinal prosthesis, would record the motor cortex signals. These signals could be decoded to drive the person's own muscles or, alternatively, to control a prosthetic arm or leg.

Augmenting Brain Function

If we can make electrical connections to and from the brain to operate prostheses, why not for enhancing normal brain function? I look at possibilities for enhancing brain function in the upcoming sections, as well as some hard questions that go along with them.

Stimulation and function enhancement

New technology is rapidly developing that will allow us to link the brain directly to computers. Microelectrode arrays with hundreds — and soon thousands — of electrodes can be mass-produced that either record brain neural activity to determine our intentions, or stimulate assemblages of neurons for signal input.

Humans (and monkeys) have already used electrode arrays implanted in their motor cortices to move computer cursors and artificial arms just by thinking about doing so. Imagine doing an Internet search simply by thinking about the information you want via a recording array in your brain connected to wi-fi. You could get any piece of information or communicate with any person on earth — just by thinking it!

Brain–computer interfaces (BCIs) may also enhance learning and brain function. Learning the old-fashioned way is hard. Getting a high school diploma takes years. Some brain researchers are working on artificial circuits that mimic the hippocampus, possibly enhancing its capability to store more information more rapidly. Perhaps external information could be downloaded into such a chip.

Your teacher, Ms. Avatar

Computers are teaching students online at all grade levels. These computers offer personalized contexts for learning that make it easier for children, people with learning disabilities, and older adults. Sometimes these computer instructors use *avatars* (computer simulations of teaching characters that students can interact with). Avatars could be created of Plato, da Vinci, or Einstein, or character combinations of these great thinkers.

Avatars may become close companions for children, adults suffering dementia, and possibly even people afflicted with psychological disorders such as depression, schizophrenia, and autism. An avatar system called FaceSay (www.symbionica.com) is designed to teach autistic children to monitor facial expressions in an attempt to improve their social interaction skills. Learning has also been successfully embedded in games in which math, science, and other subjects are presented visually in an intuitive, interactive manner.

Genetic modification

So far, genetic modification of humans has only been carried out in limited cases to repair a genetic defect. But enhancing human cognitive capacities is also a possibility. The genes that are the most interesting for augmentation are those that regulate other genes.

For example, the relative size of the neocortex is likely controlled by a small number of genes during development. Through genetic modification, this human brain area could be made larger. But should doing so be illegal? Even if the practice were outlawed in most developed countries, someone, some-where would try it. And if the genetic modulation were done by injecting into a fertilized ovum, it would produce a transgenic modification that will be in the germ line for all future generations.

Many complex questions surround this issue. Would genetically modified people be our masters, or discriminated against informally or legally? What if they were autistic savants? The technology of using genetic modification to repair genetic damage or delete disease-causing genes is likely to continue for non-disease purposes.

Simulating Brain Function on Computers

The field of making intelligent machines is called *artificial intelligence* (AI). From the point of view of neurobiology, AI can be divided into two subfields.

One subfield is concerned with enabling machines to do things thought of as requiring intelligence, like flying airplanes and driving cars, without regard for similarities between how a machine would do it and how humans would.

The other subfield of AI is concerned with mimicking human (or sometimes animal) behavior or cognition to capture some aspect of the biological mechanisms. Resemblance can range from the output or behavior only, to using models of neuron-like elements to do computations, process information, or control behavior. The dominant instance of modeling at the neural level uses what's called an *artificial neural network* (ANN), a computer simulation of interconnected neural-like elements whose connections (artifical synapses) can be modified.

Comparing brain and computer power

Humans can do things that machines cannot — in particular, tasks that require complex visual perception and manual dexterity. Machines can do things that humans cannot, like calculate pi (π) to millions of decimal places, or apply formulas to thousands of variables in milliseconds. In between these two extremes are many interesting tasks, like playing chess and driving cars, in which humans and machines today perform comparably. This overlap area is a moving target, however, because machines keep getting better at things.

A fundamental question in AI simulations of human intelligence concerns the level of comparison. No one thinks that computer chess players like Deep Blue — which calculates millions of moves in millions of potential move structures — plays chess anything like a human does. Human chess masters seem to intuit position strengths and weakness from the overall pattern on the board.

In *artificial neural networks* (ANNs) neuron-like units perform computations. These units have inputs with synaptic weights something like dendrites, and outputs with thresholds something like neural axons. If an ANN simulation plays chess, is it playing like a human? Does the ANN have spikes and refractory periods, extracellular ion concentration changes, circulating hormones, and cellular homeostatic mechanisms? No.

However, some ANN simulations behave remarkably like human brains in the sorts of errors they make and in their robustness with respect to damage of some components. ANNs set up like actual brain circuits, and then, artificially "lesioned," may even be instructive in cases of human dysfunction, such as neurological damage. Even when the goal is comparing how a machine operates with how a human brain operates, the level of comparison is a moving target, because research is showing that neurons are far more complicated than switches.

Crunching the numbers by computer and human brain

Ideas about biological intelligence often followed the dominant technology of the day — from pneumatics at the time of Descartes, to clockwork gear trains in the Industrial Revolution, to computers today. AI research goals include reasoning, learning, perception, knowledge, and behavior, such as in robotics. In some cases the goals define the technological approach, but in other cases they do not.

It may be useful to try to compare the raw computing power of the human biological brain with that of computers, even if we aren't sure at what level to do the comparison. Some of the most famous research is by the American engineer Ray Kurzweil, who compared instruction cycle rates in computers with neural firing in the human brain. For example, a computer operating at a gigahertz clock rate (10^9 cycles per second) on 32-bit words (2^5) ends up processing 10^{14} bits per second. A human brain has 100 billion (10^{11}) neurons operating in parallel at something less than about 1,000 (10^3) spikes per second, yielding also about 10^{14} bit operations per second.

We could do this calculation in many other ways, which take no account of the huge architectural differences between computers and brains. These differences are surely behind the vastly different performance capabilities between computers and brains. On the other hand, the calculations suggest that for tasks in which neither architecture has an obvious advantage, the performance may be similar.

Kurzweil and others suggest that with the rate of computer progress, sometime before 2030 all computers on earth will so exceed the capability of all humans on earth.

Downloading the Brain

Nobody lives forever, but some people like to think of ways that they could. One idea is by "uploading" your brain to a computer memory before you die. After that, either a silicon version of you could exist, or your brain could be "downloaded" to a recipient brain. Is any of this even possible?

Reading out what's in your brain

The idea of being able to "read out" the contents of your brain is an explicit analog of computer memory in which memory circuits exist that can store data written to them. These data can be recovered at any time by supplying the appropriate memory address.

Downloading the contents of human brains, however, is not so easy. Memory in brains, as the result of an adaptation to some experience, exists in the brain's architecture of neurons and their synaptic connections. Changing synaptic connections are an important form of this kind of memory. But these synaptic weights are not addressable — that is, they cannot be probed simply by supplying an address for that weight. Instead, the synaptic weights change the way the brain operates, coupling two neurons together in a slightly different way for one value of a synaptic weight versus another.

You cannot know a synaptic weight by looking at the synapse (such as with electron microscopy), and you cannot read the value of the synapse by locating a certain address. The synaptic weight is only evident by its effect on the activity of the neural network. Synaptic weights in the network are changing constantly from various causes, including internal homeostatic mechanisms. "Reading out" the effective connectivity of a neural network would require reconstructing the network completely because it is an analog computer. In the human brain, this means reconstructing nearly 100 billion neurons with over 1,000 synapses each, including the efficacy of each synapse, which is controlled by molecular mechanisms. This is, in theory, conceivable in some far future, but it's practically impossible.

What science can do now, to a limited extent, is use imaging tools like fMRI (refer to Chapter 4) to differentiate some overall patterns of activity in brain regions. This may allow us to distinguish between activity patterns — say, those evoked by a blue duck versus a red house. But differentiating between the two brain activity patterns evoked by subtly different stimuli or even imagined visualizations is far different from reconstructing how those patterns were created at the neural and synaptic level.

Better imaging technologies will surely allow more subtle brain state differentiations. Ultimately, however, reproducing an entire memory and all its links *exactly* will require reproducing the entire brain exactly.

Inserting knowledge and memories into the brain

We can insert artificial data into the brain through normal sensory channels such as vision and hearing; we do so every day with computer-generated images and sound recordings. Soon, however, we may be able to bypass these normal channels with implanted electrode chips. But the data rates for this type of information transfer will be much lower than via "normal" senses such as vision, mediated by over a million ganglion cells from each eye, transmitting to a brain system evolutionarily tuned to process that information.

Nevertheless, the ability to send information directly without using fingers to type or the voice to give commands — and without tying up our normal senses — may be quite useful. People with data transmission implants would be able to multitask all the time, dividing their attention between the real world and the digital world.

Constant, voluntary, immediate, and easy access to anything on the Internet is enormously appealing, but this technology, like others, could be abused. A more sinister idea concerns whether memories can be implanted directly into our brains without our knowing where they came from or if they're true. This idea surfaced in the subliminal advertising scare just after the middle of the 20th century (refer to the idea of priming in Chapter 12). Although it turned out that subliminal commands don't work very well, these effects could be stronger with implants. If these implants were abused, people could become like schizophrenics (refer to Chapter 17), suffering from internal voices commanding them to do inappropriate things.

Is the singularity near? Is super-machine intelligence about to occur?

Computer power and machine intelligence are increasing at a breathtaking rate. What happens when the processing capability of single computers, and the world computer network, exceeds that of single people and all of humanity? No one has any experience with this — it's currently the stuff of science-fiction movies. Like all technological advances, both good and bad may result from this development.

Part V
The Part of Tens

For a list of ten great careers for neurobiology students, head to www.dummies.com/extras/neurobiology.

In this part . . .

- ✔ Discover which parts of the brain are crucial for different thoughts and behaviors.
- ✔ See how brain science is being revolutionized by these technologies.

Chapter 19

The Ten Most Important Brain Circuits

In This Chapter

▶ Listing ten major neural circuits

▶ Seeing what these ten brain circuits do

*T*he term *association cortex,* which isn't used much anymore, arose from the idea that most of the neocortex was a non-differentiated device for learning stimulus-response contingencies. In this model, neural connectivity was random and non-specialized. Today we know that the connections between cortical areas and subcortical areas are highly specific. Damage to particular areas of the brain causes specific loss of function. After injury, plasticity mechanisms often can "rewire" the brain to overcome problems associated with the damage, but sometimes not. This chapter describes ten particularly important circuits in the brain and their functions.

The Reticular Formation in the Brainstem

The reticular formation is an ancient brainstem circuit that extends throughout much of the medulla, pons, and midbrain, and into the thalamus. It's continuous with the intermediate gray matter of the spinal cord, and is organized in a similar manner.

The word *reticular* is from the Latin for "net." Refer to Chapter 7 for more about the reticular formation.

The reticular formation consists of over 100 interconnected neural circuits that control essential body functions and life processes such as wakefulness, heart rate, breathing, and temperature. Significant damage to the reticular formation typically results in death.

Reticular nuclei in the medulla control heart rate and pain perception. Pain signals from the lower body relay in the medulla, which projects to somatosensory cortex.

The reticular formation has an important role in motor homeostasis. Motor neurons in the primary motor cortex project to the reticular formation in the medulla in *reticulospinal tracts.* These tracts control balance during body movements with sensory input information from the eyes and ears through the cerebellum.

The reticular formation projects to the thalamus and neocortex to control states of consciousness, awareness, and sleep-wake cycles via the reticular activating system (RAS). The RAS uses the neurotransmitters acetylcholine and norepinephrine (noradrenalin) that operate in an antagonistic manner to regulate state of awareness and consciousness. Cholinergic projections from the RAS to the thalamus, basal forebrain, substantia nigra, and cerebellum are increased during wakefulness and REM sleep.

The norepinephrine output of the RAS is mostly from the locus coeruleus in the pons. Locus coeruleus neurons project to many of the same areas as the cholinergic RAS system but have opposite effects. norepinephrine is high during waking and slow-wave sleep, but low during REM sleep.

The function of the thalamic reticular areas is to modulate the information projected from the thalamus to the cortex within specific sensory modalities and between different ones, depending on body state and needs. The thalamic parts of the reticular formation control important aspects of attention.

The Spinal Reflex

The *spinal reflex* is the basic unit of sensory motor integration. In this reflex, a stimulus (for example, pricking your finger) directly causes a movement (withdrawing your finger) through fast monosynaptic and polysynaptic pathways. This reflex circuit is entirely within the spinal cord, so that it occurs before your brain knows about it. The axon terminals of pain receptor neurons in your skin release the neurotransmitter glutamate onto alpha motor neurons (monosynaptic reflex) and onto spinal cord interneurons (polysynaptic reflex) to produce the withdrawal. (Refer to Chapter 5.)

These spinal reflexes can be modulated or even suppressed, however. You can, for example, override a spinal reflex if you know in advance the stimulus will occur. If you're climbing a rope, the pain in your hands may trigger a reflex to let go, but your brain, knowing it would not be a good idea to do so, may override this reflex. Overriding reflexes is essential to locomotion, which consists of deliberately falling forward (unbalancing) and catching yourself by extending one, then the other leg in a repeated cycle. Spinal reflexes also activate spinal interneurons to allow you to maintain balance while moving.

The Thalamic Relay to the Cortex

The thalamus is at the center of a neural hub whose spokes go to and from the neocortex and subcortical structures. The thalamus is not only the gateway to the cortex, but an intrinsic part of nearly all cortical circuits. Like virtually all brain structures, of course, there are two thalamic nuclei, one in each cerebral hemisphere. The thalamus receives inputs from all the senses, the basal ganglia motor control system, and the reticular formation (which I discuss in the first section of this chapter).

The output of the thalamus makes a fast, efficient link between the parietal, occipital, temporal, and frontal lobes that parallels, and to some extent, short-circuits pathways within the neocortex between different areas. This means that the thalamus is controlling the flow and processing of information throughout the brain by integrating the output of cortical and subcortical processing. This makes the thalamus more than a relay, but a true controller. Thalamic integration is essential for attention, awareness, and consciousness.

Cerebellar Modulation of Motion Sequences

The cerebellum is one of the more ancient parts of the vertebrate brain. However, unlike phylogenetically older parts of the vertebrate brain that are dwarfed by the huge neocortex, the cerebellum has increased in size with the neocortex (although not as much). The number of neurons in the human cerebellum is comparable to that of the entire neocortex.

The cerebellum modulates and coordinates motor behavior. Its extensive neural circuitry detects errors between what is "programmed" by the frontal lobes for a particular movement and what is actually executed, which depends on variables like loads and uneven ground while walking. It uses error computation to achieve correct sequences in motor behavior based on practice.

For example, with a little training you can throw a base runner out with a softball or baseball. The motions for both throws are similar, but differences in ball weight and size are crucial for accuracy. All the coefficients for doing both accurate throws are in the cerebellum whose action is called a *feed-forward controller* because it contains information about the entire sequence of muscle contractions associated with complex activities like throwing. The spinal cord is a *feedback controller* that can maintain homeostasis by using feedback to keep a limb in the same position or cycle.

The cerebellum achieves its capabilities by learning. When you first learn to throw a baseball, you have to think about what you're doing and consciously adapt to your mistakes, but eventually the process becomes automatic because the sequence has become programmed within your cerebellum.

The cerebellum plays an important role in cognition that involves spatial relations and movement. If you plan to rearrange the furniture in your house, the cerebellum is activated during this planning.

Paradoxically, the main effect of damage to the cerebellum is that although people become clumsy, they are still able to initiate and make complex movement sequences. Although this brain structure has a huge number of neurons, you can lead an almost completely normal life with a lot of damage to it. The number of neurons in a structure doesn't necessarily indicate its overall importance for other brain activity.

Hippocampal Reciprocal Activation with the Cortex

The hippocampus is part of a brain circuit that makes memories. It receives inputs from the entire neocortex and projects back out to the same areas. Within the hippocampus activation of NMDA receptors leads to changes in synaptic efficacy as part of the basis of learning and memory. The storage in the hippocampus is only a temporary stage in memory, however.

The hippocampus "plays back" a sequence of events or associations in context and activates the cortical areas that were originally activated by the event itself. This playback occurs during rehearsal and in sleep, especially during REM sleep. The result of the playback is that the memories that were stored temporarily in the hippocampus cause long-term storage back in the neocortical areas that were activated during the original stimulus.

The Amygdala Orbitofrontal Cortex Loop

Anterior to the hippocampus is another structure originally included in the limbic system, the *amygdala* (one on each side of the brain, of course). The amygdalae also interact with the neocortex in a manner somewhat similar to the hippocampus. However, unlike the hippocampus, the amygdalae are particularly involved with stimuli and memories that have high emotional salience, such as fear.

The amygdalae project extensively to the orbitofrontal cortex, as well as the hypothalamus and other brain areas associated with emotional reactions to stimuli. The amygdalae are essential for forming memories associated with emotional events, such as in fear conditioning, where a context that predicts some painful outcome becomes associated with the outcome and itself induces fear. Imaging studies suggest some differences in the function of the right and left amygdalae, but their significance is not clear.

The amygdalae function somewhat like the hippocampus in mediating the formation of long-term memories in the neocortex (primarily, the orbitofrontal cortex). The amygdalae specialize in emotional responses to contexts involving danger, such as being nervous when placing a large gambling bet. Some sociopaths have turned out to have damage to their amygdalae. Lesions to the anterior temporal lobe that include the amygdalae can produce *hypo-emotionality* (very low emotional responses), loss of fear, and *hyper-sexuality* (obsession with an excessive interest in sexual activity; known as Klüver-Bucy syndrome). Autism has been associated with changes in the amygdalae, and an association has been reported between amygdalae volume and the number of social contacts people have.

Obsessive-compulsive disorder (OCD) and post-traumatic stress disorder (PTSD) have been linked to changes in the amygdalae, particularly the left amygdala.

The Spinal Pattern Generator

The spinal cord can produce the basic rhythmic patterns for locomotion without any descending commands from the cortex. Spinal cord neuronal circuits that produce these rhythmic patterns of neural activity are called *central pattern generators* (CPGs). CPGs normally produce rhythmic patterned outputs with sensory feedback, leading to the idea that these pattern generators operated in a stimulus-reflex-movement-stimulus cycle. However, it's now clear that CPGs are capable of generating locomotion patterns without sensory feedback.

Sensory feedback does help coordinate efficient locomotion in the limbs. In a hierarchical control system, the brain normally initiates and controls the activity of spinal CPGs via descending axonal projections that constitute high-level commands — such as switching of gaits depending on immediate needs — while the spinal cord neural circuitry takes care of the details — like adjusting gait for stepping in holes or when running on slopes.

Because walking and other forms of locomotion typically involve moving all four limbs, CPGs are distributed throughout the lower thoracic and lumbar spinal cord. These circuits produce motor neuron firing patterns that synchronize rhythmic contractions of flexor-extensor muscles of the forelimbs and hind limbs. As the hind limbs move in antiphase with each other, the forelimbs move in the opposite antiphase, so your right arm goes forward at the same time as your left leg.

Top-down control from the brain takes advantage of inputs from the visual and vestibular systems. Your visual system helps to keep you from running into trees. Your vestibular system compensates for stepping in holes, and generates the proper leaning posture if you're running on a slope. Lumbar pattern generators in cervical segments are especially important for controlling your balance in these cases.

CPGs use neural circuits in which activity in half of the circuit increases while the other half decreases. This alternating phase activity is believed to be based on neural half-center oscillators, circuits of neurons that are mutually inhibitory — one leg extends while the other flexes. These oscillators extend throughout the spinal cord and receive both sensory input and cortical modulation.

The Conscious Triangle: Frontal and Sensory Cortex with the Thalamus

The thalamus, frontal lobe, and parietal lobe are almost always activated during consciousness. Moreover, their activity is also likely to be highly coupled, as coherent EEG rhythms and synchronous neural firing show. Why these three brain regions?

The lateral prefrontal cortex is the main brain area responsible for working memory, which is our mental representation of what is most important about the current situation. Frontal lobe activation is essential for abstract thought.

The thalamus links the neocortex to subcortical structures and various areas of the neocortex together. By controlling the activity of the neocortex, the thalamus appears to control what emerges from the vast amount of subconscious neural activity as conscious, accessible thought. One hypothesis is that conscious brain activity requires a time and magnitude threshold. Enough neurons must be active over a large enough region of the brain for at least half a second for conscious awareness to occur and persist.

The parietal lobe is the seat of the convergence of multiple sensory streams that allow us to locate ourselves in the world and be aware of this location. This along with the frontal lobe giving us the representation of the context of where and why we're here, controlled and coordinated by the thalamus, may be what can cross the threshold for consciousness.

The Basal Ganglia Thalamus Loop

The basal ganglia (refer to Chapter 9) are the primary controllers of behavior, using the neocortex to generate alternative motor plans and the cerebellum to carry them out. The basal ganglia receive inputs via the outer nuclei (striatum — caudate and putamen), which project to inner nuclei, mainly the globus pallidus. The output of the basal ganglia is chiefly from these inner nuclei to the thalamus, and it's primarily inhibitory to areas of the frontal lobe that generate commands for controlling motor behavior. The substantia nigra and subthalamic nuclei perform a crucial modulatory role in this system.

A common model for the basal ganglia is that of selection. The basal ganglia receive inputs about the state of the body that are translated into priorities, such as to seek food, avoid a predator, or pursue a mate. The frontal lobe executive areas generate motor programs constantly for all these contingencies. The basal ganglia select among them via the thalamus. Once selected, the frontal motor program proceeds to generate behavior with error correction control thanks to the cerebellum.

The Anterior Cingulate and Pulvinar Central Executives

The anterior cingulate cortex (ACC; refer to Chapters 7 and 8) is the anterior half of the cingulate gyrus, located above the corpus callosum and below the neocortex. It is not neocortex, but *mesocortex,* a phylogenetically earlier type of cortex that evolved as the top of the hierarchy of the limbic system. The cingulate gyrus receives inputs from the thalamus and the neocortex, and projects to the entorhinal cortex near the hippocampus via the cingulum.

The ACC controls neural processing throughout the neocortex, allocating this processing according to task demands, making it a mediator of executive function. In this sense, its function is similar to that of the thalamus. However, the ACC is particularly implicated in subjective experience associated with consciousness, particularly consciousness of pain, or even the anticipation of pain. Electrical stimulation of the ACC can reduce the perception of pain without removing the basic underlying sensation of the stimulus that is painful.

The ACC is also activated when someone is struggling with a difficult task, particularly when the person makes errors. For this function, the ACC works with the lateral prefrontal cortex that is maintaining the task demands as working memory. The lateral prefrontal cortex is holding the content of thought and the ACC is monitoring and selecting that content. The posterior cingulate cortex also interacts with the dorsolateral prefrontal cortex, but it appears to be part of the default mode of resting brain operation.

The *pulvinar* (refer to Chapter 8), a nucleus in the most posterior region of the thalamus, has widespread connections with all the neocortex. It's an important mediator of attention, particularly visual attention and eye movements associated with it. The pulvinar integrates vision and goal pursuit to generate context-specific motor responses to specific visual stimuli and ignoring irrelevant visual stimuli. If you're meeting someone at the airport who will be wearing a blue sweater, your pulvinar will draw your attention to blue, sweater-shaped objects.

Chapter 20

Ten Technologies Revolutionizing Brain Science

Many revolutions are occurring today in neurobiology. Genetic techniques are permitting scientists to modify and modulate the nervous system. With new imaging methodologies, neurobiologists can observe neural activity across the brain and within single cells. Advanced electronic technologies are enabling neurobiologists to record and stimulate neurons electrically, optically, and chemically. Many of these techniques are not only giving important insights into how the nervous system works, but also being applied clinically to deal with nervous system dysfunction. This chapter briefly highlights ten important technologies.

Optogenetics: Controlling Neurons with Light

We've known for hundreds of years that electricity can stimulate neurons, but it isn't ideal for precise control of neural activity. One reason is that because neurons always exist in circuits, extracellular electrical stimulation activates the entire circuit, with little ability to control which neurons are activated. This all changed with the development of optogenetics.

Optogenetics (refer to Chapter 4) controls neural activity by activating light-sensitive channels in neural membranes. These light-sensitive channels typically come from microbes that have evolved them to control some behavior, such as moving toward or away from light. The genes for these channels can be introduced into other animals, such as vertebrates with promoters that cause them to be expressed only in specific cell types. Applying a light stimulus to the neural tissue in these animals then activates or inhibits only those specific cells, depending on the optogenetic channel's properties.

Optogenetics allows scientists to precisely modulate activity of individual neurons in freely moving animals. In order to do this, there is currently extensive development of cell-specific promoters and micro optical stimulators to target small numbers of particular cells. The selective stimulation has not only helped to make big advances in the basic understanding of neural circuit operation but also offered insights into neurological dysfunctions such as Parkinson's disease, schizophrenia, autism, and depression.

Transcranial Magnetic Stimulation and Transcranial Direct Current Stimulation

Transcranial magnetic stimulation (TMS) and transcranial direct current stimulation (tDCS) are two types of brain stimulation. (Refer to Chapters 4 and 18.)

TMS works by creating a short high magnetic field pulse via a coil outside the head over the brain area to be stimulated. This produces relatively localized, transient electrical currents that disrupt neural activity. TMS has recently been used to treat mental disorders, like depression, by repetitively stimulating brain areas. In this use, it resembles electroconvulsive therapy (ECT) except that ECT deliberately induces a seizure, whereas in TMS seizures are deliberately avoided.

tDCS involves passing a small direct current (usually about 2 milliamps) between two electrodes on the scalp. Brain regions near the anode (positive electrode) generally appear to be stimulated, whereas areas near the cathode may be inhibited. It isn't clear how passing a small continuous current through the brain affects brain signal processing. Small electrical currents may increase neural spontaneous activity or signal-to-noise ratios because of the orientation of the neural circuit with respect to the current direction.

Most tDCS results have focused on improving some brain function by having the anode over that part of the brain. Numerous studies claim long-lasting improvements in learning or cognitive performance — from improving math scores on standard tests, to alleviating schizophrenic symptoms, to enhancing cognitive function in the elderly — from tDCS stimulation. tDCS may prove to be a powerful and simple tool for minimally invasive modulation of brain activity. The currents necessary for tDCS are typically producible with a 9-volt battery.

Genetic Disease Models: Knockouts and Knockins

Genetic mutations produce serious neurological disorders. In many cases, where and what the mutation is remains unknown, or its effect on the nervous system is unclear because the function of the protein encoded is unknown. These undiscovered factors make finding treatments and cures almost impossible. However, the sequencing of genomes in the last decades has led scientists to directly identify many genetic defects.

Genetic defects can potentially be overcome by using retroviruses to alter genes or gene expression. Retroviruses are RNA viruses whose RNA is reverse-transcribed into DNA in the host cell. The DNA that encodes the viral RNA is typically incorporated into the host's genome, after which it replicates with the rest of the host cell's DNA. Retroviruses can be engineered with sequences that knock out defective host genes or insert new genes into the host to correct for a genetic deficiency whereby an effective, necessary protein is not produced. If a gene is inserted into a fertilized ovum by a retrovirus or other means, the modification of the host will be in the germ line and passed to all future generations.

Researchers use knockin gene modification to deliberately introduce a genetic defect in an animal model, typically in mice, that is known to spontaneously occur in humans. This allows interventions to be tested in the animal model.

Brain Imaging: Optical, Magnetic, and Electrical

Until the middle of the 20th century, the only techniques widely used to study the brain were single-cell recording and electroencephalography (EEG; refer to Chapter 7). Today we have new, powerful techniques for following brain function, including optical recording, magnetic resonance imaging (structural and functional), and new electrical recording techniques such as multi-electrode arrays and magnetic encephalography (MEG). Each has advantages and limits.

The most prominent optical reporting techniques are based on fluorescent reporter dyes. *Fluorescence* is the emission of longer-wavelength light after the absorption of shorter-wavelength stimulus light. Fluorescent molecules exist that change their fluorescence in response to voltage. These dyes allow neurobiologists to record neural activity with cameras, either from many cells at once or from sub-cellular compartments.

MRI permits the structure of the brain or any part of the body to be determined non-invasively. A strong magnetic field first aligns the magnet axis of atomic nuclei in the body. Then radio frequency fields alter the magnet alignment, causing the axes of nuclei to precess (wobble), producing a rotating magnetic field detected by the MRI scanner that can be used to construct an image of the scanned area. Functional MRI (fMRI) uses changes in the amount of hemoglobin in a given brain areas (blood flow) or its amount of oxygenation (blood oxygen level dependent [BOLD]) to give an index of brain activity in a particular area. Structural MRI images can have millimeter resolutions, while fMRI resolution is on the order of centimeters for most scanners.

A more recent technology, MEG measures the small magnetic fields associated with current flow in the brain. It has moderately high spatial resolution, approaching fMRI, with simultaneously high temporal resolution like the EEG. Multi-electrode recording arrays have hundreds — or soon thousands — of individual recording electrodes, each one of which can record the activity of one or more neurons. These electrode arrays can also be used to stimulate neurons in some configurations.

Interfacing Brains with Computers

The nervous system consists of (1) neurons that mediate sensory inputs, (2) more neurons that process those inputs, and (3) neurons that produce behavior through muscle contractions or modify behavior by releasing hormones and other neuro-active substances.

For sensory inputs, the most successful artificial replacement at the neural level has been the cochlear implant hearing aid (refer to Chapter 18). Neural hearing loss most often occurs with damage or death of the auditory hair cells in the cochlea that transduce sound pressure waves into firing in the auditory nerve. Total conductive loss and neural loss can be substantially alleviated by cochlear implants, which are linear stimulation arrays surgically threaded into the cochlear spiral with electrodes that stimulate the auditory nerves directly.

Artificial vision efforts have not been as successful as those for hearing because the input to the visual system has far more neurons in a much more complicated arrangement. Efforts have been made to stimulate retina and visual cortex, but at best only tens of distinct pattern elements have been achieved, which is far too low for clinically useful vision.

On the output side, efforts have been made to overcome paralysis, such as results from spinal cord injuries. These include recording motor command signals from cortex, relaying these past the neural axon break, and stimulating muscles directly, or muscle motor neurons. These techniques are improving, but at present most are unreliable and don't produce subtle movements. Similar research is being done on controlling prosthetic limbs in amputees.

Deep Brain Stimulation

Many neuroscientists are surprised by the significant positive effects on a nervous system — containing billions of neurons — that can be achieved by stimulating the brain with as few as two electrodes. This is happily the case for what's called *deep brain stimulation* (DBS; refer to Chapters 17 and 18).

Deep brain stimulation was first tried for Parkinson's disease according to the idea that if the output of a single, small brain nucleus (the substantia nigra) was deficient, perhaps just elevating its output artificially with current pulses that increased neural firing would compensate for its low output. This turned out to work. The results of deep brain stimulation have led to new ideas about how the basal ganglia system works.

Some patients who have had DBS for Parkinson's disease have also shown reduction in symptoms from unrelated causes. Chronic pain has been alleviated via stimulation of the periaqueductal and periventricular gray zones and several thalamic nuclei. Some treatment-resistant depression has also responded to DBS via stimulation of the cingulate gyrus, nucleus accumbens, striatum and thalamic areas.

A major advantage of DBS is the lack of side effects that usually occur with pharmacological treatments. It's also easily and immediately modifiable and reversible.

Multi-Electrode Array Recording

Microelectrodes (refer to Chapters 4 and 18) arrays allows scientists to record from a large enough percentage of neurons in a given brain region to begin to deduce neural circuit operation. They also allow relatively selective stimulation of small numbers of neurons. A few microelectrode stimulating electrode arrays have been implanted in paralyzed humans to allow direct neural control of computer cursors. Some primate experiments have yielded impressive results with brain control of prosthetic arms.

Developments of microelectrode arrays are likely to be powerful and rapid, following the massive world technology push toward bigger, faster, more powerful, and less energy-consumptive computing chips. These may permit far more complex and competent prosthetic devices than those that currently exist.

Fluorescence and Confocal Microscopy

In order to understand the nervous system's structure and how it works, you have to be able to see it. Fluorescence microscopy, which is also used in non-living sections, can image living cells in brain slices or even intact animals. It works by irradiating either an artificial fluorescent dye put into the cells, or a fluorescent reporter made by the cell itself (by adding the DNA sequence coding for the reporter to the cell's genome).

Some fluorescent dyes can show different colors in different cell types. Others can show neural activity by changing fluorescence with membrane potential or by changing fluorescence according to the concentration of ions like calcium or sodium.

A particularly promising branch of fluorescence microscopy is two-photon confocal microscopy. This involves pulsed laser irradiation at high infrared energies so that two photons are simultaneously absorbed by the fluorescent reporter. The reporter then fluoresces as though it had absorbed a single higher-energy photon. The advantages of this technique are better localization of the absorbing area, lower the background, and less damage from infrared radiation of the tissue than occurs with traditional fluorescence irradiation. Confocal microscopy is often able to resolve single synapses, previously only possible with electron microscopes. It can also scan large brain areas revealing many neurons and their activity.

Advances in Electrophysiological Recording

Single neuron recording electrodes can be extracellular or intracellular. Extracellular electrodes have a sharp, pointed conductor such as a wire or carbon fiber that is insulated along its entire length except for a small region near the tip. When such an electrode is placed near a neuron generating action potentials, the extracellular current flow can be detected and amplified, giving access to the firing pattern of that neuron. Extracellular recordings can be very stable, lasting for days in tissue preps, or even months in awake behaving animals. Advances in multi-electrode recording in behaving animals and large microelectrode arrays with hundreds of electrodes are occurring rapidly.

But extracellular recording cannot reveal much about what inputs the neuron receives and how these integrate to produce its activity. For this, you need intracellular recording (refer to Chapter 4). The two main types of intracellular recording are sharp electrode and patch. *Sharp electrodes* are glass tubes (micropipettes) heated in the middle and pulled apart so that the glass necks down to a very sharp tip, which still is open. Laboratory pullers routinely make such electrodes with tips smaller than the resolution of light microscopes. These micropipettes can be filled with a conductive salt solution and inserted into single neurons by which various currents mediated by ion channels in the neuron can be monitored. Such recordings are typically stable for a few hours at most.

The problem with sharp electrode intracellular recordings is that they are noisy — with an impedance well over 100 megohms — and injecting current into the cell is difficult. An alternative intracellular recording method uses a patch pipette. This is a pulled glass tube like the sharp electrode, but with a much larger tip and lower impedance (4 to 12 megohms). This tip is placed against the cell membrane, where a seal is made by suction.

The patch pipette seal is very stable, and the impedance seen through the electrode jumps from a few megohms to gigohms when the seal is first made. At this point several different types of recording can be made, such as membrane channel recordings and "loose" or "cell-attached" patch recordings that allow very high signal to noise monitoring of neural spike activity. Voltage clamp recordings are also used to determine ion flow through various membrane channels at any command holding potential desired.

Patch pipette recording has revolutionized our understanding of single neuron function. It can typically be learned in six months by a dedicated graduate student, and yields stable, low-noise recordings that last for hours.

One caveat is that in the ruptured membrane patch-clamp recordings the contents of the neuron are typically replaced by the contents of the patch pipette, so that the osmolarity and constituents of the patch pipette must be carefully controlled so as not to kill the neuron.

Tissue Culture and Brain Slices

Although recording from neurons in anesthetized or even awake animals is possible, it is difficult, and usually only extracellular recordings are possible. Prior to the last quarter or the 20th century many neurobiologists turned to invertebrate preparations such as the squid axon to learn about basic nervous system function because these preparations could be kept alive in the laboratory dish.

This has now completely changed. Isolated mammalian brain slice preparations can be kept alive for eight hours or more. Tissue culture preparations, grown from immature neurons over weeks and months, are even more robust.

One of the most revolutionary developments in neuroscience has been the ability to "back-transform" adult cells into pluripotent stem cells that can differentiate into functional neural tissue. This permits culturing neural tissue models from cells of a patient with a genetic defect whose origin and mechanism are unknown. Recordings from these tissues may reveal the mechanisms behind the dysfunctional neural connectivity or activity underlying their difficulties. The tissue culture then also provides a way to test pharmacological treatments to cure the disease. It is important to keep in mind that knowing the locus of a genetic mutation behind a neural dysfunction does not automatically translate into a treatment regime because the function of the protein encoded may be unknown and embedded in a complex regulatory system whose operation is poorly known.

Tissue culture also lessens the need to use so many laboratory animals in testing. Although virtually all neurobiologists accept animal testing as necessary, using fewer animals would cost less and be more efficient.

A final issue concerns transplants and tissue repair. Progress is rapidly being made in constructing three-dimensional tissue cultures that perform the functions of entire organs, like portions of the kidney or pancreas. Making such organs from one's own cells would mean that transplanted organs wouldn't be rejected by one's own immune system. Plus, we would have no need to harvest embryos for stem cells. Researchers envision transplanting externally grown single cell types, such as retinal photoreceptors to replace dead ones in a patient's eye who has gone blind. In other cases, entire, externally grown organs or brain structures may be transplantable with advances in tissue culture technology.

Index

• D •

• E •

HIV, 311
hnRNA, 28
holistic processing, 178
homeostatis
  automatic nervous system, 119
  body function regulation, 141
  nervous system, 14
homunculus, 149, 219
horizontal section of brain, 161–162
hormones
  cell components, 35–36
  female and male brain differences,
    181–182
  growth-regulating, 122
  hypothalamic-releasing, 141
  multicellularity, 10
  oxytocin, 122
  somatostatin, 122
  vasopressin, 122
human brain. *See* brain
human intelligence, 1
hunger, 279–280
Huntington's disease, 21, 311, 319
Huxley, Hodgkin (Nobel Prize), 11
hydrocephalus, 306
hyperosmia, 225
hyper-sexuality, 361
hypnogram, 138
hypogeusia, 231
hypoglossal nerve, 131
hypoglossal nucleus, 127
hyposmia, 225
hypothalamic-releasing hormones, 141
hypothalamus
  body function regulation, 140–141
  circadian rhythm, 137–140
  insula (insular cortex), 141–142
  nervous system, 14

● **I** ●

IB (intrinsically bursting) pyramidal
    neuron, 297
IGF (insulin-like growth factor), 346
illness, neurological, 44–46
imitation, 263–264

immediate memory, 240–243
implantable technology, 22
inactivation process, resting potential, 58
indirect pathway basal ganglia neural
    circuit, 148
infero-temporal cortex, 200
inflammatory myopathies, 313
inhibitory neurotransmitter, 71
initiation, transcription mechanisms, 28
inner segment, photoreceptor, 187
inner-speech consciousness, 282
instinct and adaptation, 233–234
instincts
  educated, 281
  quick reaction, 280–281
insula (insular cortex), 141–142
insulin-like growth factor (IGF), 346
intelligence
  adaptive behavior, 276
  artificial, 350–352
  brain size factor, 278
  emotional, 278–281
  IQ differences, 278
  language, 276–277
  meta, 277
  performance components, 277
  processing speed, 278
  reflexive behavior, 276
  social, 276–277
  super-machine, 354
interneuron
  and circuits, 79–82
  classes, 298
  transforming information, 43–44
interphase, 26
intrinsically bursting (IB) pyramidal
    neuron, 297
intron-mediated enhancement, 30
introns, 29
inversion, chromosome mutation, 45
ion exchanger, 51
ion movement, 52–55
ion transporter pumps
  cation chloride co-transport ion pump, 52
  sodium-calcium, 52
  sodium-potassium, 50–52

• O •

About the Author

Frank Amthor is a professor of psychology at the University of Alabama at Birmingham (UAB), where he also holds secondary appointments in the UAB Medical School Department of Neurobiology, the School of Optometry, and the Department of Biomedical Engineering. He obtained his undergraduate degree in Bioelectronic Engineering from Cornell University, and PhD in Biomedical Engineering from Duke University. Frank has been an NIH-supported researcher for over 20 years. He has also been supported by the U.S. Office of Naval Research, the Sloan Foundation, and the Eyesight Foundation. His research is focused on retinal and central visual processing and neural prostheses. He has published over 100 refereed journal articles, book chapters, and conference abstracts.

Frank's career has been devoted to understanding neural computation, both for its own sake and for the sake of making neural prosthesis that restore and augment human function. His specific research has been to investigate complex neural computations in retinal ganglion cells, the first locus in the visual system of highly specific and nonlinear analyses such as motion and directional selectivity. The investigative techniques Frank has used include virtually the entire suite of single-cell neurophysiological techniques, including single-cell extracellular recording, sharp electrode intracellular recording and staining, patch clamp recording, optical imaging with both calcium and potentiometric dyes, dual electrode recording, and, most recently, microelectrode array recording. His current research interests involve further translating basic research on the retina to the development of neural prostheses, both for the visual system and for other disabilities.

Frank is currently Interim Director of Behavioral Neuroscience in the Psychology Department at UAB. He has taught extensively on the nervous system, from genetics and ion channels, to neural function, to gross anatomy, in courses such as Behavioral Neuroscience, Cognitive Neuroscience, Perception, Sensory Information Processing, Cognitive Psychology, and Vision Science. He has written two other books: *Neuroscience For Dummies* (Wiley) and a science-fiction novel called *The Phoenix War* (Sam's Dot Publishing).

Dedication

To my wonderful wife, Becky, and to Philip, Rachel, and Sarah, for being the world's best kids and now the world's hope for the future. Thanks also to my parents, Agnes and Ryder, and my stepfather, Jim, and to all my teachers who thought I was someone worth investing time in.

Author's Acknowledgments

This book owes its existence to my agent, Grace Freedson. I thank my acquisitions editor, Anam Ahmed, for working with me to develop the framework for the book. Special thanks go to Heather Ball and Elizabeth Kuball, who together made the book readable. I thank them for their kind diligence. I also thank my technical editor, Kelly Dougherty, who corrected many mistakes working on a very early draft of the book. The mistakes that remain are, of course, my responsibility, and I encourage readers to email me at amthorfr@gmail.com when they are found.

Publisher's Acknowledgments

Acquisitions Editor: Anam Ahmed

Project Editor: Elizabeth Kuball

Copy Editor: Elizabeth Kuball

Technical Editor: Kelly Dougherty

Project Coordinator: Phil Midkiff

Cover Image: © iStockphoto.com/Yakobchuk

Special Help: Heather Ball